# A SURGEON IN NAPOLEON'S GRANDE ARMÉE

*To my wonderful family and Carlota, for your love and generous support.*

*And to Peter, Joe, and all my friends, for your company, which has punctuated my work with so many happy times.*

# A SURGEON IN NAPOLEON'S GRANDE ARMÉE

## The Campaign Journal of
# BARON PERCY

## CALUM JOHNSON

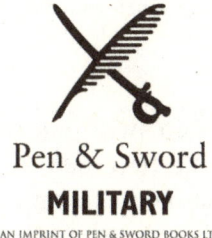

Pen & Sword
**MILITARY**
AN IMPRINT OF PEN & SWORD BOOKS LTD.
YORKSHIRE – PHILADELPHIA

First published in Great Britain in 2024 by
**PEN AND SWORD MILITARY**
An imprint of
Pen & Sword Books Ltd
Yorkshire – Philadelphia

Copyright © Calum Johnson, 2024

ISBN 978 1 39904 425 7

The right of Calum Johnson to be identified as Author of this work has been asserted by him in accordance with the Copyright, Designs and Patents Act 1988.

A CIP catalogue record for this book is available from the British Library.

All rights reserved. No part of this book may be reproduced or transmitted in any form or by any means, electronic or mechanical including photocopying, recording or by any information storage and retrieval system, without permission from the Publisher in writing.

Typeset in Times New Roman 11.5/14.5 by SJmagic DESIGN SERVICES, India.
Printed and bound in the UK by CPI Group (UK) Ltd.

Pen & Sword Books Ltd incorporates the imprints of Pen & Sword Archaeology, Atlas, Aviation, Battleground, Discovery, Family History, History, Maritime, Military, Naval, Politics, Social History, Transport, True Crime, Claymore Press, Frontline Books, Praetorian Press, Seaforth Publishing and White Owl

For a complete list of Pen & Sword titles please contact

**PEN & SWORD BOOKS LIMITED**
George House, Units 12 & 13, Beevor Street, Off Pontefract Road,
Barnsley, South Yorkshire, S71 1HN, England
E-mail: enquiries@pen-and-sword.co.uk
Website: www.pen-and-sword.co.uk

or

**PEN AND SWORD BOOKS**
1950 Lawrence Rd, Havertown, PA 19083, USA
E-mail: uspen-and-sword@casematepublishers.com
Website: www.penandswordbooks.com

# Contents

Introduction .................................................................................... vi

1799 – The Army of the Danube and the Campaign in Helvetia .......... 1

1800 – The Army of the Rhine and the Campaign in Germany ........ 40

1805 – The Austerlitz Campaign ................................................... 51

1806 – The Jena Campaign ........................................................... 57

1806 (continued) – The Polish Campaign ...................................... 80

1807 – The Campaign of Eylau .................................................... 107

1807 (continued) – Dantzig ......................................................... 171

1807 (continued) – Friedland and Tilsit ....................................... 209

1807 (continued) – From Tilsit to Berlin ...................................... 242

Appendix .................................................................................. 291

Select Bibliography ................................................................... 302

Acknowledgements ................................................................... 305

Index ....................................................................................... 306

# Introduction

I first became aware of Pierre-François Percy while researching Napoleonic logistics. Percy's testimony challenged my preconceptions about the path-breaking success of Napoleon's military administration. This impression was founded on sayings only loosely attributed to the French sovereign (for example, 'an army marches on its stomach'), and the legacy of a man who certainly considered logistical innovation, even if it only partly succeeded in improving the plight of his soldiers. A competition to invent a way of storing food, which led to canning, or the tree-lined boulevards that once shaded columns of troops marching in intense heat, and which now offer respite to strollers and car passengers: these examples draw a compelling picture of a leader concerned with the welfare of his men on campaign. In this introduction, I hope to explain a little of the value of the *Journal*, both as an experiential account of a fascinating, chaotic and devastating period in European history, and as a historical resource that tests, at times, the prevailing historical narrative.

Before considering the *Journal* itself, it is first necessary to provide a brief overview of the life of its author. Of all the figures to have emerged as pivotal during one of history's most fascinating and turbulent periods, the name of Pierre-François Percy (1754–1825) is one of the less well known. Chief surgeon in the armies of the Directorate and under Napoleon, Percy earned the title of Baron from the latter in 1810. His name is inscribed on the Northern pillar of the *Arc de Triomphe*. Yet his life and contribution to military surgery have been relatively underexplored, and his legacy has paled in comparison to the career of his colleague Dominique-Jean Larrey. This absence from the historical narrative is, I believe, unfounded, and I hope to demonstrate here why he deserves more recognition.

Percy was born on 28 October 1754 in Montagney-lez-Pesmes, in the Haute-Saône *département* of Bourgogne-Franche-Comté in eastern France. The house where he was born is today on the *Route de Motey Besuche*, and bears a plaque recognizing the surgeon as Baron of the Empire and Member of the Institute. His parents were Claude Percy, himself a military surgeon, and Anne Gaillemin, the daughter of a local farmer. If the village today seems rural and remote, surrounded by fields and sheltered by woodland, it must have felt even more bucolic in the eighteenth century. Percy grew accustomed to, and fond of, this countryside, and nature remained one of his passions throughout his life.

As a young man, Percy was sent to study in Besançon, the capital of the Franche-Comté region, where his family expected him to train as an engineer. Attracted instead to surgery, he had to overcome the resistance of his father who, having served with Tallard's infantry as a *chirurgien-major*[1], had retired resentful and disillusioned. Percy was a gifted student and a prolific writer. In 1775, he was admitted to the doctoral examinations of the Faculty of Medicine in the city, and became a doctor in medicine at the age of 20. From there, he went to Paris to continue his studies and was taken under the wing of the French surgeon Antoine Louis (1723–1792), life secretary of the Royal Academy of Surgery. The following year, Percy enlisted in the *Gendarmerie de France*, where he joined the Scottish Company as an *aide-major*[2] in Lunéville. It was the beginning of a three-decade military career, in turn under a king, a revolutionary government and an emperor. In August 1782, he was appointed *chirurgien-major* to the Berry cavalry regiment, and joined his brother, a clergyman, in the northern city of Béthune before being posted to Strasbourg.

A central theme in Percy's career is the marriage between the practice of his craft and the study (and later teaching) of its theory. While serving in the French Army, Percy entered, and won, the Royal Academy of Surgery's annual competition in 1785, 1786 and 1788. His dominance was so complete that the Academy requested that he stop competing. According to Percy's eulogist Marie-Jean-Pierre Flourens (1794–1867), Perpetual Secretary of the Academy of Sciences from 1833, this measure was taken 'to rekindle a little of the general competitive spirit that such sustained successes were threatening to extinguish'.

In January 1789, with revolution brewing in France, Percy was appointed surgeon-in-chief of Flanders and Artois. Three years later, he became consultant surgeon to the Army of the North and continued to move posts for the next

---

1. Senior surgeon of a regiment. Equivalent to first class.
2. Surgeon acting as an assistant to a *chirurgien-major*. Equivalent to second class.

decade, leading the health service for the armies of the Moselle, Germany, Mayenne and the Rhine, the planned invading force against England, as well as co-directing the famed Val de Grâce military hospital in Paris. On 2 February 1804 (12 *Pluviôse*, Year XII), he was appointed surgeon-in-chief and inspector-general of the Grande Armée, Napoleon's imperial army in Europe.

Devoted to his profession for much of his early life, it was only in 1802, in the tenth year of the Republican calendar, that Percy married Rosalie-Claudine Wolff. She was the daughter of a lady whom Percy had treated in Strasbourg. He was 47 and she was 43. The couple would never have children, but there was clearly a great deal of affection between them, and Percy writes in the *Journal* of his relief at hearing that his wife is safe and well. On his way to Potsdam, for example, Percy remarks: 'I met the *commissaire* [who] told me that he had taken my wife to Wurzbourg, where he has left her in good health, although afraid of the partisans: this good news gave me the greatest pleasure.' Concern for his wife was a familiar theme in Percy's correspondence, and following his retirement he wrote in a letter to a former colleague that his wife was ill and that 'if I had lost her, I would have followed close behind'. In fact, Rosalie-Claudine Percy outlived her husband by fifteen years, dying in Villevaudé on Christmas Day in 1840. She had remarried after Percy's death, to the military intendant Aimé Auguste Jean François Berger de Castellan (1774–1855). Madam Percy shared her husband's altruism, bequeathing 10,000 *francs* to the commune of Villevaudé for poorer inhabitants who were suffering from illness. Moreover, she was active in the village in her old age, and helped to found a *bureau de bienfaisance* (charity bureau) – a religious charity organisation – which remains today under the guise of the commune's *centre communal d'action sociale* (CCAS, Communal Centre for Social Action). In 1829, she gifted the village its church clock, which, at 7.00 pm on 1 October, brought regular timekeeping to its residents for the first time.

Percy's notebooks begin in 1799, during the French campaign against Austria in Germany and Switzerland. It is best left to the surgeon himself to describe the events of the subsequent years, although there is value in highlighting some of the key moments for which Percy was present. When General Jourdan's health deteriorated during the campaign in Helvetia (Switzerland), it was Percy who persuaded him to leave for Strasbourg and accompanied him there. In 1800, Percy also convinced General Moreau to sign a convention with the Austrian general Kray, protecting medical officers, hospitals and patients under an act of neutral inviolability. The idea had its roots in a similar agreement signed in 1743 between Generals Stair and Noailles in the War of the Austrian Succession and contributed, in the mid-nineteenth century, to the foundation of the Red Cross.

In 1807, Percy witnessed the horrors of the pyrrhic French victory at Eylau and the devastating chaos of its aftermath. From there, he attended the siege of Dantzig (Gdańsk). He had regular audiences with Napoleon himself, and was a relentless advocate for modernization and regularization of the military health service in these meetings – although his ideas and suggestions often fell on deaf ears. Following the capture of Berlin and Gdańsk, and the French victory at Friedland, Percy was also at the meeting of the rulers of France, Russia and Prussia – Napoleon, Alexander I and Frederick William III respectively – at Tilsit, where they would sign the peace treaty that brought active hostilities to a close in the War of the Fourth Coalition (1806–1807).

Percy's final campaign was in 1809, and he was made a baron after the Battle of Wagram. After his retirement from active duty, the surgeon returned to Paris and devoted more time to his two peacetime passions: teaching and horticulture. Glimpses of each can be found in the *Journal*, in Percy's desire to share his knowledge with his colleagues and readers, and his fascination with his surroundings. During a period of relative peace in the early years of the nineteenth century, Percy had bought his country residence, Petit-Bordeaux, close to Villevaudé and just east of Paris (a sign of the French capital's growth, the commune is now almost a suburb, located equidistantly between Charles de Gaulle airport and Disneyland Paris). The country mansion was on the *Route de Lagny*, and there is today a *Rue de Percy* just south of Villevaudé, which meets this road. At his country home, he grew vegetables and raised a flock of sheep, which he had brought to Petit-Bordeaux from Spain.

Percy found it difficult to navigate the changeable and uncertain politics that beset France in the years that followed his retirement. He rallied to Napoleon upon the latter's return from Elba, and was appointed surgeon-in-chief for the campaign that culminated at Waterloo. As a consequence of such public support for Napoleon, Percy was forced to retire as inspector-general of the medical service of the armies during the Second Restoration and his movements were subject to constant suspicion. Indeed, he was summoned by the Minister of Police more than twenty times before Louis XVIII, with whom he enjoyed a mutual respect, having worked as a consultant surgeon during the First Restoration, intervened personally.

As Percy approached the fiftieth anniversary of his doctorate in medicine, his health deteriorated markedly. Shortly before his death, as he left his country residence to return to Paris, he wrote below a Latin inscription on a gate to his property that read 'While I breath, I hope' a riposte in the same language: 'I hoped, and I was mistaken to have hoped.'[3] In December 1824, he read the eulogy at the funeral of his colleague Deschamps, but his voice could hardly be heard. He remarked that 'the air seems to be unable to reach my lungs'. He resorted to jalap, a purgative that had helped him in Poland when he had suffered from a severe cough, but on this occasion it served only to aggravate his illness. He had little to fear from death, having witnessed the passing of friends and colleagues among the hundreds of corpses that littered the battlefields, ambulances and hospitals of the campaigns in which he had participated. Indeed, by the end, he embraced death and talked about it freely, claiming that 'this conversation is as pleasant to me as if I were walking in a garden planted with roses'. A devout man – he kept a bible by his bedside and had the habit of reading it daily – Percy was reconciled to his fate.

Pierre-François Percy died on 18 February 1825 and was buried in the vast Père Lachaise Cemetery in Paris, in the graveyard's eighteenth division.

Percy's was a varied and difficult life, and its challenges and opportunities shaped his character. He was industrious, had several professional and personal pursuits, and was evidently respected by his subordinates and his superiors. Moreover, the *Journal* portrays him as complex, compelling and contradictory. Percy's notebooks give the impression of a man with an acerbic humour and a sharp temper, who was confident but self-aware, and who married his sense of duty and vocation with a fascination for history, culture, nature and religion.

Several individual moments from Percy's life distil these aspects of his character. For example, in 1793, the National Convention decreed that medical workers would have to be judged worthy of their position. Each medical officer received a sealed envelope that they were to take to their local council and, under the supervision of two members of the *société populaire*, they would answer the questions it contained without notes or preparation. True to its egalitarian principles, the Convention ordered that Percy take this test, despite his growing renown. Unimpressed, he published the answers he had provided before the council of Bouzonville, prefaced by a sarcastic remark:

---

3. In Latin, '*Dum spiro, spero*', to which Percy added '*Speravi, spe erravi*'.

'Here I am, waiting. It is a question of knowing whether I will be found fit to keep a job in which I have surely done a great deal of harm, if indeed I lack talent, in the three years, almost, during which I have been exercising its difficult and important duties, and whether it is by mistake or for good reason that the army and the generals have granted me their respect and their confidence.'

One of the requests was to suggest a series of questions to ask medical officers. In response, Percy continued disdainfully:

'The commission, knowing how little it costs the mind, how easy it is to set questions, wanted to turn me into an examiner for a moment, no doubt to give me a rest and to let me catch my breath; I thank them for this kind thought.'

Among the questions he proposed was the following:

'Who is the leader he [the medical officer] must obey among the great number of individuals who claim the right to command? What are the questions that have been put to him at different times by visitors, examiners, commissioners, inspectors, agents, delegates and representatives of all kinds, who have in turn summoned, assembled, harangued, exhorted and threatened the medical officers without ever having taught them anything?'

This episode highlights two aspects of Percy's character that are pertinent in the context of the *Journal*. One is Percy's caustic humour. Interspersed among the descriptions of destruction and horror that form the greater part of the *Journal*, there are occasional flashes of wit or sarcasm, often directed against an administration that Percy finds to be deficient and heavy-handed.

The other facet of Percy's character is the surgeon's awareness of his fame and ability, which, among several other competing factors, has implications for the way we view the *Journal* and its reliability. An uncomfortable tension between ambition and humility pervades the *Journal* and Percy's other writings, as well as others' impressions of the surgeon. It is a conflict highlighted by Flourens in his eulogy to Percy. Eight years after the latter's death, Flourens set to describing the surgeon's character and contributions to the study of medicine. Flourens's panegyric reveals Percy's charity and, seemingly by contrast, his lust for fame:

> 'In this noble and superior soul, the passion for doing good was always bound-up with the passion for glory and science; and perhaps never has it been better appreciated than by his example, that this love of glory and science is still just the love of humanity, viewed from another perspective.'

Percy, too, understood the position to which he had risen. In a letter to his sister in 1809, upon hearing that he had been made a baron, he wrote:

> 'You will have heard that His Majesty has deigned to name me a Baron with an allowance of one hundred thousand *francs* ... Here is a boy from Montagney who has found his way reasonably well. Tell our mother, and only her, that her Pierre-François has good *brequillons*[4] and that he is a baron of the Empire and a knight of the Crown of Bavaria, etc.; but that will not prevent him from being Pierre-François, son of the poor Claude Percy.'

This echoed a sentiment that the surgeon had first described at Tilsit, as he came across the three monarchs returning from a military parade:

> 'Our Emperor was kind enough to greet me in his turn, smiling as usual, and perhaps they deigned to talk for a moment about their humble servant. Poor father Percy! If you were alive and could see your Pierre-François treated with such distinction by the most important rulers in the world, what would you say?
>
> '... I am far from being open to pride. I am far more susceptible to astonishment, and how could I not be surprised and almost ashamed of the reputation that I have acquired, of the universal benevolence accorded me, of the rank to which I find myself elevated, of the fortune that I have made; finally, of that which

---

4. *Brequillons* refer literally to small pieces of wood, logs or sticks, but Percy implies here that he has amassed great wealth.

I am and that which one thinks of me? Heaven has blessed my work; I have fulfilled my duties and my role as an honest man and a zealous citizen; without intrigue, without means unworthy of a sensitive man, I have been successful. Far from having the talents of the late J.-L. Petit,[5] I had his simplicity and his love for our art, and, always while seeking the small things, the great things sought me out.'

Despite Percy's fame in his own time, his legacy does not compare to that of Dominique-Jean Larrey, his compatriot and his junior by around twelve years. Larrey was the surgeon-in-chief to the Imperial Guard for the period during which Percy was in charge of the surgical service of the Grande Armée. Although sometimes depicted as rivals, their aims were often aligned. Both recognized the importance of assisting the wounded more quickly, since the chances of saving the life of a wounded man diminished as time passed. As his *Journal* mentions, Percy developed the concept of a *wurst* – a horse-drawn ambulance designed to carry surgeons and medical supplies more quickly to the battlefield, to provide swift and direct first aid. The idea was never introduced because of the reluctance of the military administration, who felt that giving medical officers horses would set a dangerous precedent. Instead, it was Larrey who saw his creation put into action. His *ambulances volantes*, or 'flying ambulances', were intended to transport the wounded away from the battlefield more quickly, so that they could receive medical attention at a field hospital.

One famous point of divergence is in the two surgeons' approach to amputation. Larrey was a staunch advocate for fast amputations, both in the time taken to perform the operation itself and in his promotion of immediate amputation for certain kinds of wound, such as comminuted fractures and shattered limbs. It is claimed that Larrey personally performed more than 200 such operations in a single day at the Battle of Borodino (7 September 1812) during Napoleon's ill-fated invasion of Russia. As instances in the *Journal* show, Percy was more conservative, and evidently wrestled with the difficult gamble of amputation: if a limb could be saved, it would afford the wounded man a better future and hopes of a total recovery; however, if amputation was delayed and later required, the chance of survival was significantly reduced.

---

5. The French surgeon Jean-Louis Petit (1674–1750).

Larrey ultimately succeeded Percy as surgeon-in-chief to the army in 1812 as Percy's health, and in particular his eyesight, began to deteriorate. Nonetheless, when Napoleon returned from Elba, the returning general reappointed Percy to his former role. Larrey fared better under the Restoration and published his own memoirs; he also had a son, Félix Hippolyte Larrey, also a renowned medic. His legacy has therefore outshone Percy's, since the latter faded increasingly into the background following Napoleon's second exile, leaving nothing publicly to attest to his abilities.

Indeed, it was almost a century before Percy's notebooks from his campaigns were introduced to the public. Nothing better represents Percy following his death than his *Journal* – of all his writings, the one with the greatest potential to reach and influence a broader audience. The *Journal* recounts the surgeon's experiences in the campaigns in which he was an active participant between 1799 and 1809. The *cahiers* ('notebooks') that compose the published edition trace his journeys, duties and observations in several conflicts and across several countries, including Switzerland, Germany and Poland. His startling first-hand testimony also describes some of the most pivotal moments of the campaign, from key battles such as Jena-Auerstedt, Eylau, Friedland and the siege of Gdańsk, to the meeting of the three monarchs at Tilsit. And yet it is a complex text, serving several often-competing aims, and born of obscure origins. Its readers must be alert to both its value and its challenges.

Percy's *Journal* was first published in 1904 by the Paris-based printing house Plon-Nourrit et Cie. The French historian Émile Longin edited and introduced Percy's account, and the biography provided before the present translation draws extensively on Longin's profile of the surgeon, although it aims to take a more distanced approach, since Longin's own introduction is, at times, as much hagiographical as historical. In the early twentieth century, Plon-Nourrit published several works of French history, particularly concerning notable characters of the Napoleonic period (1799–1815) and the Second Empire (1852–1870). Longin was himself a prolific author of histories, writing predominantly about the Franche-Comté region of eastern France, where Percy was born.

Percy's contribution to the history of Napoleonic conflicts has been largely unexplored; where his *Journal* has been cited, it has tended to be from a purely surgical perspective. The purpose of this preface is to present the nature and significance of the *Journal*, which is a uniquely vivid and immersive account of the period.

A central feature of Percy's notes is their hybridity. The *Journal* is simultaneously full of humour and of grief, and woven from a sometimes-jarring blend of factual observations (descriptions of places, numbers of wounded, distances) and emotive details. The *Journal* combines at least three genres: military account, medical notes and private testimony, with each reflecting a different readership. On the one hand, the *Journal* was not published during Percy's lifetime, implying a limited, familial audience. Private readers may have understood some of the idiosyncratic references found in the *Journal* and they could take interest in the daily movements of the surgeon. There is also a focus on the deeds of people close to Percy; he occasionally mentions his brother, and closely follows the heroics of Pierre-François Wadeleux, his nephew (the son of his beloved sister, Anne) and namesake, who became an aide-de-camp to General Lecourbe.

On the other hand, non-publication says nothing of the intention to publish, and the *Journal* contains hallmarks of the didacticism found in surgical notes of the Napoleonic campaigns, including those of Larrey. Although I can find no evidence of an *ordonnance* requiring senior surgeons to keep a logbook in the period, the *Journal* may have been intended for a broader readership, including military superiors and junior surgeons. In his later life, Percy, as a professor, would certainly have had cause to draw on his experiences to frame his teaching and justify his approach. Interestingly, Percy just once addresses the 'dear reader' directly – an outlier in an account that otherwise implies, but never formally acknowledges, the potential for publication. Ultimately, the *Journal* found this public among Plon-Nourrit readers interested, as their contemporaneous catalogue suggests, in the Napoleonic conflicts.

This varied audience lends the *Journal* a polyvalence, and it contains features typical of expressive, informative and operative texts, to borrow from the taxonomy of text-types expounded by the translation scholar Katharina Reiss (1976). Indeed, the autobiographical genre is primarily expressive, a kind of literature, and Percy's *Journal* includes detailed descriptions intended to contextualize and inspire interest in the events it describes, both pre-publication for a narrow, specialist (or private) audience and, with the release of Longin's edition in 1904, for a general but informed public. In this sense, the *Journal* is a kind of travel diary, a narrative journey through the history, culture and nature of the places that Percy visits, from the traditional dress of German peasants and the tribes of the Caucasus, to Jesuit coffins in a former castle of the Knights Templar.

The text also serves an informative purpose, aiming to establish facts of the campaigns with precision. Injuries are described in scientific detail, and Percy records dates, locations, distances and patient numbers meticulously. As one reviewer, the French archivist and historian Pierre Caron, noted of the *Journal* in 1904:

> 'It constitutes, for the history of military surgery, a first-class source of information: numerous are the passages relating to exceptional cases of trauma, operational procedures, treatment of the wounded and sick, and the pharmacopoeia of the start of the [nineteenth] century. It also provides, on the life of Napoleon on campaign, in the bivouac, some particular details to remember. Finally, … it offers a strikingly realistic picture of the internal state of the Army of the Rhine, and especially the Grande Armée, from 1805 to 1809.'

Lastly, Percy's writing has an operative goal, attempting to convey his perspective to convince readers of his surgical and administrative abilities, and to divert criticism away from his actions. This aim, as we have seen, is only partly successful, for the *Journal* presents Percy as a complex and conflicted man, or, in the words of Caron, an 'intransigent character tempered by a great deal of kindness'. Thus, the *Journal* constitutes an integral aspect of Percy's legend-building, enacted by himself and his commentators, and imitated by many key Napoleonic characters, including other medical officers such as Larrey. However, the persuasive function of the text is not merely a tool of self-mythology; Percy opines on his colleagues and their condition, about Napoleon's strategy (although he is unfailingly respectful and obedient to the emperor), and about the character and qualities of generals, officers and administrators.

The *Journal*'s form similarly reflects this mixture of functions and styles. On the one hand, the text contains very long sentences with few connectives, a style reminiscent of the work of nineteenth-century French novelists such as

Zola. On the other, pronouns are frequently omitted, lending the work a note-like abruptness. The language is evocative and emotional, either a reflection of its author's feelings or intended to foster empathy with a future reader.

Narrative and opinion can be valuable historical sources, but if the *Journal* is to be used as a means for more objective study – for example, on the condition of the French Army, the state of logistics or the practice of military medicine in the period – it is important for the reader to form a judgement on the accuracy and reliability of Percy's testimony. That decision must be a purely personal and instinctive one, based on several competing factors, some of which I will attempt to expound. In fact, issues of reliability relate both to Percy's account (for example, the extent to which he may have selected or altered his own recollections) and, in the absence of his original manuscripts, the potential for intervention by others involved in the publication of the *Journal* in 1904.

Journals, as one of several texts that fall under the umbrella of autobiography, have long been a source of fascination for historians and enthusiasts. However, their reliability, and thus their utility as evidence for historical studies, is much debated. Autobiography is a means of telling a story from one's own perspective – a narrative that posterity may otherwise record differently. They have formed a substantial body of sources since the period of the European Renaissance, and the practice of documenting one's recollections only increased in the Napoleonic age, as literacy rates throughout Europe climbed and veterans of all ranks began to record their memories of the campaigns in writing. As with all perishable artefacts, the proliferation of autobiography is supported by the greater ease by which one can obtain and protect written records from a period close to our own.

The explosion of military autobiographies engendered a number of incompatible accounts, many written long after the events they describe. In this context, it is necessary to distinguish between different kinds of autobiography. We may settle on the definition of a journal as autobiography written during (or in the immediate aftermath of) the event that it recounts, rather than retrospectively. This immediacy is likely to be the most trusted form of autobiography, since works written with greater detachment – what we might call memoirs – may benefit from their author's capacity to consider the portrayal of an event that best suited their purposes. Thus, memoirs offer more scope for manipulation and distortion, omission and fabrication. Journals, despite their immediacy, are of course not immune to the author's self-interest, due to an inherent process of auto-censorship – a practice born of a writer's fear of disclosing details that could affect their own reputation.

As far as it is possible to speculate, Percy's *Journal* avoids some of the pitfalls of autobiography. Percy wrote almost daily, in close spatial and temporal proximity to the situations he describes. Indeed, Longin, the *Journal*'s original editor, wrote in his introduction:

> 'Among the heroes of the Napoleonic epic, there are hardly any who ... stole some hours of rest in order to recount the day's events. It is only much later that, taking the quill, most consider consecrating the leisure time that peace granted them to retelling their glorious rides across Europe.'

Longin certainly had a stake in the reliability and uniqueness of Percy's *Journal*, and stood to profit from its commercial success. Nonetheless, contemporary reviewers lent their support to his attestation. Caron suggested that the *Journal* possessed an 'incontestable authority', having been written 'more or less daily' and 'by no means ... for publication'. As we have seen, this claim is little more than an assumption, and aspects of the *Journal* suggest that Percy was indeed conscious at the time of writing of the possibility that his words might reach a broader readership.

Irrespective of Percy's intentions, the *Journal* only appeared publicly eight decades after the surgeon's death, and in its public absence, others had the opportunity to manipulate the surgeon's legacy and his testimony. Indeed, the early historiography on Percy is riddled with personal connections that blemish the illusion of objectivity in the work of the surgeon's commentators. Charles Laurent's *Histoire de la Vie et des Ouvrages de P. F. Percy* ('History of the Life and Works of Percy') was the only significant work on Percy to appear before the *Journal*'s publication. Laurent was Percy's nephew. Published only two years after the surgeon's death, in 1827, the *Histoire de la Vie* wove many of Percy's writings into a biography, and Laurent incorporated several extracts from the *Journal des Campagnes*. Laurent did not harbour any illusions of objectivity; he overtly stated that the purpose of his history was to 'raise a monument' to Percy, highlighting his genius and generosity. Laurent was also a surgeon, and his familial and professional ties to Percy consolidate this motive.

Longin's introduction assumes a similarly admiring tone, and he claims in this preface to have lived in Percy's childhood home in Montagney-lez-Pesmes. Moreover, Longin knew Percy's relatives intimately, and he speaks of having asked them about the location of the original notebooks that he had been unable to uncover:

> 'I came to discover [the *Journal*] in Egypt ... . I sincerely thank Mr. Charles Laroche [Percy's grandnephew], an engineer for the Suez Canal Company, for the good grace with which he allowed me to publish the manuscript that he possesses.'

How Laroche came to possess the manuscripts is unknown; living a century after Percy, he could not have known the surgeon himself. An engineer called Charles Laroche did indeed work on the Suez Canal and died in 1936, though this says little of the manuscript's whereabouts. Their invisibility in the historical record makes Longin's typed edition the principal version of Percy's original notes, and, to any practical extent, it must be treated as an original in its own right. In Longin's edition, the *cahiers* are compiled chronologically, with chapter headings placed between workbooks relating to distinct campaigns. As well as accidental distortions or errors, the act of typing out Percy's handwritten notes gave the editor an opportunity to alter their content, remove any supplementary notes made on the original scripts or incorporate other comments into the main text where they were once afterthoughts. The modifications are impossible to quantify, but they must be presumed to exist, to the impoverishment of Percy's testimony. Nonetheless, the evidence available appears to attest to the near-accuracy of Longin's edition. Although there are minor discrepancies between the passages of the *Journal* that Laurent cites in his history and the version of the *Journal* reproduced by Longin, these are predominantly grammatical, and do not alter the sense of the extracts. They are likely differing interpretations of the handwritten manuscripts. Moreover, Longin's overt interjections are minimal. He employs only sparing footnotes, designed to inform rather than influence the reader. This clarification and contextualization is distinct from the text itself.

Longin's one unavoidable intervention is to highlight omissions, caused by the loss of pages from the *cahiers* that Percy used. Although Longin notes that several workbooks are missing across the campaigns, he does not consider the gaps considerable. There is one significant exception, with implications for how historians use the *Journal*, when Longin interjects to highlight a break in the text:

> '... the third notebook is unfortunately lost. The narration restarts with the fourth notebook, only after the day of 21 February. There would therefore be a complete gap from the 17th until the 21st if the chief physician Dionis du Séjour, librarian of the Technical Committee of Health, had not been very keen to make known to the physician inspector-general Dujardin-Beaumetz that the National Library possessed an extract from the *Journal des Campagnes* relating to the Battle of Eylau. Indeed, one finds there, in the "French Manuscripts" under the number 12315, an original manuscript of eighteen pages *in-quarto*, without an author named, listed as belonging to M. Monteil, and acquired on 3 May 1837 by the State. It is entitled *Notice chirurgicale sur la bataille de Preuss-Eylau* ['Surgical Notice on the Battle of Preuss-Eylau']. The author presents this text as "an extract from the journal that Baron Percy held strictly and that his friendship for us has seen him entrust to us".'

Longin then transcribes two pages from this document, to complete the entries for the missing dates. However, this account is in the third person, and mentions Percy by name, so it cannot be drawn directly from the original manuscripts, as its author claimed. It is, at best, a reworking. Longin suggests that the document's author must be Laurent, because of his familiarity with the subject and with Percy. Laurent's potential authorship means that the *Notice* assumes many of the same pitfalls as the *Histoire de la Vie*. The *Notice* is neatly presented with a wide left margin for edits, which suggests it may itself have been revised. Nonetheless, with the original *Journal* scripts irretrievable, historians must treat this handwritten extract as the most reliable reproduction available.

The anonymous author – perhaps Laurent – also transcribes an earlier extract from the *Journal*'s original manuscripts. Describing the aftermath of Eylau, the *Notice*'s excerpt is consistent with Longin's *Journal* edition, except for some very minor discrepancies. As in the case of the *Journal* and *Histoire de la Vie*, such differences are plausible misinterpretations of Percy's original handwriting. The congruity of extracts reproduced in Longin's *Journal*, the

*Notice* and Laurent's *Histoire de la Vie* lends weight to the reliability of the 1904 edition.

Having established the factors at play in the *Journal*, its content and its provenance, it is possible to consider how Percy's testimony can influence the historical narrative. The value of the *Journal* is partly in its experiential testimony, which sheds as much light on the daily life of the army as it does on the world-changing events that Percy witnessed. Irrespective of the reader's instinct concerning the reliability of the *Journal* in any objective sense, the text remains a fascinating portrait of the subjective feelings and experiences of a surgeon in Napoleon's army, and a document of its author's disposition, actions and observations.

One interesting aspect of Percy's account is how he bridges the divide between officers, administrators and 'the ordinary soldier'. Some autobiographies of the period were written by officials who might have been motivated by a desire to justify their actions and secure their legacy. Others were written by regular foot-soldiers, whose insight into the conditions of military life is invaluable, but who lacked a broader awareness of the decisions that influenced their lives on campaign. Percy's rank and role placed him in a select group of the most senior officials of the French Army and allowed him privileged access to Napoleon (and Jourdan and Masséna before him), and often the military leaders of France's adversaries. And yet Percy existed simultaneously within and outside the army, lending his testimony a degree of detachment that allowed him to be both informed and honest about the issues facing the army as a whole. Part of the *service de santé*, he stood outside of the principal military hierarchy and was ultimately powerless, despite his appeals to Napoleon and his administrators, to affect the situation of the soldiers from a logistical perspective. For the officials involved in army supply, they had cause to justify, or even mask, the problems they encountered, or indeed created. As a legacy for a wider audience, it would demand a remarkable display of impartiality and humility to record one's own failings in one's autobiography. Therefore, somewhat counterintuitively, Percy's greatest authority may be in his perceptions of army supply as a whole – not in his observations of the health service, in which he played a direct role. He chose the location of the hospitals, directed and assigned the surgeons, but was unable to affect the strategic and, in general, administrative decisions that governed the lives of thousands of French men (and some women) on campaign. Where it concerns the army's surgical service, he is deeply protective of his surgeons, defensive of the conditions of the patients and consistently unwilling to acknowledge the flaws in his own decisions. He directs his admonitions towards administrators – *commissaires* and *ordonnateurs* – and yet he is extremely reluctant to judge the actions of his subordinates or his leaders; despite the abhorrent conditions that he describes, his refusal to speak against Napoleon is noteworthy.

Contemporary reviewers of Longin's edition were the first to consider how Percy challenged traditional interpretations of Napoleonic logistics. Caron proposed that Percy's notebooks 'evoke the deplorable state of logistics, the marauding, the incessant pillaging, tolerated by Napoleon'. A year later, an Anglophone commentator, H.M. Bowman, added that the *Journal* revealed the French Army's 'bad administration of supplies'. Yet, the *Journal* has rarely contributed to the debate surrounding logistics; indeed, it failed to make a broader impact even in its own time. Writing just three years after the *Journal*'s publication, the British civil servant and military historian Francis Loraine Petre remarked that 'in organising his armies, his supplies, his finances, and his lines of communication, Napoleon never surpassed his efforts in 1806 and 1807'. Moreover, scholars have tended to regard Napoleonic logistics as an extension of strategy, and given Napoleon's almost unblemished record, at least superficially, in the major battles of the campaigns – for example at Jena, Eylau, Friedland and Gdańsk – the foundations that he laid to achieve these victories have often basked in the same historiographical glow. Percy's *Journal* emphasizes the variability of the army's preparation and supply, both according to geography and across the chronology of a campaign. Most astonishing is the manner in which supply lines collapsed in the aftermath of key battles and in the wake of peace, as the army began to withdraw.

The Grande Armée often employed a system of requisitioning. Historians variably posit requisitioning as an architect in the rise of more modern war methods, an archaic system that evidences how strategy had begun to outstrip logistical capacity. On the one hand, Napoleon's desire to conduct warfare based on decisive and rapid movement against armies, rather than protracted sieges against key fortifications (with the exception of Gdańsk), required the creation of a more flexible supply method, capable of providing for armies moving swiftly across vast distances. Requisitioning carried the risk of exhausting a community's resources, but this implied threat encouraged the army to continue their advance. The policy also reduced the army's dependence on baggage, allowing it to move without its cumbersome brakes. The revolution in agricultural methods in Europe in the eighteenth and nineteenth centuries meant that rural surpluses were increasingly common, making requisitioning more reliable. Percy's interest in his natural surroundings means that he followed the harvests closely. He was frequently amazed by the ability of the land to support an army of thousands of men and animals, and struck by the indelible impression left by these invaders on rural communities and their livelihoods.

Other scholars have viewed requisitioning as a necessary consequence of Napoleon's ambition and desire for speed – the last resort given the limited number of wagons and the poor standard of roads. Again, Percy testifies to these failings, bemoaning the lack of vehicles to carry equipment and medical supplies, and witnessing provisions, carts and people lost to potholes, muddy pools and impassable waterways. Ultimately, a reliance on requisitioning left the army at the mercy of its hosts, the terrain and the climate – and as the army pushed further into poor country, this way of living became increasingly untenable.

Percy's greatest challenge to historical perspectives concerns supply administration. The influential Israeli historian Martin van Creveld states that the *ordonnateurs* and *commissaires*, who managed the levying and supply of resources, formed 'an unrivalled administrative machine' that oversaw the organization of receipts for the reimbursement of local populations at the war's conclusion. At the onset of the 1806 and 1807 campaigns in Germany and Poland, Percy attests to the efficacy of the requisitioning system. On 27 November 1806, for example, Percy states that 'the *commissaire* is the amiable Catuellan, a charming young man from Rennes, who has had us given good white bread and mutton for three days'. Three months later, another *commissaire* orchestrated a similarly smooth levy, and complications in the earliest months of the campaign are infrequent.

The state of logistics deteriorated after the Treaty of Tilsit, signed on 8 July 1807. The peace agreement brought a halt to fighting, but the French Army was still in Poland and required food and accommodation during its steady return to France. By 23 July, Percy records that efficient administration of supplies had disintegrated:

> 'Besides, it is the same story in almost all quarters; everywhere people steal with as much audacity as impunity; the officers steal; some *ordonnateurs* will leave Warsaw, Wloclaweck, etc., with half a million *francs* that they have plundered; they sell the magazine stores; they make deals with the suppliers, etc.'

Administrative corruption was one contributing factor in the collapse of military supply, but the peace also reduced the urgency with which the army moved, meaning that soldiers stayed for longer in the places they visited, increasing their burden on local populations. Percy's *Journal* gives a voice to the communities faced with the challenges of supplying a vast army – a perspective that is easily lost in tactical histories without a human face. Percy shows the distinction between requisitioning and pillaging to be ambiguous, with protracted stays in a town or region quickly draining the local population's excess resources. Near Guttstadt, for example, Percy remarks that a young girl needed bread, not money, which would have no value in a village left wasted by the passing French and Russian soldiers. He reflects that 'this poor village is absolutely devastated. So are all those through which we have passed.'

Percy is particularly aware of the issues of supply that affected the medical service. He recounts instances of surgeons using knives and craft saws for amputations, and he frequently laments the lack of cases for surgical instruments, lint for dressings and *infirmiers*[6] to perform the basic duties of care to the wounded, such as transport and cooking and distributing broth. Scholarly descriptions of the French Army's medical service have tended to downplay such shortages, depicting the campaigns as, at worst, unremarkable for their time, and at best medically and administratively innovative. Indeed, Percy is inadvertently complicit in portrayals of a well-functioning medical service in the French Army. Alongside Larrey, their ideas and improvements, only sometimes implemented, create an illusion of modernization in the period. And yet the French medical service was neither ahead of its time nor even ahead of its contemporaries. Following Eylau, for example, the mortality rate for French wounded was between two and three times worse than that of the Russians, and throughout his *Journal* Percy is full of praise for the training and status enjoyed by his Prussian counterparts. Disease, exploitation and inexperience only exacerbated the lack of supplies. Corruption, in particular, is a difficult object of study given its clandestine nature. Largely hidden from the historical record unless later exposed, personal accounts such as Percy's provide a qualitative, subjective means of filling this historiographical absence. While Percy felt powerless to unmask those involved in corrupt administrative practices to his superiors, he was compelled to provide examples in his notes, whether with or

---

6. Medical orderlies employed to give help to wounded soldiers on the field, and to assist in hospitals.

without the knowledge that they may one day be shared publicly. Percy paints the directors of the hospitals at Marienbourg and Kustrin as 'contemptible' and worthy of execution, and yet he understands that nothing will be done to end the abuse, for 'His Majesty knows it, he swears, loses his temper, and the wrongdoing continues.' The negative effect of peace is again evident in the deterioration of hospital conditions and the attitudes of administrators; indeed, Percy's accounts of corruption all appear after the peace treaty signed at Tilsit. In Kœnigsberg, the effect of peace was especially evident in late July 1807:

> 'Everything is being loaded on to ships, and there is an immense wealth of boats, grains, flour, wine, brandies, rum, rice, etc., in the port; the army will have some of it; the *commissaires* and storekeepers will have a lot more of it. What thieves! There was a serious question of shooting several of these gentlemen and some directors of the Warsaw hospitals convicted of theft, maladministration, and corrupt practices of all kinds; peace suddenly changed the mood, and the Emperor, who wanted them to be executed, has forgotten this matter. These crooks stole nearly half a pound of meat from each patient every day, not to mention everything else: craven, barbaric, sinister murder, worthy of the cruellest death.'

The risks and the opportunities of the *Journal* as a historical source are multiplied by the process of translation, since recreating Percy's account in a new setting, marked by a foreign language and a foreign culture, adds an additional layer of inevitable, if unintentional, manipulation, while also introducing a new and different audience to the surgeon's perspective.

Translation is an act of ventriloquism; the words of the original are modulated with the ambition of achieving perfect resemblance, but the result is merely similar, never the same. Therefore, translation is, by nature, an imperfect art, and the search for a complete rendition of Percy's words is consequently doomed to fail, given the differences of language, of readership and of cultural context in which the original and a translation are produced. Therefore, translating the *Journal* entailed a series of decisions, the results of which were designed to balance the competing tensions, so often insoluble, between readability, accuracy and retention of the original's idiosyncrasy. The aims of the following paragraphs are to describe some of the problems that arose from these rival objectives and to explain the choices made, not as a justification, but rather for the reader's awareness. Most importantly, it should be recognized that this translation is not a single, perfect portrayal of Percy's testimony and the motivations that underpin it, but rather one of a multitude of possible interpretations, each with its merits and each acting on the text in subtle but far-reaching ways. Indeed, it is hoped that being conscious of the imperfections of the translation is the first step to mitigating their unintended impact.

Central to my approach was a belief that the translation should capture something of Percy's unique voice, his singular position and the remarkable time in which he lived and wrote – an epoch of startling grandeur and destruction. The content of his *Journal* often makes for an uncomfortable reading experience, and the complexity and awkwardness of the translation strives to support that effect textually, rather than introduce an artificial fluency that contradicts or mediates it.

The *Journal*'s polyvalence, and the need to reproduce its multiple functions in the translation in similar but differing ways (determined by the requirements of a culturally and temporally distinct readership with different professional backgrounds and reading objectives), gives rise to several complex and sustained translation challenges.

One of the greatest practical challenges is the question of place names. Percy refers to the towns through which he travelled using the names by which he knew them at the time – a mixture of French equivalents (for example, German towns with the suffix '–burg' often become '-bourg') and, in other cases, the names given to a place by its contemporary occupants (most noticeable is the use of Prussian names for towns in modern-day Poland). In this way, Percy consciously or unconsciously adopts a translation strategy of his own, known as orthographic adaptation, just as English speakers may unquestioningly use 'Rome' for the Italian capital Roma and 'Munich' for the German city of München. One potential solution was to use the indigenous, modern names for all the places that Percy visits: the Polish-language name for settlements in Poland, German-language names for towns in Germany, and so on. This would have made Percy's journeys more readily traceable, by using the toponyms that appear on modern maps – a significant practical advantage. However, this strategy also presented two clear disadvantages. On the one hand, the insertion of modern place names shatters the illusion that is necessary to immerse an audience in the narrative, reminding readers that they are reading about past events from a temporally and culturally distinct perspective. Much like the anachronistic presence of a car or mobile phone in the text, if Percy were to refer to a settlement by a name that he could not have known and would not have used at the time, the belief that one is reading the original would be shaken. Furthermore, on a pragmatic level, not every hamlet through which Percy passed can now be identified, even with the aid of a map and by extrapolating from the distances and contextual details that the surgeon provides. Some have been absorbed into larger towns (for example, many of the places to which Percy travelled in the vicinity of Warsaw have now become suburbs of the city itself). Without modern equivalents for every settlement, the principle of consistency that such an approach could offer becomes invalid.

An alternative strategy was to retain the names that Percy knew and used, a method that would ensure consistency with the original *Journal*, but that would make it harder for a reader to follow his journey. Moreover, this strategy would mean moving away from the names familiar to modern Anglophone readers; for example, Warsaw would become 'Varsovie', Vienna would be rendered as 'Vienne' and Jena, the site of the famous battle, would keep its French name of 'Iéna'.

Despite the respective advantages and disadvantages of these approaches, I chose perhaps the least consistent of all the options, using Percy's own spellings in most cases but, where a clear orthographic equivalent exists in Anglophone culture, I adopted this toponym in preference. Therefore 'Warsaw', 'Mainz', 'Vienna' and 'Jena' are all preferred to their French alternatives. This strategy is subjective and imperfect, but aims to provide the greatest accuracy without sacrificing clarity.

Place names are indicative of a broader challenge: how to translate the various forms of linguistic specificity presented by the *Journal* and, more precisely, culturally, temporally and domain-specific items. The most complex translation challenges combine multiple forms of specificity; for example, military grades are particular to a culture and an epoch, while certain components of medical, military or transport equipment are described using terms that are both archaic and specialized. These forms of lexical specificity are typically inextricable, and mediating them means searching for the origin point of several converging axes. Moreover, the issue of linguistic specificity must reckon with two generally competing aims; that is, to render the original as comprehensibly as possible, to facilitate understanding, while also maintaining some of the historical and cultural flavour of the original, which serves to ground the *Journal* in its time and remind the reader that Percy was writing in French more than two centuries ago. This contextualization also supports the persuasive and expressive aspects of the original text. The strategies that I have adopted in attempting to mediate this tension can all be considered conservative, since the goal of retention was considered paramount to avoid undue alteration or loss.

I found several resources invaluable in identifying, defining and translating culturally and, in particular, temporally specific items. First, the *Dictionnaires d'autrefois* – a free, online search engine that compiles entries for the search term in several key historical French dictionaries – was an essential asset. Most useful for this translation were the fifth and sixth editions of the *Dictionnaire de l'Académie française*, published in 1798 and 1835 respectively; the two dates fall within Percy's lifetime and are therefore likely to reflect how contemporary French speakers understood his language.

A second key resource was *A French-English Military Technical Dictionary*, by Cornelis de Witt Willcox, published in 1917 by the United States Government Printing Office. Although its use calls for some caution because of its American-English leaning and more than a century of distance from Percy's writing, it contains many phrases lost from modern dictionaries as technologies of war have advanced. I found it a useful prompt and a comprehensive guide to military terminology.

The most fundamental and impactful translation decision was to decide what to translate, and consequently what to omit. There is a strong argument for the inclusion of Percy's campaigns in Spain in a translation for an Anglophone audience, given that Britain was a key actor in the region. However, it is precisely because this translation's readers are likely to be comparatively unfamiliar with the campaigns in Germany and Poland that Percy's experience of these wars is a valuable resource. Longin's original introduction has also been omitted, but many of its salient elements have been summarized earlier in this preface. Of the parts that remain – indeed, the majority of the 1904 French edition – care has been taken to include every detail of the original. As previously noted, the absence of the original manuscripts means that this translation perpetuates the omissions in Longin's edition; ellipses signal these gaps in the narrative, breaking its flow but serving, also, to remind the reader of the *Journal*'s provenance and subjectivity.

Indeed, Percy's diligence in keeping notes throughout his campaigns creates an inevitable risk of loss, of being hurried or interrupted. Every imperfection in the text attests to the difficult conditions in which its author was immersed, and about which he was writing.

A principal aim of this translation is to encourage its readers to read the original. Both paper facsimiles and digital copies in French are readily accessible – the *Journal* can be found in the digital library stored at https://www.archive.org. However, for those who would prefer to read in English, this edition represents an imperfect alternative, designed to render Percy's testimony accessible to a wider audience, including to scholars who may use it as a valuable personal experience of the period. The greatest value of Percy's *Journal* is its details, its unique perspective and the range of the author's involvement in several campaigns throughout Europe. Although Percy is not alone among his contemporaries in lamenting the appalling conditions that beset the army on campaign, his account hints at a frustration among the misery and an understanding that this fate was not inevitable, rather a consequence of fundamental shortcomings. For historians interested in the military logistics of the period, Percy's *Journal* provides a model for a new methodological framework that shifts such studies away from complex statistical analyses towards experiential accounts. Percy's *Journal* avoids many of the dangers associated with retrospective memoir-writing, and of the risks that remain, a journal's subjectivity can be its asset. In full appreciation of the precautions that such an approach must consider, it has much to add to an established historical field in need of rejuvenation.

Above all, it is necessary to remember that Pierre-François Percy was a real man with quirks and qualities, flaws and failings. His testimony includes his tiresome grumbles about the heat, his quips to colleagues and adversaries, his complacency and his sweeping prejudices – particularly stark to a modern reader. However, one flaw that he did not possess was naivety, and his *Journal* displays a remarkable self-awareness. Percy judged himself before his audience had the opportunity to reflect on his actions, and for all that he believed in his talents, he was not afraid to reproach himself – for taking a spur left on the ground during a chaotic retreat or for succumbing occasionally to the temptations of the pillage.

His *Journal* tells us much about life on campaign and the state of the Napoleonic armies during his time, but it also tells us about *his* life, rendered vivid as much by the everyday as by the remarkable and the terrible.

I hope you enjoy reading Percy's *Journal* as much as I enjoyed translating it, and I would welcome any comments or suggestions.

Calum Johnson<br>January 2023

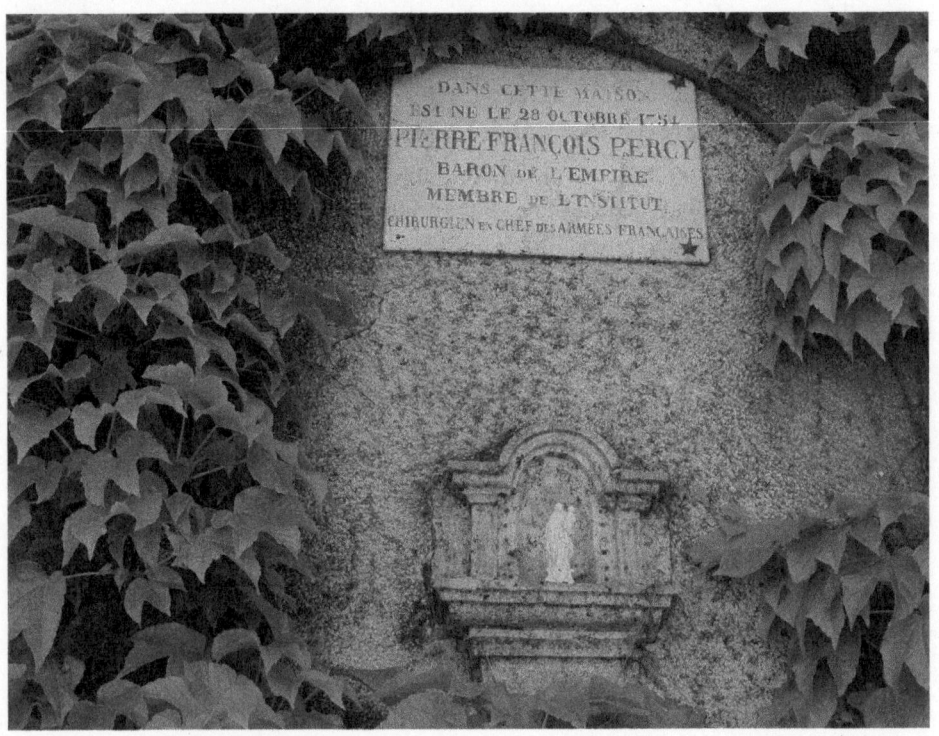

# 1799 – The Army of the Danube and the Campaign in Helvetia

With the Emperor[1] having failed to reply to the invitation made to him by the Executive Directory to send back Russian troops recently taken under his pay, and the plenipotentiaries of Rastadt[2] constantly resorting to new ways of stalling and delaying, the army received orders to hold itself ready to march, and General-in-chief Jourdan organized it as follows.

Contradictory plans were deliberately disseminated to confound speculation and to allow us to cross the Rhine without warning. The precise day remained known only to the generals. Jourdan, to exploit people's curiosity more fully and to deceive the spies, threw a large party on 10 *Ventôse*, during which nobody could detect the slightest hint of the journey being planned. In fact, we were even led to believe that the murmurs of peace or of armistice that were coming from the Empire might be well-founded. Meanwhile, during the night of the 10th, there was a movement of troops so considerable that already by five o'clock, in the morning, despite the bad weather and the poor visibility, more than 15,000 men, with the entire headquarters at their head, were at Kehl and on the road to Offenbourg. Eighteen thousand others passed through during the day with the baggage and artillery.[3]

---

1. Percy refers to Francis II, the Holy Roman Emperor from 1792 until the dissolution of the Empire in 1806. He remained Archduke of Austria until 1835.
2. The Second Congress of Rastatt, held in the town from 1797, was intended to negotiate a peace between the French Republic and Holy Roman Empire following the War of the First Coalition.
3. Longin: 11 *Ventôse*, year VII (1 March 1799).

Around midday, we had the *corps ambulance*[4] leave, intending that it would march with the vanguard; it was only composed of six caissons, instead of the twelve or fifteen that it was supposed to have; but given the usual shortage in our magazines and the lack of interest of the majority of those who are involved in the administration of hospitals, we considered ourselves lucky to have been able, through importunity and action, to procure even these limited means for ourselves. In total, the six caissons were carrying only 100 sets of straw bedding and implements in equal measure, an amount that would hardly be enough for 150 injured men, for we cannot have two patients on each bed – that is, the straw mattresses – because amputees and those patients who have fractured their extremities must sleep alone. Admittedly, the vanguard requires fewer provisions than the divisions or the ambulances, which must be quite well equipped to support the needs of the establishments along the route and to set them up as the army advances.

Following the ambulance of the vanguard were marching on foot, as is customary, the surgeons of all grades attached to the ambulance service. The officers had not had time to secure a horse for themselves and the younger men did not have the means for one, yet they were all dressed in new clothes and their uniforms shone with new and distinctive embroideries that identified their rank and role. They should have been afforded a *wurst*[5] of mounted gunners to transport them wherever the company is going, and in particular so that they can arrive more quickly and more fresh on the battlefields, where ordinarily the surgeons on foot only arrive after they have run and hurried more or less across the ground, which wears them down, leaves them breathless and renders them, as a result, barely fit to help the injured. The proposition that I had made to our generals of giving to my colleagues of all divisions, and especially of the vanguard, this type of agile, light wagon, which ten individuals can comfortably straddle, and the explanation that I had made to them of the distinct advantages regarding the security that one should draw

---

4. The term 'ambulance' is used to refer to the medical service during and in the immediate aftermath of battle. An ambulance was typically a temporary field hospital that provided first aid and dressings, treated the most serious wounds and prepared the transportable wounded for evacuation.
5. A type of French wagon introduced by Percy during the Revolutionary Wars. It was loosely shaped like a sausage, hence its name, with a long, thin central segment that the surgeons could straddle. This central part was generally a closed box for storing equipment, with a padded seat on top and footboards along the sides.

from it, the promptness and the improvement of the service, pleased them so much that it was immediately arranged that several of the aforementioned *wursts*, unharnessed, would be put at my disposal. The harnesses were made eagerly and with pleasure by the senior officers of the artillery who were charged with this task, but the ambulance crews were required to provide the horses and it was this that posed an obstacle to our project. The horses were not refused; but the hindrances, the defeats and the excuses all multiplied, and the *wursts* taken from the arsenal for the respite of the surgeons and the well-being of the injured returned to where they had come from, because it had been dangerous, perhaps, to make a show of giving vehicles to the medical officers, those whom a system of ill-will, oppression and humiliation has for a long time condemned to be covered in dust and mud. It is considered preferable that they go on foot and that they are unhappy; otherwise, some administrators say, they would become too insolent.

The surgeons of the *corps ambulance* of the vanguard were the citizens … ,[6] of the 1st class; Chapotin and Schal, of the 2nd class; Masson, Henry, Prat, Bury, Beaumont the younger, Jacque, Verrier, Vitrac, Paperet. It is worth noting that, among these surgeons, four of them spoke German: it is a forethought that cannot be neglected when one makes war in Germany; it facilitates the service, communications and contributes greatly to helping the medical officers to get by. On the lightest and best-harnessed wagon was: firstly, half a case of cut cloth, with a case of amputation instruments for the service of the sub-division, which the *corps ambulance* of the vanguard is always obliged to carry more or less at the front; secondly, a big case also full of cut cloth and containing a case for amputations and one for a trephine[7] as well.

After the ambulance of the vanguard came that of the second division of the army. Five badly drawn wagons were carrying everything: still only a hundred sets of straw bedding and a single case of linen and surgical implements. Next to these wagons, on which they were allowed, with some difficulty, to leave their small bags of clothes, were ten surgeons marching on foot, mixed in with the carters and the *infirmiers*, their heads lowered, their hearts sorrowful, doing their best to hide their fine buttonholes and wishing for the honour of their art that those passing by would take them for anything other than medical officers.

---

6. The first set of names, for the surgeons of the 1st class, were lost to Longin, the editor of the 1904 edition of the *Journal*. His own footnote says 'the names have remained blank'.
7. A surgical instrument used to remove an area of tissue or bone, typically from a person's skull.

Only their leader was on horseback. It was the citizen Lauzeret, of the 1st class; his colleagues on foot were ... .[8]

The third division followed close behind and resembled the others in every sense. The surgeons who constituted its service were the citizens Capiomont the elder, of the 1st class; Guyot, of the 2nd class ... .

We made our way towards Gengenbach and entered the charming valley of the Kinzig. Nowhere is more picturesque, more curious, than this valley: we are travelling along it, always with the river to our right or our left, and a chain of mountains, which offer the most delightful spots and views. Fruit trees lend shade to the buildings scattered here and there along the slope. The waters of the Kinzig roll, howling, over enormous stones. The wind continually stirs the pine trees on the top of the mountains; it is an astonishing and unrelenting noise. The rocks hang like precipices above the track, which is magnificent. This valley is cold; however, our soldiers are in good health, thanks to the kindness of the general, who does not leave them to bivouac. It only takes one night of bivouacking for hundreds to come down sick, so crisp, fresh and sharp is the air. The river contributes significantly to this singular freshness. Nowhere, in the whole valley, is more than a musket's range in distance from one mountain to another, and the stream flows through the middle. We have had, during the eight days that we have spent in this wild place, only a few cases of fluxion and ophthalmia.

On the 14th, it was decided that an evacuation hospital should be established in Offenbourg: the citizen Roussel, of the 1st class, was immediately sent to this city to be put in charge of this service; he was given Bourgeois, Alix, ... as assistants.[9]

From Gengenbach we went to Haslach, a small town surrounded by a modest wall, in the middle of a small valley crowned by mountains.

The same evening, the 14th, we stayed the night in Hornberg, another small town, more insignificant still than the previous one, overlooked by mountains as far as the eye can see. On one of them is a castle of little importance, where we found only a single cast iron cannon that had been nailed closed; some veterans from the area of Furstemberg were guarding it.

On the 15th, we were ordered to establish a hospital for 150 patients there. Its lodgings are beautiful: in each room, there is either a stove or a pan, and

---

8. These names are lost.
9. Longin: Name left blank.

eight patients can be placed there. The water is excellent there; it comes from one of the neighbouring mountains, which is twenty-four *toises*[10] higher than the one on which the castle is built.

An order was given to the citizen Latour to send without delay, in his charge, all the caissons of equipment that were requested of him more than a month ago. There was an order to oppose the removal of 6,000 standard weights of medicines intended for the Army of Helvetia from the pharmacy magazine. I sent a request to the *commissaire des guerres* Tailleur to put at my disposal the twelve horses made available to him by the headquarters for the three promised *wursts*.

The citizen Marchand, acting as agent-general, has left Strasbourg penniless. When the question arose of setting up the hospital in Hornberg, as it was not possible to have bread, meat or any other foodstuff on credit in that town, he was reduced to asking the *commissaire*-general Vaillant for 50 *louis* in advance or as a loan, something unheard of at the outset of a campaign! At least 50,000 pounds would have been necessary just for the service to run adequately.

We stayed in Hornberg, where we were piled on top of each other. Having needed to go to the headquarters on the evening of the 15th to the 16th, I suffered a fall when I entered this shack. I would have preferred to stay a quarter of a mile away from the headquarters; it is not so bad there and you live more freely; but we had to sleep on straw, in a large room where there were seven officers from the light artillery and their eight servants, all also on the straw. These citizens' supper had been noisy; everyone had drunk a little too much, such that during the night, since we lacked a suitable receptacle, they left in procession to satisfy a need that the large quantity of very light white wine that they had consumed caused to return with every passing hour: from which one can judge whether our night was pleasant and calm. I will not speak of the salacious intentions of some who did not sleep at all; nor of the snoring of those who, more happily, slept off their wine in peace; nor of the outbursts, as many unsophisticated as intellectual, of those who stayed awake and those who slept. There you have it: what one might call a night at war. Thankfully, Brigadier Lagastine, leaving on a reconnaissance mission to Freudenstadt, 9 leagues from Hornberg, left me his bed in the town.

---

10. A unit of length equal to approximately 2 metres. It was used in France from the twelfth to the nineteenth century.

General Ernouf, who had also gone to Freudenstadt, a fortified town near the Kniebis, was so cold there on 16 *Ventôse* that he all but died with his entire escort. On passing through Rutzenaw (others say Rupessaw), he was interested in seeing the spring of sparkling water that can be found in this region; he tasted it and found it very pleasant. It is indeed sparkling and has a taste not found in water of this type, which ordinarily has a bitter flavour and leaves an acidic taste in the mouth. It is very similar to what in some countries is called '*piquette*';[11] it has something wine-like and refreshing about it; in large amounts, it purges very well and, if one drinks it in small doses, it makes one urinate abundantly and restores one's digestive functions. A salt is extracted from it that is much sought-after in the area; it is a perfect purgative at a dose of one and a half ounces. It costs 24 *kreutzers*[12] per pound; 100 quintals[13] are produced per year. The water only holds a small quantity of it in solution; it has been necessary to establish fascines for measurement, as in the salt works of Turckheim, etc. This salt deliquesces easily; the interior of the factory is covered by it, giving it a whiteness comparable to snow.

Speaking of snow, 6 inches of it fell on the night of the 16th to the 17th. This night caused the bivouacs a great deal of harm; the men and animals were very badly affected; several men fell ill. Around noon, the sun was so fierce that the snow melted quickly. It fell again during the night of the 17th to the 18th; most of our brigades were bivouacking, which made them very uncomfortable.

On 16 *Ventôse*, a hospital was set up at Hornberg castle, where several of the sick were immediately taken, those to whom billets[14] in the town had been given while they waited for the hospital to be ready. Parot, of the 2nd class; Oberlin, Astoque, of the 3rd class, ran the service there.

We left Hornberg on the 18th for Villingen, 6 long leagues away. The road is well maintained, but it is mountainous and exhausting for the wagons and the people on foot: it is an unrelenting climb and the track is extremely steep. Villingen is a rather pretty town; it is built in a regular pattern in the shape of a cross. It has four gates and four main streets leading to them; the houses

---

11. Now used to describe cheap wine, '*piquette*' was originally a slightly alcoholic drink made from diluted brandy.
12. Minor coins issued by many German states.
13. A unit of weight equal to 100kg or 220lb.
14. A '*billet de logement*' was an order to an inhabitant of a town to provide lodgings for passing soldiers.

are painted in different colours, but generally with little taste, and on almost all of them one sees images of saints or princes; the fountain that marks the point where the four streets meet is worthy of note thanks to its statue of Charlemagne armed to the hilt. I stayed and slept for two nights in a wine merchant's house. It snowed all night from the 18th to the 19th; the bivouacs suffered greatly; and yet, not many fell ill. There will be a hospital in Villingen and the service will be entrusted to Normand, 2nd class, and to Versel and Boudeville.

The road from Hornberg to Villingen, which I said was beautiful but very hilly, runs between forests of fir trees, the greenery of which is delightful in winter. One can see trees as tall as 48ft that have a diameter of 18 inches even at their thinner end. Next to every reasonably sized house is a mill or water saw; the water flowing from the mountains lends itself willingly to any use that one wants to make of it, and an industrious man can manage it with enough skill; he makes his own mills. It is rare to find more than two houses together on the road and off to the sides; they are scattered across the small valleys and surrounded by furrows and stretches of meadow that, together with the fruit trees, suffice for the needs of these gentle and simple people. The country folk have preserved the patriarchal customs; the men are dressed in hessian and wool; they wear their hair long and flowing, with a fur cap and over it a small felt or straw hat decorated with pompoms and ribbons; there are no buttons on their clothes, nor on their gaiters, but hook-and-eye fastenings; their breeches are held in place by elegant braces, these being the only luxury they know. The women have long plaits, and their little hat is always adorned with pompoms and placed over their ear; they wear corsets decorated with coloured ribbons stitched into the seams and they lace themselves from top to bottom, which crushes their chest; their red and black skirts hardly cover the knee; they always have red woollen stockings and shoes with iron heels. The area's production is limited to excellent potatoes, from which one typically makes this meal: they are usually cooked in water; then one holds one of them in one's left hand and bites into it. With one's right hand one draws curdled or fresh milk, which is drunk with a spoon to moisten the potato in the mouth. Rye, very little wheat, a small number of oats and a great deal of turnips – there you have the wealth of this region. They earn a little money for themselves by selling some of the farm animals that they raise and the planks of fir that they saw in their own mills.

In Villingen, we found a rather nice place for a hospital. It is the convent of the *Cordeliers*.[15] Before, during General Moreau's campaign, this building was used as an asylum for the sick; but when the enemy suddenly seized the valley of the Kintche and Villingen, the hospital fell into their hands along with the medical officers and workers, who were taken to Heidelberg and then returned; the surgeon-in-chief was the citizen Bailly, who had his wife and son with him. After us, the Austrians also turned this monastery into a hospital; they kept it until they retreated, leaving there only bedsteads and some spoiled provisions; we returned there on 19 *Ventôse*. We will be able to place 200 patients in it. The Imperial soldiers had placed boards over the cobbled floor of the church, which is very beautiful and very large, and ordinarily had a hundred beds there. We will not have the same fortune because the supply administration has established its commissary in this very church, where it has its ovens and its kneading troughs: if they had been allowed to do it, they would have taken the finest rooms for their magazines and the lodgings of their workers. In this way, the building has lost the better half of its resources, and instead of the 400 patients that we might have been able to treat there comfortably, only about 200 can now be accommodated.

It was established in principle that no sick people would be allowed to cross the Rhine again and that all would be treated on the eastern bank; exceptions would be made only for those who had lost a limb or whose illnesses and injuries were likely to last more than six months. Two years ago, we witnessed how much abuse the evacuation on the western bank gave rise to; the sick, once they arrived in France, did not return and, under the pretext of illness, a crowd of soldiers crossed the river to return home; from this blunder stemmed the continual weakening of the army.

There will be several lines of hospitals. Offenbourg, Hornberg and Fribourg will form the final line, after which there will be no more evacuations. Between Villingen and Fribourg there will be a hospital where the evacuated patients will be able to spend the night and arrive in Fribourg the following day. I would have liked the administration to send for some provisions from the magazine at Colmar in order to establish the hospitals in Fribourg and Villingen and that, in turn, they would transport the supplies of the now-abolished hospitals in Toul, Thionville, Verdun and Longwy to the eastern bank, which would have greatly enhanced the service; but it is in their nature not to risk anything and to spend

---

15. The religious Order of the Franciscans.

the least possible, such that the country must supply everything; and so we will continue to see the linen and other effects of the unfortunate inhabitants removed and it will be easy for the administration to make enormous profits.

The army took the name of the Army of the Danube on 19 *Ventôse*.

The headquarters is still in Villingen as of the 23rd.

The 3rd Division (Saint-Cyr) has established a small improvised hospital in Rotweill, to which it has already sent several patients.

It was asked whether the surgeons would be paid fairly while on a war footing: 'Yes,' came the reply, 'that is, if by *fairly* you mean *rarely*.' Indeed, they are paid *rarely*, and in their case all they have known is that footing.[16]

Such is the state of suffering in which the hospital service finds itself that yesterday at the headquarters there was not the slightest aid for three or four sick people who had gone there to request it: no supplies, no food, no *infirmiers* anywhere; *infirmiers*, because they are not paid and are mistreated when they go to ask for their due. The hospitals behind the lines at Toul, Verdun and Longwy have been taken down; why have the equipment and personnel not been sent immediately beyond the Rhine? This measure would have spared us a lot of trouble; but Marchand maintains that we must risk nothing in the face of the enemy; in other words, we must take everything from foreign peoples and then send large bills to the government; is a bad woollen blanket thus more precious than so many objects that we are not afraid to bring?

To make a success of our service in Germany, it is absolutely necessary to have workers who speak both languages: I tend to place two or three in each division; they are required for the establishments and the evacuations.

On 22 *Ventôse*, since the army had moved to the right to be closer to the Army of Helvetia, it was necessary to abolish the hospitals established in Villingen as in Hornberg and Offenbourg; the patients from the first were immediately evacuated to the second, which in turn had to transfer them to the third, and from there to Strasbourg. The resources and personnel from these three hospitals had to be transferred immediately to Schaffhausen, where there will be a large establishment; the medical officers will meet in this town, and from there they will go to those towns in the forest where it will have been necessary to place the hospitals.[17]

---

16. The original wordplay rests on the orthographic similarity in French of the words *guerre* ('war') and *guère* ('hardly').
17. Longin: Rheinfelden, Laufenbourg, Sackingen and Waldshut.

On the 23rd, we were in Engen, a town that has become famous for the pillaging to which it was subjected for three days during Moreau's retreat, *quaeque ego miserrima vidi*;[18] I found it more beautiful and cleaner than it was then.

On the 24th, it was ordered that there would be a corps of 6,000 flankers under the orders of General Vandamme, who would move in front of Stokach and have an ambulance sub-division.

We were obliged to leave in the care of the magistrates of Villingen eight patients who could not be transported when the hospital of this town was abolished, all of whom were affected by catarrhal peri-pneumonia. Having met the citizen Gouvion, who was accompanying a convoy of some other sick men, halfway between Villingen and Donaueschingen, I made him turn around in order to leave them in the latter of these towns and to hand them over to the magistrate, who gave him a receipt for them in the proper way. In Geisingen, where we arrived on the evening of the 23rd, 5 leagues from Villingen and 2 from Donaueschingen, the sick who had gone there in the hope of finding a hospital were similarly handed over on receipt to the magistrates, and we are thus reduced to helping. This was how our fathers behaved in their wars because they lacked ambulant hospitals; the ancients, both Roman and Greek, did the same; but then no entry register was kept and the government did not pay the agents-general of hospitals.

The small image that heads the letters of the agency in question consists of two horns of plenty (for it alone), opposite which are, on one side, the head of Minerva with the inscription *Minerva*, and, on the other, an ancient bust with the inscription *Aesculapius*. A bad comedian once suggested that instead of these busts, they should put there those of Mercury and ... and that they should make several holes like those in a watering can in the bottom of the horns to show how the money pours out or to resemble the barrel of the Danaids.[19]

Our *wursts* were finally brought thanks to the diligence of citizen Willaume, each one harnessed to four horses; I had the satisfaction of seeing all three

---

18. Percy quotes a line from Virgil's *Aeneid* that means 'those terrible things I saw'. However, the full line, to which Percy might have been alluding, reads 'those terrible things I saw, and in which I played a great part'.
19. In Greek mythology, the Danaids were the fifty daughters of Danaus, the king of Libya. Married to the fifty sons of Danaus's brother, Aegyptus, all but one killed their husbands on their wedding night. When they died, the daughters were condemned to fill a pierced basin with water. The myth now represents a futile, never-ending task.

of them well equipped with surgeons and enjoyed the astonishment of the columns that were passing alongside them.

On the 26th, I arrived in Stokach, 4 leagues from Engen. The day was beautiful and the sun was quite fierce. The road, lined with forests, provides charming views and one meets several wealthy and well-built villages. Along the way, I saw many bushes of rose campion, anemone; its beautiful violet calyx and the novelty of this first sign of spring are a pleasure. The region is full of mountains and the road suffers for it; there are constant slopes; also, at various points, one comes across a post on which is nailed a tinplate picture representing a wheel under which a child is placing an iron wedge; it is to signal that one must jam the wheels, subject to a fine.

On leaving Engen, the view plunges to the left onto a valley full and large enough to field 20,000 horses in battle; General d'Hautpoul had stopped his reserve there, composed entirely of cavalry, and for nearly four hours it had been there to await its billets; these halts are too frequent and harm both the horses and men. Finally, the column was roused and we marched with it to the first villages.

I spent the 27th and 28th in Stokach.

I had the satisfaction of meeting my colleagues of the 2nd Division, those of the 1st, and those of the reserve in Stokach; the citizen Bottin, in charge of the latter, returned home to Phalsbourg on the 28th. The surgeons of the new corps of flankers came to find me there, Spach, Jaëgre, Vitrac and Verrier; they have been sent on secondment from the *corps ambulance* of the vanguard, which was in Krumbach on the 26th, and joined the flankers just after Mösskirch. They had, for all their service equipment, only a small case of instruments, half a pound of clotting ointment and a bag full of bad linen, and yet they could have 2,000 wounded from one day to the next. And this is how the great agency serves! The *commissaire* Varion, who is with the vanguard, knowing that there was very little to help the wounded, was not willing to give either a caisson or any straw bedding, or to share the lint with the corps of flankers; but General Vandamme, who is his superior, will certainly know how to get what is lacking.

The evacuation line will pass through Tuttlingen, Stokach, Geisingen, Stühlingen, Waldshut, Sackingen and Rheinfelden. In Stokach there is a very pretty building, where we found sixty beautiful bedsteads and to where the town has sent us almost as many provisions; this morning, the 28th, there were thirty patients, but they will be evacuated today, except for three who could not be transported, so that, if necessary, we can place 100 wounded there; I have entrusted its service to the citizens Gouvion, Gardeur and Drapier.

The night of the 26th to the 27th was excessively cold; the wind was to the northwest; the sky was foggy; it had only frozen slightly. The bivouacs suffered a great deal, and the entire force, which had been on the move since four o'clock in the morning that day, was extremely uncomfortable. In the evening, the wind changed to the southwest; the following night was milder; it rained a little. Not many fell ill.

On the 26th, from five o'clock in the morning until five o'clock in the evening, our generals were all on reconnaissance; they found at Pfullendorf, and further on at Ueberlingen and in the surrounding area, Austrian posts commanded by senior officers with whom they spoke. They assured them that they were extremely reluctant to fight, that the entire Imperial army was hoping for peace; one of them did not want to withdraw until he had received a written statement from General Jourdan explaining the reasons why he was being asked to do so; his request was met with laughter and he left with that. Ueberlingen was full of *émigrés*, whom the town was ordered to send away, on pain of military execution if any were found there, as well as a single deportee, during the army's next arrival.[20] One of the former dared to present himself before the general-in-chief and ask him what was to be done with him: 'Who are you?' Jourdan asked him. 'I am an *émigré*,' replied this reckless man with a sort of pride. 'An *émigré*!' said the general and those who surrounded him immediately, 'so you've come to be shot?' And they chased him away by the shoulders.

And yet we did not have orders to restart the hostilities; we made good ground, but it was because the enemy was retreating of its own volition. Masséna was fighting in the canton of The Grisons and Jourdan had not received any news from the Directory since that of the 10th. On his return from reconnaissance, a messenger arrived from Paris. The general hastened to open the packages; everyone paid close attention; we did not dare to breathe. I was there and, like the others, I was burning with impatience to know whether the orders were for peace or war. The general announced to the heads of division present that we would stay together until the positional work was finished, that they had become more important than ever and that from tomorrow we could expel all the Imperial troops that we might find before us.

---

20. *Émigrés* were opponents of the French Revolution who had fled France.

The next morning we left for Pfullendorf. During the night, I saw to our hospital in Stokach so that, if we fought, we could place the wounded men there. While we lack supplies, tools – everything, in fact, that an active army needs – these items are rotting or have already spoiled in great quantities in the premises of the hospitals abolished four, three and two years ago, in Pont-à-Mousson, where there is still, at this very moment, an attendant called Chalon; in Bergzabern, where we found a case of instruments a month ago, etc. What administration! To see the indifference, the lethargic idleness of everyone in charge of such affairs, when one speaks to them of the hospitals, one would think that a sick person, that a wounded person, ceases to be a man when he can no longer be a soldier. All of the administrations are backed and supported; this one is abandoned; one meets only cold hearts when one looks to awaken the humanity and arouse the solicitude of those in charge. We resemble those priests whom tradition and edification granted to the dying or the sick: they hardly cared whether they set them on the road to salvation, or whether they provided them with some consolation, whether they helped them to bear death with less resentment; perhaps even did not think them capable of such generous care, but they were needed, because then everyone would have cried out if they had not seen a Capuchin monk by the side of some unfortunate who was on the point of breaking, or a curate beside the bed of a dying patient. It is not the soldiers who think this way: there are general officers in the armies who are full of respect for the surgeons; Saint-Cyr and Lefebvre are among them. I heard the latter protest in his frank and military tone against the injustice and meanness of those who took the horses away from the surgeons of the demi-brigades. He said pleasantly one day when the general-in-chief and his general staff, in the middle of which I found myself, were on a high plateau from which we were looking down on the troops going into battle: 'I should like to be like the devil who took Jesus Christ up the mountain. Yes, if I had the virtue of Astaroth, I would go at once to look for all the members of the medical council and would say to them: "See for yourself, you wretches, if a surgeon with a bag on his back can, having travelled 6 leagues, rescue the wounded calmly and with ease."'

Yesterday, the 29th, I arrived in Pfullendorf (*Julii Pagus*), the most irregular city that has ever existed; it has suffered so much, two-and-a-half years ago and since our withdrawal, that we should be surprised to have found so many resources still there. When I arrived, I found the main headquarters, that of General Lefebvre and that of General Souham; everyone there was living on top of one another. The citizen Willaume, who had arrived before me, had saved a small room for me with the same physician with whom I had stayed during General Moreau's retreat.

On the 29th, at eight o'clock, in the evening, General Jourdan returned from reconnaissance with the generals Ernouf, Daultanne and others; they had visited a large stretch of country from past Ueberlingen to beyond Mengen and had met the enemy regularly. While dismounting, General Jourdan dictated the battle orders for the following day. He had decided, on the way, to attack on all fronts; this order meant in essence that the vanguard would chase the enemy before it as far as possible beyond the stream at Ostrach; and that the other divisions would do the same on the fronts where they found themselves respectively; namely, the first division under the orders of Férino in the vicinity of … , the 3rd under the orders of Saint-Cyr in that of …, and the corps of flankers towards Mengen.

I will never forget that General Jourdan, signing each copy of the aforementioned order intended for the leaders of the vanguards and divisions, said aloud: 'My heart strikes me whenever I sign such documents. For how many unfortunates am I signing a death warrant! No court ever condemns so many at the same time.'

The next day, the 30th, I left with the citizen Willaume for Ostrach, where the vanguard was, the skirmishers from which were already engaging those of the enemy. At nine o'clock in the morning, the ambulance of this vanguard had still not arrived, because it had only been informed a little late. In the meantime, we dressed a few wounded, who were led to us in the village where we had dismounted after taking a look at the arrangement of the troops. One of those wounded (he was a Waëtché hussar[21]) had received a sabre blow that had cut his cheek away from the cheekbone and a portion of the upper alveolar process[22] that supports the two molars; the cut began at the left temple and ended, crossing the lips obliquely, on the right side of the chin; the flap of skin was hanging down and left a quite considerable hiatus; it was necessary to put three stitches there. Another received a sabre blow that cut through his nose and the protruding portions of both cheeks, which created a terrible flap: he was a sergeant leading the 4th Hussars. Other injuries included: a shot from

---

21. I can find no record of the Waëtché hussar regiment, but it appears again elsewhere in Percy's account.
22. The bone that surrounds the tooth sockets.

which the musket ball entered above the external angle of the eye and was, in all likelihood, lost in the maxillary sinus; a gunshot through the pelvis; and a lance blow from an uhlan through the stomach of a *chasseur* from the 1st Chasseurs.

The wounded, numbering ninety, were partly housed in the civil hospice in Pfullendorf, with others in a building next door. They will be evacuated this morning to Stokach, but what an evacuation! These unfortunates are half-exposed because of their injuries; their uniforms are sodden either from the blood or from a poultice, and there is not a shred of blanket to give them for the journey. When they arrive in Stokach, there will be hardly any straw for them, and no bedsheets. The town of Pfullendorf has supplied provisions and 50 ells[23] of dressing cloth; it has also provided some *infirmiers*.

At eight o'clock, the baggage trains had started to file through the town and retreat, which caused us alarm about the results of the battle. It is surely the case that the uhlans and the Austrian skirmishers started to attack our men at three in the morning; there were many of them. The first injured arrived in Pfullendorf at nine o'clock.

Among this baggage, it is notable that there are a large number of wagons, and they are always the best harnessed, on which women ride with small children. It should be forbidden for all women in this position to follow the army since they can only be harmful to it. These wagons, arbitrarily reserved by one person or another and which are so badly needed to follow the ambulant hospitals, should be returned to their true destination by strict policing: now that we have 150 wounded to evacuate, vehicles are scarce and only wagons loaded with women or carrying a soldier who has made himself its owner are found on the roads.

At ten o'clock, the army withdrew, not being able to resist the enemy with so few soldiers, who outnumbered it four-to-one. The fighting had been very fierce on both sides until that time and, despite our disproportionately small force, our men had held back the enemy since three o'clock in the morning; but eventually we had had to yield to them. The retreating soldiers returned through the woods, which are 2 leagues long: I am referring to the retreat of the vanguard. Our ambulance was obliged to withdraw too, which it only did

---

23. An ell is an archaic unit of length typically used to measure fabrics. Its length varied throughout north-western Europe, but was equivalent to approximately 45 inches. The word 'ell' (French '*aune*') is derived from the Latin word '*ulna*', and was originally the length of a human arm.

late, because of a lack of vehicles to transport the injured; we had to leave many of them in the hands of the enemy. Many were thrown on the *wursts*, gun carriages and artillery caissons. I saw an artillery driver, whose left leg had been blown off by a cannonball, sitting on the front of an ammunition caisson, holding his thigh with both hands and the naked stump writhing, the flaps of skin flailing with each jolt of the wagon; he was shouting to the two drivers: 'Gallop! Quickly, quickly!' Not able to stand such a spectacle being given to the whole army, I had him carried to the side of the road, where he immediately fainted. Those who passed by, believing him dead, said: 'There goes another one.' 'No, no,' he replied, 'I am not dead.' I had left the citizen Bury, a surgeon of the 3rd class, with him to have him loaded on to a wagon, if one passed by; but this medical officer was forced to flee like the others. A number of the wounded died on the way; those who managed to make it to Pfullendorf have been dressed, had their operations, received some food and have been evacuated immediately to Stokach.

The general-in-chief had a horse killed from under him. General Lefebvre was shot in his left forearm, the musket ball entering below the thumb and getting lost somewhere much further down. Having met him as he was returning in his carriage, with the citizen Masson, of the 3rd class, going before him, I wanted to go back, but he did not consent; the citizen Lauzeret, of the 1st class, who saw him on his arrival in Pfullendorf, removed the musket ball from him, which had run the length of his radius. There are some injuries of the greatest severity. I was going to amputate the wrist of an infantryman when the citizen Willaume, of the 1st class, realized that the musket ball, which had ripped and shredded his whole hand, had also torn the tissue and muscles from his lower abdomen, such that his intestines were now protruding with only the peritoneum to hold them back: I did not want to perform an operation that a complication so terrible had rendered fruitless. I was likewise going to amputate a foot that was completely torn to shreds by a biscayan;[24] but the heel bone and the Achilles tendon were ripped off, and the subject did not appear to be able to cope with the two operations. A musket ball opened the femoral artery at its middle part; his leg was immobilized; the blood was no longer flowing; I postponed any operation.

---

24. A high-calibre cast-iron musket ball, fired from a long-barrelled musket. They were also included in rounds of grapeshot.

While we were at our busiest with our dressings, four Austrian officers came to me, one of whom spoke good Latin, and all four wounded. Having been dressed, the one who spoke Latin begged me so urgently to find a wagon for him that I answered his prayer; he showered me with blessings. They had a squadron surgeon of the Waëtché hussar regiment with them, taken prisoner at the same time as them; I kept him with me to have him sent back to his corps.

At four o'clock, the wounded stopped coming. The number of those who passed through the hands of the surgeons easily reached 1,200. It is said that the day cost us 3,000 men, as many dead as wounded and out of action.

The soldiers withdrew in a slightly disorderly way, but at the end of the wood, everyone found their corps and gradually the units were reformed. The cavalry reserve immediately occupied the high ground outside Pfullendorf and the artillery placed itself in front; there was a fierce bombardment, which lasted until four o'clock; the enemy were not able to drive us from our high ground, where the vanguard, the 2nd Division and the reserve are spending the night in bivouacs, which will be cold. The enemy holds the wood, which they have taken from us, and where they are seeking cover. Their artillery is well served. A cannonball came to kill, only 20ft from me and the citizen Lagastine, the beloved horse of this officer of the engineers; the enemy was firing on a group of trimmed hats, in the middle of which was the general-in-chief.

We had nearly 300 wounded men in the abbatial house, 375 in the market building and just as many in the civil hospital. There was no lack of linen; the town provided a lot of it, but there are no stretchers, no *infirmiers*; there were some of them with the vanguard. Three stretchers were lost and the *infirmiers*, through their cowardice, did all sorts of foolish things; they wanted several times to cut the horses' harnesses to flee more quickly, and they took the caissons far away on three occasions.

At seven o'clock in the evening, there were still 125 wounded, as many Austrian as French, in the three buildings. At eight, having been warned that during the night we would be leaving, we again evacuated around a hundred of them, and, as we had treated our prisoner surgeon well, we tasked him as we left with the care of those who remained, almost all of whom were genuinely impossible to transport; I wrote him a request in Latin, which was translated into German for him, in which I tasked him with passing on my greetings to de Mederer, Joackim and Eckhard; I think he will take good care of our remaining wounded.

At eleven o'clock in the evening, I left for Stokach, 5½ leagues from Pfullendorf; it was the most beautiful night in the world; I arrived at nearly two o'clock in the morning. It was 2 *Germinal*.[25] Already all the wounded from the previous day had been evacuated, some going to Schaffhausen, others going to Geisingen; those who arrived after me, and who had been the last to be evacuated from Pfullendorf, were sent to Schaffhausen, where a hospital had been hastily established to receive them; the citizens Deguerre, Fischer and Bientz were sent there.

Having thrown myself on a bed for an hour, I continued on my way to Aach, where the military headquarters was to go. I was the first to arrive. The 2nd Division was before Aach, with its ambulance placed not far from it.

The next day, the 3rd, we went to Engen, from where the administrative headquarters had withdrawn the same morning in order to go to Geisingen. General Jourdan took great measures around Engen to stop any enterprise on the part of the enemy, who were marching on our heels; we thought that they may even try to take our headquarters, which would have involved a great deal of audacity. We did not sleep peacefully that night from the 3rd to the 4th; yet we heard nothing; it has been quite cold and unfortunately our troops, who were very tired, had, on the heights where they were bivouacking, neither enough wood nor enough food; the latter was lacking rather more than the former.

This morning, at seven o'clock, the enemy skirmishers fired on the road from Aach. The battle began at this point a quarter of an hour from Engen, where we were eating breakfast peacefully; the call-to-arms was sounded; everyone left the town. Arriving at the last house in the area, on the road to Geisingen, and having heard the cannon and musket shots on all sides, I took the decision to stay and have the surgeons I had with me stop; a wounded man came to us from the direction of Aach, and told us that he was not the only one; this warning prompted us to seize the large inn, The Star, to make an ambulance from it. We already had a few wounded there, but we were lacking everything. The *wurst* of the surgeons of the ambulance sub-division of the 2nd Division was a full league from Engen: I had it return, and five surgeons with it; but food, brandy and wine were all missing. From the balcony of the house we saw a cart-driver passing with six horses, and a dilapidated wagon on which there were a few bags of salt, a crate of dried pears mixed with sliced

---

25. The seventh month of the Republican calendar, corresponding to late March/early April.

dried chestnuts, at the bottom of which was a cheese wheel, plus two small casks. We had two empty wagons, but no horses: I had those of the cart-driver stop. He had probably unloaded in Schaffhausen and was returning to some unknown place. I only wanted his horses and, indeed, I immediately had them harnessed to our two wagons, on which the citizens Hostein and Verner rode to go to gather and bring back the wounded who were on the heights; but when I looked in the crate, I found the things that I have just mentioned and, on catching a scent from the barrels, I realized that one was brandy and the other wine; I therefore seized everything, and never have these items arrived at a better time; we were able to refresh our wounded and provide a service to many Frenchmen, generals and others, who were dying of hunger and thirst in the middle of the fields. Someone ventured to say that this cart-driver was being awaited by the Imperials, that this cargo was for them and that it was by mistake that it found its way to Engen: this was the pretext for seizing it and our man, accused from all sides, still thought himself fortunate to be let off with the loss of his wine and his other foodstuffs.

At midday, we had only twenty wounded, despite the dreadful fighting that had been taking place all morning. One of them, an Austrian, was brought by five of his prisoner comrades, having been shot through the stomach from back to front; a portion of the omentum and his intestine were coming out; the continual urges to move his bowels and the hiccups, foreshadowing certain death, moved us to isolate this unfortunate man. Another from the same corps had a fractured left leg with comminution[26] of the bones; more than twenty splinters were removed, and I took the opportunity to make felt the necessity of large incisions and of the communication established largely between the entry and the exit to pass the fingers there freely, which must meet; the citizen Lauzeret operated. One infantryman had a broken right thigh in its upper part; the musket ball had not exited. Another long lecture on the need for deep incisions in such cases; the citizen Lauzeret in the meantime made similar ones; they are frightening, because the muscles swell immediately and it is necessary for the scalpel to disappear, so to speak, into the wound, but eventually one must reach the bone; once it was reached, splinters were removed in the middle of which the musket ball was found cracked and covered with sharp edges; the wound did not bleed.

---

26. A fracture into several fragments.

On the evening of the 4th, in the fear that, with the army coming to withdraw, we would be obliged to abandon several wounded men who could not be transported, we ordered twelve peasants to carry to the Capuchins of Engen, with stretchers and in their arms, five individuals so seriously wounded that it would not be possible to transfer them any further. Only three wounded remain at The Star Inn, where we had established the ambulance, one of whom was paralyzed in his lower limbs when his spinal column was hit by shrapnel, and another having received a musket ball close to the bladder; these two were catheterized this morning, the 5th, and the urine of the latter was streaked heavily with blood. The third, a sergeant major of the 83rd, was shot through the chest, slightly above the xiphoid cartilage, which plunged him into the most dreadful anguish. This man is of noble birth: he is aware of his condition, recognizes that he cannot survive this incident, but he is dying full of spirit.

5 *Germinal*. – Yesterday, after our men made some advances on the enemy, whose prisoners informed our generals of their forces, resources and positions, it was decided by the general-in-chief that we would attack them this morning on all fronts. I dined with the general, who seemed to me to be distant and sad; he could only eat a little soup before he went to throw himself on a bed, having given the order to set off riding at two o'clock in the morning and to be given a fairly strong guard, for, since he is staying in the town, it would have been possible to see him fall into the hands of the enemy, had they known about this circumstance. The fodder was distributed yesterday at eight o'clock; the brandy and bread were handed out at midnight. At five o'clock this morning, the first shots were heard. Since yesterday evening we have had no more cut cloth; the *commissaire* Souvestre, in charge of the service of the 2nd Division that was going to provide it, and behind which we found ourselves, told us several times that he had sent to the quartermaster of the ambulance of this division, who had remained in Geisingen, the order to come without delay with one or two caissons loaded with linen, splints, etc., and to bring with him some *infirmiers*. We were waiting for him impatiently this morning; he had not arrived by nine o'clock. I have written to him in a most insistent way, speaking to him about responsibility: it is two o'clock in the afternoon and we have not yet seen him; has he received these orders and notices?

In any case, having had no help from the *corps ambulance*, which was still positioned behind the lines, the sub-division with its *wurst* found itself in a most difficult predicament. All the medical officers that constitute this ambulance have been in Engen since yesterday; they slept on the floorboards at The Star Inn, and at daybreak they began to cut up linen and prepare themselves to receive the wounded. At half past five, they began to arrive. I hurried to send three wagons and two surgeons behind the fighting line; they soon came back filled; they returned up to five times, each time freshly loaded. Then, since our forces had gained ground and were too distant, it was necessary to send the *wurst* with three surgeons and an *infirmier*; then the division became a *corps ambulance* and the service of the *wurst* was a subdivision. We lacked linen, we were running low on everything; the inhabitants brought us everything, even the curtains of their windows, but nothing was cut, and one can judge the difficulties in which one must find oneself when it is necessary to cut the linen up while making dressings and performing operations. There was no lint either: it was replaced by tow and flax. I saw two infantrymen hitched to a small cart on which they were taking back their wounded comrade. Others carried an injured man on a stretcher made of branches and on their shoulders; others, on muskets tied together with their handkerchiefs, barrel against barrel; they passed two muskets linked in this way under the backs of the knees and, with two others similarly tied, they carried the torso, by means of more handkerchiefs or a bread bag passed under the armpits and through the loop of which they had slipped their musket. Finally, others carried them on their shoulders, as children are usually carried; they had only their legs and thighs on their shoulders; comrades walking behind them carried their arms and their torso.

The day of the 5th bought us more than 500 wounded from the vanguard and the 2nd Division. Several died on arrival at the ambulance. The citizen Cohorn, major and aide-de-camp to General Decaen, was shot in the short toe extensor muscle of his left foot: the incision that I made did not help me to find this foreign body and it was necessary to give up on extracting it; he left immediately for Schaffhausen, from where he will go to Strasbourg. Several foreign officers, all able to speak Latin, also arrived with more or less considerable wounds. In general, our troops endured a terrible hail of musket balls and shrapnel from very close range. I amputated the thigh of an artillery driver who had been hit in the knee by a 3lb cannonball. A *grenadier* arrived with thirteen sabre blows, several of which caused lesions to the skull and one that cut the angle of the lower jaw, the lateral muscles of the neck, the jugulars and, according to the citizen Lauzeret, the carotids, which I could not believe; this wound was frightening; one could have lost one's hand in it; we made three stitches there. This young man, full of valour and courage, had already been cut down and disarmed when a Barco hussar,[27] to whom he had even given his watch and his money, treated him cravenly in this way. Another *grenadier* arrived with seven sabre cuts, one of which was absolutely the same, but less deep than the previous one: again, it was a Barco hussar who committed the cowardly act; the *grenadier* had surrendered and lowered his musket. An Esterhazy hussar[28] arrived with his ear and cheek, and the full alveolar process, slashed. A sergeant-major of the 2nd Half-brigade was hit by a musket ball that entered at the level of the xiphoid cartilage to the left and exited at the same height 8 inches back. This extremely resolute man was in terrible anguish; he could hardly breathe; he could see himself dying. I spoke of this earlier. Since his wounds were exposed, he breathed in and out through their openings with a frightening noise. He died at midnight with his diaphragm open. A sergeant of the 7th who was hit in the shoulder by a 7lb cannonball arrived with a wound so wide and in such a state of weakness that all we could do to reassure him was to apply some cloth to it.

Our *wurst* still has not returned and it is six o'clock in the evening. The enemy, who had this morning repelled the centre of the army, have been pushed back in turn; they are, it is said, beyond Stokach. The division to the left and the one to the right have also sustained considerable losses and have caused much larger ones still for the enemy. The day of the 5th has cost us 1,500 wounded. We have continued to take prisoners; at least 300 have passed through Engen today.

Our poor surgeons are very weary: since half past five in the morning they have not stopped working or running behind the line to collect the wounded; they have had twenty complicated fractures to dress, which alone have cost ten hours of time; the large operations came next, and then the innumerable and incessant dressings that it has been necessary to make; that of a *grenadier* with thirteen sabre blows took an hour and a quarter. We have evacuated to Geisingen, where the administrative headquarters is: at the moment, there is a surgeon of the 1st class there, the citizen Willaume; four of the 2nd class, Gaillardot, Laisné, Gouvion and Jouvenot; several of the 3rd class, including the surgeons from the hospital previously established in this town, so they

---

27. A regiment of the Austrian cavalry, perhaps named after the officer Vincenz von Barco.
28. Taking their name from Paul Anton Esterházy, the Esterhazy hussars were a French regiment composed of Hungarian soldiers and refugees.

have been able to sufficiently serve the wounded that have been evacuated to them. It was necessary to fill the barns, and the wounded were cold. The state of suffering in which the wounded find themselves after a battle is a great obstacle to recovery: if they were warm in winter and were not burned by the sun in summer, the injuries would be less troublesome. Several comminuted fractures of both thigh and leg were improved after making deep incisions and extracting the splinters: they were evacuated during the night. It would be desirable that such wounded were never evacuated, but how can we provide for their treatment, once the army leaves? Hospitals are indeed left behind; but a few sick people in isolation can hardly be left.

Six *carabiniers* with sabre wounds came during the night. During the day, they had charged against the Imperial *cuirassiers* and, having wanted to aim as usual, without thinking of the cuirass that these soldiers conceal under their jackets, they were unable to hurt them. In a second charge, they used their sabres and caused a lot of harm.

On the 6th, it was quiet: the enemy had lost more than four leagues of ground; General Souham had chased them beyond Stokach. The military headquarters was due to go to Aach; our *wurst* is there; all of our wounded have been evacuated. The weather is superb: it is warm and the nights are quite mild. It is rare to see a finer springtime; but this beautiful season is lost on the unfortunate country where men make war. Nature seems to take part in the unhappiness of the inhabitants: mutilated trees, devastated hedgerows, fallow land trampled by the fighters, ruined houses, nothing feels the soft influence of spring; the fields are deserted; solitary ploughs wait there in vain for the oxen that the soldiers have eaten or the horses that they have taken with them. The birds still sing around the houses, but men are crying there; they give themselves over to the pleasures for which the season inspires in them the appetite and the need; the unhappy inhabitant sheds tears as he sees his wife and his children, whom he will no longer be able to provide with bread. At any rate, spring does not exist in regions that are the theatre of war; the philosopher can come there to think; the lover of nature must keep away from it; the former will draw sombre pictures from it and will be able to set out great ideas there; the latter would moan and be too unhappy there.

Of the 500 wounded who came to us yesterday, about forty died overnight. An Austrian officer, young and handsome, succumbed to a wound in his lower abdomen. Most Austrians have the portrait of a woman over their heart: when our soldiers do not take it from them, they console themselves of their wounds and their captivity by kissing this dear portrait; those who speak Latin say: '*Est carissima imago bene amatae.*'[29] The soldiers, and more often the sergeants, have rings on their fingers and some small piece of home given to them by their lover: it is a great sorrow for them when they are taken away from them; I therefore recommend that these items be respected, their possession having a moral influence on these unfortunate people.

One sees here the dead, the dying; one hears the cries, the groans of those who are suffering, the screams of those on whom we operate; it is as if nobody heard them. Everyone passes by, goes and comes; each thinks of his own safety, his own affairs. They walk over the battlefield, count the bodies, speak of it as if one should never run risks; this apathy, to which all the philosophy in the world could never drive men, is fortunate for the military.

Would you like your wounded to be well looked after on campaign? Have them carried to the capuchins and, in general, to the poorest convents; the rich monasteries will treat them less well. I warn my successors who make war in Germany that I have had much to complain about regarding the Abbey of Sainte-Croix, in Augsburg. The capuchins of Engen and the Franciscans of Saulgau have shown themselves to be excellent.

The citizen Maréchal, surgeon of the 2nd class, head of the sub-division with the *wurst*, slept this evening near the source of the Aach River in the same bed that Prince Charles[30] had slept in the previous night.

At one o'clock on the 6th, we began to withdraw: General Souham lost all the gains of the previous day; the 6th Dragoons suffered greatly, the 1st also. They are starting to file past.

On the 7th, the 2nd Division and the vanguard arrived on the heights of Villingen. Never had the soldiers appeared to me so exhausted. All along the column, there were only yawns; I did not hear the slightest expression of joy or gaiety; they were marching half-asleep; the cavalry slept atop their horses; a number of infantrymen fell because of drowsiness and exhaustion; the roads and ditches were strewn with men overcome by the insurmountable need for sleep; the officers and generals were suffering from it too. This region is drained; our troops are in a very bad way here.

At six o'clock in the evening, snow started to fall in large flakes. It was so heavy that we could not see one another more than ten steps ahead. On the

---

29. Approximately, 'it is the dearest image of my beloved'.
30. Archduke Charles of Austria, Duke of Teschen.

heights before Villingen, we have a small number of cavalry and infantry, which does not make our stay in this town very secure, but we will run the risks; the generals-in-chief are there; their horses are still saddled. The enemy was not yet at Donaueschingen at four o'clock in the evening; they are not hurrying to pursue us; they only want to make us pass back over the Rhine; it remains to be seen if they will succeed in that regard. It is said here that the Austrian general Hotze has seized Schaffhouse, from where he will have pressed on as far as the forest towns, which means that our hospitals will have fallen into his hands. General Bellegarde is going to chase Masséna from Switzerland: this news seems to me apocryphal.

Yesterday, the 6th, I left Engen at eleven o'clock in the evening, having finished everything that concerned my service: I left citizen Delorme in this town, to take care of twenty-two Austrians and seven Frenchmen who remained there sick, and I gave him an order accordingly. Above the Austrian soldiers' room is a captain from this nation who was shot in the thigh. This man, aged 50, speaks Latin wonderfully; he wanted to stay in Engen; we consented to it, in return for a signed acknowledgement from him; he was so pleased with us and with citizen Delorme that he was planning to obtain the approval and gracious welcome of the generals of the Imperial army for him. This captain is called Metzig.

The night was extremely dark; we could hardly see; we had to pass by the side of the artillery pieces and caissons, on a narrow road, at the risk of causing a lot of damage. I arrived very numb in Geisingen at one o'clock in the morning. Luckily I found an open barn; the musicians of the 4th Hussars had put their horses there; I placed mine there and next to them some straw was spread out for me, onto which I threw myself after I had something small to eat.

This morning, the 7th, I left Geisingen at half past five. The 2nd Division was marching out of the town. I had been told that the headquarters was at Löffingen, 4 leagues from Donaueschingen: I was going there and passed near a small town called Hüffingen, without planning to enter it, when, having asked an inhabitant if there were any French people in this town, he told me that more than 300 wounded from this nation had arrived there yesterday during the night, and they had not yet left. I therefore entered and, having seen a crowd in the distance, I judged that it was there that our injured were likely to be. I found a surgeon called Fayet at the doorway to a large building serving as a barracks for the soldiers of the Prince of Furstemberg. He was making the wounded file past one-by-one and giving each of them a glass of wine and a hunk of bread; they were then loaded onto vehicles, and when all those who were transportable had been processed in this way, the convoy, composed of thirty-three wagons, left under the supervision of citizen Contal, of the 3rd class, who had arrived in the army that very day. I made a requisition order to the bailiff for twelve wagons for the remaining patients, whom I have placed under the protection and responsibility of the town; I left to care for them the citizens Fayet and Toussaint, who must have had plenty of trouble obtaining the transport for the injured in question after I left. It was agreed that the Austrians would stay: I found a *felcher* who tended to them. As I was returning from there having learned that only the sick and the artillery crews were passing through Frülingen, Neustadt and Fribourg, I met General Compère, whom twenty-four peasants were carrying in turns on a stretcher. A musket ball has broken this general's leg; he is going to have this wound treated by Laroche, his friend, in Huningue; citizen Capiomont, head of the *corps ambulance* of the 3rd Division, where General Goulu was, is accompanying him.

I arrived at Villingen at one o'clock, having made 18 leagues since yesterday at eleven o'clock in the evening and having seen more than 700 wounded on different routes, thrown on wagons, without an escort, dying of cold, because they are not given blankets and they are completely naked or covered with uniforms soaked with blood.

I must not omit to report that, in the battle of the 5th, the general-in-chief had taken up such a good position with General Saint-Cyr that the division of this general was set to capture the rear of the archduke's army, which would have routed this force and allowed a lot of men to be taken. Unfortunately, two battalions ordered to reinforce the left wing arrived late, because they were 3 leagues away, and the cavalry reserve only charged after it had received the order to do so for a third time, which resulted in General d'Hautpoul, to whom this order was given, being sent back behind the lines.[31] Still this cavalry, including the two regiments of *carabiniers*, charged badly; they broke rank and ran away with their tail between their legs. General Jourdan flung himself behind them to rally them; he held his plume in his hand while shouting: 'Here is the rallying point. Halt, halt!' The fleeing horsemen were also shouting 'Halt!', and yet they spurred on even more. So failed this most beautiful plan. General Jourdan thought he would be crushed by the deserters,

---

31. General d'Hautpoul was court-martialled in Strasbourg for failing to charge on time, but was acquitted.

and if unfortunately he were to be knocked from his horse, he would have fallen into the hands of the enemy.

It is believed that the source of the Danube is at Donaueschingen. It is the aristocracy of the Prince of Furstemberg who placed it at the foot of his castle. The actual source is near Villingen: four streams – the Brieg, the Brag, the Brug and the Brog – converge to form this great river, and all four neighbour Villingen; all that is presented in Donaueschingen for the source of the Danube is a small spring, which feeds a modest stream.

On the 7th and 8th, it was cold and snowed, which made our bivouacking troops extremely uncomfortable. On the 9th, the snow intensified, but the weather grew milder: we have had few falling ill. The thermometer was between two and three degrees below zero on these three days. Villingen, which Marshal de Tallard spoke about at much too great length in his letters, is an insignificant town, overlooked on all sides, but surrounded by a good wall and with a second interior surrounding wall separated from the first by a deep ditch; one must light a fire there all year round; this region is very cold. On the 9th and 10th, it froze.

Yesterday, on the 9th, in a reconnaissance mission that was made by the generals, it was found that to the left of Villingen there was not a man to protect the headquarters and that if the enemy had known of this oversight, which had persisted for two days, they could have taken the general-in-chief and the entire general staff. This large error or big misunderstanding was remedied by having a part of the 2nd Division return and by stationing it in front of Villingen, ensuring that the left was well covered. Ignorant as I was to this circumstance, I slept undressed like the two previous nights and lived in the greatest security. Yesterday, during the same reconnaissance mission, the enemy showed themselves at the entrance to the second village on the route from Geisingen, three-quarters of a league from here. It is presumed, given the inertia with which to all appearances they are continuing and because of the rest that they are giving us, that they have taken forces over the Neckar and that they have plans on that side.

The general-in-chief wrote a letter on the 8th of this month to the Minister of War in which he invited him to take the swiftest possible measures in order that the hospital agency can serve usefully: he said that an administrator appeared at the headquarters, who may have some understanding of the service, but who, being deprived of all means, of all resources, has only been of very minor assistance since the start of the campaign. He added: 'The wounded would have been left without help, if it were not for the zeal, above all praise, of the medical officers.' I have informed the heads of all the services of the endorsement that the general-in-chief has given us, inviting them to make every effort to justify the faith that he has in us and to deserve further expressions of satisfaction from him in the future.

On the 9th, at three o'clock in the afternoon, I left Villingen with the citizen Flosse, who was ill, next to whom I took a seat in General Ernouf's carriage. It was extremely cold. Since the headquarters must be evacuated the following night and the troops before it must withdraw to take up a position in front of Hornberg, I took advantage of the opportunity. The countryside was covered with snow 5 or 6 inches thick in several places; the thermometer was 10 degrees below zero. We again saw the houses, so calm and beautiful, that line the road and whose inhabitants had spoken so highly of the French when they were advancing. What a difference! The houses were pillaged, lain waste to, and their unfortunate families were on the run. The greedy soldiers, because they were hungry; the cowardly and cruel *vivandiers*;[32] above all the women, who had thrown themselves on the army's rear, had left nothing there: oxen, cows, calves, poultry, everything had been devoured; the nearby bivouacs had been the devastating final straw. It is a truly dreadful sight to see a thousand families, not so long ago peaceful and happy, plunged suddenly into adversity and need.

On the 10th, 11th, 12th and 13th, we stayed in Hornberg. The general-in-chief has made every effort to protect himself there from attacks by the enemy. General Férino has been sent along the road from Neustadt and he is guarding the route from Fribourg and the Saint-Pierre Valley. Souham has his division around Hornberg, where the vanguard also is, under the orders of General Soult, Lefebvre having been wounded. Saint-Cyr is on the Kniebis and is occupying Freudenstadt, and Vandamme's corps of flankers is defending the gorge of Fricksthal and the twenty-four farms. We have made abatis[33] from trees nearly half a league in depth. Therefore, we are safe here and the communications are well established, but we are dying of hunger; the hay is running short and the troops do not have any brandy.

---

32. A sutler or camp follower, who sold provisions to the soldiers.
33. A line of defence formed from a row of felled trees laid on a battlefield as a kind of rampart. The branches face outward, against the enemy, and are sharpened to deter advances.

## 1799 – The Army of the Danube and the Campaign in Helvetia

The snow is covering the land at a depth of 6 inches; the thermometer is very low; the cold is glacial. The number falling ill is increasing.

It is believed that the enemy, who are not appearing in the vicinity of Villingen, where they have only 600 men, and who are showing themselves more or less in the area of Rottweill, are marching to the right towards the Neckar and Philipsbourg; we do not know their designs.

The Army of Observation has just been merged with that of the Danube: if this measure had been taken earlier, the Archduke's army would be no more. I have heard it said several times to General Jordan that our successes in Helvetia mean little for the reason we declared war, which is to overthrow the Emperor; that it was absolutely necessary to defeat the Archduke resoundingly once or twice and throw him behind his entrenchments at Ulm; then to have a part of the Army of Italy, that of Helvetia and our own follow.

During the disorderly passage of the army, the deserters and the equipages through Fribourg, on the 6th and 7th *Germinal*, all the French who were in this town, even the garrison, ran away, based on the rumours of the impending arrival of the enemy that were circulated by those deserters and the peasants. Only the surgeons did not leave their post; they had 700 wounded at the time; the citizen Rousset was in charge of them. Some surgeons not making up the service of the hospital in this town allowed themselves to be swept along and fled like the others, but after a few hours, the shame brought them back to their colleagues.

On the 13th, at five o'clock in the evening, the enemy pushed their scouts very far, both towards the area of Fricksthal and to that of Triberg. From this move, it was predicted that they would attack in the morning, and the headquarters in Hornberg was on the alert all night, except perhaps for me, who slept undressed and very well.

The next day, at half past five, I went to see the general-in-chief, whom I found booted and dressed: he had suffered all night and could neither open his eyes nor speak without feeling nauseous. I decided that he should go to Strasbourg, from where we are only 16 leagues away, and where he truly needed to go to avoid a serious illness that was threatening him. At half past seven, we left. At eleven, we arrived in Gengenbach, where he ate a broth at the abbey, and at two we were in Strasbourg. I put him on a diet of chicory water, to use cream of tartar and to take baths. Soon he had recovered.

Halfway there we met an extraordinary messenger who brought him the authorization he had requested from the Directory to go to explain himself before it on topics concerning the army and several generals. This news calmed him a lot; but, when he saw that by a decree attached to the aforementioned authorization, Masséna was to command the two armies in the meantime, he suspected that he would not return.

On the 14th, the enemy, just as we had expected, attacked Triberg and thought they would surprise the headquarters of the 2nd Division, then commanded by General Goulu; they had a lot of trouble escaping; the peasants had led them down little-known and unguarded lanes. The retreat of the 2nd Division set the tone for the rest of the army.

When I left, I had given the order to have my caisson taken to Haslach; my packhorses followed just behind; on the 15th, they arrived in Gengenbach and on the night of the 15th to the 16th, they arrived at one o'clock in the morning in Strasbourg.

On the 20th, General Jourdan, whom I had been caring for since the 13th, left for Paris, leaving the main command with General Masséna, who had arrived the day before.

On the 21st, the army was organized into central, left and right portions: the two divisions with Bernadotte, headquartered at Manheim, composed the left; the corps of troops under General Souham at Kehl, Offenbourg and Kork were the centre; and the right was headquartered at Bâle. This latter wing is the strongest.

On the 22nd, we were summoned, as we had requested, to the *commissaire-in-chief* in order to decide on the means of assuring the service. The agent in charge had left for Paris; he was represented by the young Marchand. It was decided that the ambulances would be resupplied and increased by a third; that there would be only three large *corps ambulance* each able to provide two sizeable sub-divisions; that following behind the headquarters, a well-stocked magazine would be in operation from which one could draw at all times, whether to establish evacuation hospitals or to replace the items consumed by the *corps ambulance*; that there would be in each of the aforementioned corps two evacuation clerks, a greater number of workers and sufficient *infirmiers*, plus a cutler, laundrywomen, etc. Marchand promised to provide all this, but we are not counting on it. He assured us that a thousand sets of bedding were arriving from Paris, which I refuted for the reason that to carry a thousand sets of bedding one would need ten large wagons and that for three years not a single cart carrying hospital supplies has been seen on the roads. It was decided that the chief medical officers would have a caisson carried by four horses.

On the 17th, we had a similar meeting with the citizen Schiellé, *ordonnateur*[34] of the 5th Division: it was agreed there that the hospitals of the Children of the Homeland in Strasbourg, Molsheim and Ensisheim would be re-established, which took place immediately.

On the 23rd, I published the honourable and congratulatory letter written, on behalf of the general-in-chef, by the citizen Vaillant to the army's medical officers, regarding the zeal, great endeavour and courageous devotion that they had shown during the course of the campaign. Already, General Jourdan had expressed in a letter to the Minister, dated the 8th, his great satisfaction with the manner in which these medical officers served.

On the 18th, I received the longest and most impertinent letter from the medical council: I replied to it on the 19th and did so only by deriding these buffoons.

On the evening of the 23rd, we received orders to leave with the headquarters for Bâle.

On the 24th, citizen Mouron, the Inspector-general of Hospitals, arrived in Strasbourg, sent by the health board on the most urgent order of the Minister, who had been persuaded that the service was in the most deplorable state and that the wounded we had sustained were crowding the hospitals and almost without help for lack of resources. Citizen Mouron ensured the opposite when he arrived; he spread money and revitalized the service; we have obtained more *infirmiers*, evacuation clerks and many of the resources that we were lacking from him.

On the 29th, I left for Huningue. As I passed through Neuf-Brisach, I saw at the hospital several wounded, with whose condition I was satisfied. Upon entering into a room, I heard plaintive cries: it was a flute-like voice, which I recognized immediately as that of a poor tetanus sufferer. I went to the bed from where it came and found there a young infantryman with an amputated leg and taken by trismus for the past two days; I prescribed *mochlique*;[35] I do not know what its result was. Already three had died from this terrible complication. In Colmar, tetanus is causing the greatest ravages. I advised citizen Morel to turn to *mochlique*; he wanted to use antimonial copper.

Arriving in Huningue, I saw in the room of citizen Laroche, the surgeon in charge of the hospital, General Compère, wounded on the 4th *Germinal* with

---

34. A military administrator charged with ensuring adequate food and equipment supplies.
35. A strong laxative.

the flankers corps: the musket ball that entered through the internal face of his tibia, below the tuberosity, exited at the same height on the external part of the leg, detaching, without fracturing, the fibula. I saw it dressed twice: the wounds are healing beautifully; but there was considerable damage and the loss of tissue is very great. The whole cylinder of bone is missing across a stretch spanning four finger widths; the splinters are rattling; there is quite a lot of pus but it is healthy. I think that this brave man will recover. There was a humoral complication: emetics and laxatives used appropriately have remedied it. The pain and fever are mild; he is able to sleep and has an appetite; everything indicates a happy recovery.

I accompanied General-in-chief Masséna on 29 *Germinal* to the wards of the hospital in Huningue. Seeing him and hearing his words of consolation delighted the wounded; he was satisfied with the service and heard the patients praising the surgeons with pleasure.

In this hospital there is an infantryman from the 25th Line Infantry, who received a musket ball in the lower part of the tibia, which split the bone more than 8 inches higher: it was necessary to find the wound that I identified perfectly; he is well. Another had his arm ripped away very close to the joint: the head of the humerus remains; the wounded man is faring well; however, the aforementioned head of bone should have been extracted, as it is always a significant obstacle to healing. Another has been hit in the vertex by a musket ball, which has split, leaving half of it outside the body and with the other half having introduced itself under the skull: paralysis of the left side of the body; trephine; extraction of the foreign body; high hopes for recovery. Another, who had his calf pierced by a 3lb cannonball: a thin stretch of teguments is making a bridge between the entry and exit of the cannonball; it has partially healed. A mounted gunner's calf was torn away by a cannonball: his recovery is very advanced. An infantryman, the external condyle of whose left knee was blown off and the kneecap crushed, is expected to recover. Citizen Cohorn, injured in the fighting at Aach, on 5 *Germinal*, by a musket ball that had entered through the muscles of his left foot, is doing extremely well. He has not had a single complication and the wound has almost entirely healed, from which I am inclined to conclude that the musket ball, which I had looked for in vain and that I believed to be lost, was redirected by the tendons, which it struck, and that it returned by the same path that it had taken when it entered, for how can one believe that it is still in his foot when he has so little pain and so few complications?

# 1799 – The Army of the Danube and the Campaign in Helvetia

On 1 *Floréal*, I arrived in Bâle and lodged with *M.* Bourcard senior, the former burgomaster: an excellent house.

From the day after my arrival, I began the search for premises for a hospital. I was advised to take over the hall of the Margrave of Baden, a large and superb house. I saw it; it suited us and it was agreed that it would be made ready to receive our sick. But despite our exhortations, they were not able to enter until the 18th of the month; even then, they found only tattered 5-foot-long mattresses and scraps of blankets there. Capiomont, the younger, was appointed its chief surgeon, with Tainturier, Mougeot and Petit-Mangin.

During my stay in Bâle, I received a response from the medical council to my reply: in it, they dared to talk to me about honesty and generosity, and their letter, quite short, badly written but bulky, cost me twenty-two *sous*. I sent it back to them with this note:

> 'Citizens, you who in all things show so much honesty and generosity, put some more of them into the postage of your letters. This one, which I am sending back to you, cost me one franc and ten cents this morning, and you must feel that it is hardly appropriate for a poor subordinate to bear such expenses on behalf of his supreme chiefs, and that, since he is exposed to their admonitions, they should at least be free. I do think that after the effort that the epistle must have cost you, you may have had some lapses. Please do not have any more of the same, I pray you; otherwise, I may have some of my own in turn, and mine would cost you much more dearly than the price I paid for yours.
>
> 'My greetings and respectful obedience.'

On the 13th, I left for Zurich, where General Masséna, with all his general staff, had headed two days previously. I had seen in Bâle the botany professor Lachenal and the professors Socin and Mieg the uncle; I liked the nephew of this latter, a young physician, a lot.

In Rheinfelden, on the Rhine 3 leagues from Bâle, I found the surgeons Bourdet, Maillard and ... , who had come from Moelhin, where they had been unable to find premises for a hospital, to search for them in this town; we found them there together. Sixty straw beds were placed there to receive the evacuations that will likely be taken to Bâle from Kœnigsfelden.

I went to Brugg, where Dr Zimmermann died, and within musket range I found the hospital in Kœnigsfelden. It was, at the time of Calvin's reforms, a huge monastery for men and women; a large wall separated them. Since then it had been turned into public granaries. It was in the church of this convent that the old dukes of Habsburg, descendants of the House of Austria, were interred; their bodies were removed twenty-eight years ago on the orders of Joseph II and his mother.

In this building, one can see the room or cell where Agnès, daughter of Albert who was assassinated by his ward Jean, lived. The painted stained-glass windows of the choir of the church, which today is the hospital's magazine, are of the greatest beauty and well preserved. There were 800 sick, 500 of whom were wounded, and only ten surgeons, three of whom were very weak. I saw amputees who were doing quite well and fractures that seemed certain to heal there; but, in general, the casements in the rooms are too narrow and too far apart, although there are openings on both sides, the ceilings are too low and the rooms too segmented, too far from one another. There is little cleanliness, with dirty and badly kept supplies. The building is invaluable and could be a great resource. Baron, of the 1st class; Schal, of the 2nd.

From this hospital to that in Rheinfelden there are 7 full leagues and quite bad roads, and in this region oxen pull the wagons. Thus, there is no possibility of evacuating from one to the other in one day. It was therefore necessary to establish a staging post in Hornhausen or in Frick to accommodate the evacuated patients for one night.

I arrived bright and early in Baden, famous for its sulphurous thermal waters, which are a very short distance from the town and where there are some rather beautiful inns. I found there two types of public pool, not covered, except one that has a partial roof; in the latter rises a 12-foot column, which is the body of a pump; around the capital is a gallery, to which one climbs by a ladder; the pump is started, and the hot water rises and falls into a reservoir placed on the capital, which is pierced with four holes where as many shaped iron gutters are inserted, along which the water flows and forms the shower. Directly below where it falls, in the bath, are four seats on which the patients are seated to take the shower. In general, these baths are not very elegant, but cleanliness is important there. Each inn has ten or twelve baths, which one must descend several steps to enter.

The area surrounding these waters must have provided the idea of using them for lepers and sufferers of venereal diseases. A confinement centre has also been established half a league from Baden, in the abbey of Wettingen, from where these sick people go under good escort and in good order to bathe in turn in Baden, in a tank below the small town, where they do not trouble the bathers and are not seen by anyone. They live as if in barracks, except that they have only one cooking pot; they help themselves and they have been given only one surgeon of the second class and two of the third class. The sufferers of venereal diseases, 250 in number, are on one side of the house and the lepers are on the other; they do not go to the baths at the same time; a kitchen has been established for those with venereal diseases.

In Baden there is a barracks where soldiers rendered vulnerable by their infirmities are sent with board and lodgings to take advantage of the thermal waters; they are kept there so as not to distance them too far from the army. Indeed, Luxeuil and Bourbonne, where many would prefer to go, are full, or will be full within a fortnight. We obtain the same results and we save the Republic a lot of expense, not to mention that we do not weaken the army, these men gathered together in the number of a few hundred being able, at the first strike of a drum stick, to take arms and be useful.

On the 13th, I was in Zurich. The ambulant hospital was established when the French entered the old *renfermerie*:[36] the building is very bad and the very expensive repairs that have been made there, to make it larger, have not made it any more salubrious. No-one with a significant injury has recovered there, not one amputee; the wounded survive there for ten or twelve days, then they contract hospital fever and succumb. The majority of the rooms only have windows on one side; the latrines contaminate more or less all of them; the courtyard is a stinking cesspit. Each day since my arrival, six or even ten men have been lost there.

After the attack of Feldkirch, where the army of Helvetia had sustained 2,000 injuries, who were all evacuated to Zurich, there have only been five surgeons for twenty days at the hospital of this town, each with 400 wounded to dress and on whom to operate. Moreau, of the first class, who is only 22 years old, has distinguished himself, as has Robert, his assistant, by an extraordinary diligence. At the same time, there were only the same number of surgeons at Kœnigsfelden for still more patients. Thus, everywhere we were lacking them, except in the Army of the Danube, where I had the ability and prudence to recruit some for myself.

---

36. A hospital.

The majority of the thigh amputees were dead by the twelfth day, after complaining for a long time about an intense pain in the hypochondrium[37] and in the stump of the thigh with the hip bones; the latter, upon opening up the corpse, is nearly always found to be permeated by or even full of pus. Be wary of patients with matte white and dry teeth, especially if the hospital is unsanitary: they nearly always die of hospital fever. Black tongue, burning cheeks, moist and gungy eyes and dry, tough hands: bad symptoms.

With the citizen Willaume having succeeded Moreau and having often visited the hospital with him, we had taken the decision to have the most seriously wounded descend every day on a stretcher into the garden, into the hallways, into the air, into the light: they almost all pulled through. Air and light! Nutrients, essential antidotes.

From Zurich, patients are evacuated by boat on the Limmat: it takes only four hours to arrive at Kœnigsfelden, such is the speed of the river; the sick board within a pistol's range behind the hospital, which is very convenient. We would have certainly desired to have a better building for a hospital, but it has been impossible to find one. Only one was suitable: it was the superb orphanage, but it was deemed unnecessary to request this asylum for the unfortunate children whom the generous compassion of the inhabitants and of some founders took in and looked after decently. The administration of this house is a model of good economy and commitment.

On the 16th, the wounded coming from the region of The Engadine arrived. They had travelled almost 50 leagues in the extreme cold, in the rain, and having only encountered two staging posts, which even then were very poorly supplied. They had been taken across land to Lake Wallenstadt: they had been boarded onto boats at this lake; then they had made the land journey that it was necessary to make to reach Lake Zurich, where they boarded again.

Those who were only lightly wounded will pull through; the others are already thin on the ground. Admittedly, because they were wounded in a state of misery, having fasted or having lived on only the most foul bread; having fallen prey to the bad weather of the seasons for eight or nine days of evacuation, their dressings not having been changed more than once; after being allowed to engage in all sorts of excesses or negligence during the journey, after so many unfortunate setbacks, it was very difficult for us to save them.

---

37. Located in the upper part of the abdomen.

On the 14th, a battalion of the 76th Half-brigade was ambushed by the rebellious mountain people in the town of Schwitz, the latter massacring 100 infantrymen or officers, among others the commandant and two captains; a great many were wounded in the defence that took place when they could run to arms. The peasants of this canton were all armed, some with good muskets, some with bad ones; others with maces, etc. This weapon is familiar to them and it is terrible; those whom it hits all die from the many holes that the spikes, with which this murderous implement is bristling, make in the skull; they call it a *comb to groom the French*. All the wounded were evacuated via the lakes and arrived on the 17th.

Since the rebels had caused the death, in terrible agony, of more than 100 of our men who were taken prisoner at Dissentis, 6 leagues from Coire, a detachment drawn from General Ménard's division was directed to march against them. The young Burcke, aide-de-camp to General Masséna, was invited to lead this force, which was to punish those responsible and avenge the death of our unfortunate comrades. The rebels, to kill their victims, had invented the most inconceivable tortures.

Each commune that revolted came to claim a number of prisoners proportionate to its strength; they argued over them and they wanted to see who could make theirs suffer the most. They had taken two pieces of cannon and they were armed with the muskets that they had taken from our men. We pursued them vigorously; a bridge they were guarding was destroyed along with the two pieces of cannon; 1,500 perished, their weapons in their hands. The village of Dissentis and the abbey were reduced to ashes, from where the monks, leaders and those who stirred these revolts had fled, except for two who were shot while trying to evade the flames. During the fire, 300 more individuals who had hidden in the houses, or whom the hope of forgiveness led to the feet of the avengers, were killed. We had 115 wounded. This expedition took place on the 18th.

General Soult, on the other hand, was sent on the 13th to fight the rebels in the surroundings of Lake Lucerne; they fired several fierce salvos at him, just as he was about to disembark, and he had 110 wounded, who were evacuated to Lucerne. Following his corps of troops marched the ambulance of the vanguard, whose leaders were the citizens Chapotin and Frillot.

On the 15th, the enemy surrounded the famous fort of Luziensteig, the key to Italy, and took it along with the entire 14th Half-brigade and all of the artillery; there were few injuries. Since then General Lecourbe has found himself cut off and was forced to fall on Bellinzona.

On the 19th, General Soult, at the head of a corps of troops previously composing the vanguard, marched against the rebels of Schwitz, who had burned Altorf and who were overrunning the surroundings of Lake Lucerne. These people were led by a man named Schmidt, a former Swiss officer in the service of France. They had constructed wooden cannon 12ft long, 4 inches in diameter, and able to fire five or six shots each, fully ringed in iron and mounted on hastily made gun carriages; they had twenty-five of them, which were to fire a hundred shots or more.

The first one exploded on the first shot; the others fired, but badly. They also had entrenchments made of bales of cotton, muslin, cloth and silk, behind which they fought. With their leader having been killed during the first French salvo, they took flight and 200 of their men were killed; not a single prisoner was taken; the soldiers took enormous spoils. Such was the ignorance of these rebels that instead of firing on the French before they disembarked and while they were still on the boats, they had waited until they were ashore.

To disembark, there was only a narrow area, where a single boat could land; even there the ground was silty. With experience, they could have showered Soult's whole corps with musket fire.

On the 26th, the enemy captured Coire, Mels, Sargans and Wallenstadt. We had some wounded, among others an officer, whose crural artery was caught by the point of a sabre (at first it was thought, but the outcome proved otherwise): no complication.

General Soult has marched against the rebels of Schwitz. His troops disembarked on the 19th, at the height of Seedorf, and turned towards Attinghausen by following the two banks of the Reuss. The others disembarked to the left of Fluelen and moved ahead of Bürglen in order to cover the valley of Schachenthal.

On 1 *Prairial*, the enemy seized Saint-Gall, which they entered without any resistance at four o'clock in the evening. We left supplies and belongings there. The sick have been saved. When a wagon that was taking six of them, including two officers, overturned, one of these officers, who had barely recovered from a fractured arm, broke the same arm again; the other similarly broke this limb.

On the 2nd, the enemy advanced on Winterthur. On the 3rd, fifty hussars were cut down in a little wood near this town by other enemy hussars lying in ambush.

On the 4th, the headquarters left for Aarau.

On the 5th, General Masséna moved ahead of Winterthur at three o'clock in the morning, crossed the line occupied by the division of General Ney and gave battle. The enemy resisted until five o'clock in the evening without losing an inch of land, and at this time they started to withdraw; but only in order to take up better positions further back. We had 700 wounded and more than 200 dead. On the 6th, they restarted, and at eleven o'clock in the morning they engaged in fighting that lasted until the night. General Masséna had formed a corps of *grenadiers*, believing that with these brave men he would repulse the enemy; they were cut to shreds and shot down. This day there were a thousand wounded, nearly all *grenadiers*, *chasseurs* and *carabiniers*.

On the 7th and 8th, they were still fighting. Yesterday, on the 8th, it was necessary to abandon Winterthur and retreat to Zurich; there were still a lot of injuries; we have taken 1,500 prisoners. The hospital in Kœnigsfelden, where I was, received 3,000 wounded in four days. They have been taken to Bâle via Aarau, where there is a little hospital, and via Hornhausen (a bad staging post) and Rheinfelden, where there is an evacuation hospital.

# 1800 – The Army of the Rhine and the Campaign in Germany

Today, the left wing under the orders of General Sainte-Suzanne found itself before Kehl at five o'clock in the morning. The attack was broad and simultaneous; the enemy held for some time, but has lost 300 men from the Swabian militias and around 100 prisoners of their own; the major of the 1st Mounted *Chasseurs*, the young Dubois of Crancé, was killed.

On the same day, the centre, under the orders of Lieutenant-general Saint-Cyr, passed through Vieux-Brisach, found almost no resistance and then continued to Fribourg.

The reserve and the right wing marched at the same time.

Today, the 10th, the headquarters is in Säckingen; Moreau, who slept in this town, is leaving for Waldshut where General Delmas's division is.[1] Saint-Cyr is near Saint-Blaise. Lecourbe has made great progress on his left.

Yesterday, I saw 200 prisoners of war pass by and found seventy-five wounded at Rheinfelden, including one with a fractured leg.

An ambulance will be established at Säckingen in the old building known as the barracks. This town offers few resources. There is a noble chapter, whose ladies are very well raised, courteous, speak freely of their beloved God and provide plenty to eat.

Here, I spoke to the generals Dessolle and Moreau about the inviolability of the hospitals and gave them the article that I had translated from the German gazette *Allgemeine Zeitung*. They were struck by reading this text and did not hesitate to adopt its principles, promising to take the initiative in such an

---

1. Longin: General Moreau, named commander-in-chief of the Army of the Rhine, started on 5 *Floréal*, Year VIII (25 April 1800) the brilliant campaign in Germany that finished with victory at Hohenlinden and compelled the Austrians to make peace with France (1801).

honourable cause. I made General Moreau feel how worthy it was of him and of the French nation to propose to General de Kray such a moving convention, so apt to fix the eyes of philosophy and to prove the philanthropic principles now professed by the French. I did not forget to speak to him of his own glory, to which this beautiful act would add a new lustre; I went as far as to tell him that winning a battle would perhaps do him less honour, and cited to him Stair and Noailles, who had been immortalized by this convention in the campaign of 1743. General Dessolle seized this opportunity with enthusiasm and General Moreau invited him to write a letter to de Kray. It was worded as follows:

> 'It is time, General, to reduce as much as it is within our power the horrors and disasters of the war, and the wounded, these honourable victims of the war, particularly deserve all our interest, all our solicitude. I therefore have the honour to propose to you that we regard hospitals as inviolable and never hold the wounded who will be found there as prisoners of war.'

The letter was signed and it was agreed that on the next day it would be sent to de Kray.

I left Säckingen with Simonet, the agent in charge of the hospitals. The column was making its way to Laufenbourg. The road is very bad; we encountered 200 prisoners and fifty wounded accompanied by a surgeon; the bridge at Laufenbourg was broken, otherwise we would have followed the left bank of the Rhine, where the road is excellent. Very close to this town is a rapid descent; everyone was jamming the wheels of their wagons; our coachman chose not to take this precaution. The shaft of the carriage was too short; the horses struggled to hold themselves back and, feeling the shaft on their hocks, began to buck, casting off the strap or support that links the front wheel axles with the rear wheel axles. The linchpin broke off in turn; the spooked horses would have thrown us into the Rhine were it not for a low wall that stopped them. While the coach was being repaired, we walked towards Waldshut; it was 3 leagues away. I was lent a horse but we made this journey on foot. It was the 11th.

During the day, a hospital was set up in the beautiful building of the bailiwick. This house can hold between 160 and 200 patients: good casements, good rooms, a good kitchen and a well-enclosed courtyard, with water. Delightful view: one can see Brugg, and only 4 leagues must be made in order to evacuate to the large hospital of Kœnigsfelden.

A pontoon bridge had been established a quarter of a league away. I left that same day in General Dessolle's carriage; it was going to Neubourg, a few leagues away. We found a substantial column of our troops and the whole cavalry reserve, which forced us to alight and walk for an hour to the town. On the right upon entering, on the hill, is a beautiful castle, rarely inhabited and offering the greatest resources for a hospital; it can house 400 patients. The cellars are superb; wine had been drawn from them for more than 15,000 men to drink, and the granaries had provided grain for the same number. Dinner was ordered for twenty officers. The two sons of the bailiff speak French: when they learned that General Dessolle was to come that very evening to the castle, have dinner and sleep there, they did everything possible to prepare, and at eight o'clock dinner was ready; but an order was received that announced that the general would not be coming and that it was necessary to go to join him. Nonetheless, we still ate dinner, and we invited the first starving soldiers that we met.

From two o'clock until seven o'clock in the evening, the fiercest bombardment could be heard beyond the mountains, to the left of the town.

Outside the town, I found an ambulance bivouacking under the lime trees: I had it leave, since it was more than 5 leagues from General Leclerc's division, to which it was attached. I was even more surprised to find the surgeons of this division a bit further away, led by citizen Duplessy: they excused themselves on the grounds of the ill will of the *commissaire des guerres*, who had refused them any means of travelling, and as this *commissaire* came to pass by, I strongly reproached him for his conduct, which could have compromised the service. Everything was moved on at once. Fortunately, this division had still had only some minor skirmishes.

This morning I proposed to General Moreau that he form with the general-in-chief of the Austrian Army the same convention that was created during the campaign of 1743 between General Stair, for the English, and Maurice de Noailles, for the French, so that the hospitals, as well as the wounded, sick and hospital workers, are immune from harm.

He promised me that he would take care of this important subject without delay, so appropriate for adding to his reputation as a great general that of a human hero and philanthropist. I am awaiting the outcome of this process impatiently.

22 *Prairial*[2] – On this day the *commissaire*-general was given: firstly, the summary of the surgeons retained despite their dismissal; secondly, that of surgeons not mentioned in the statements of the minister on 22 *Ventôse*; and thirdly, that of the *sous-aides*[3] drawn from the battalions and army corps by order of the general-in-chief, dated 17 *Floréal* and published in the army's orders. I had attached a rather long letter that it was necessary to send verbatim to the minister.

23rd – Among the 250 wounded that I visited at the hospital of Saint-Esprit in Memmingen, I noticed several leg amputees who were doing well. Only a mounted gunner was having dizzy spells and was very weak, as a consequence of the blood that he had lost; his wife, luckily for him, had followed him to the army; she cares for him with a lot of affection. I had him vomit lightly: he felt better for it. Two arm amputees (amputated five days ago) were walking in the courtyard. One sergeant had had two toes blown off by a cannonball or a biscayan and the bones of his metatarsal had been broken away and badly stressed: his foot was going to be amputated. I opposed it; I am sure that he will recover; I had the dangling flaps of skin cut away, the splinters of bone taken out and the foot covered with a poultice. I was shown to a man whose whole leg was gangrenous, cold and as hard as marble: he still had good vision and strength, and his disposition was peaceful, apathetic; he felt the need for amputation. I sent for a retractor in order to operate myself in the presence of four surgeons from the Val-de-Grâce,[4] one of the 1st class and the others of the 2nd class. The injured man was placed on a chair, I told the others to make the compression and to arrange the instruments near me, and I made the incision. The artery gave way; I had them compress it; it gave again. I placed the retractor, which was held badly; the section of the bone was difficult; there was still a lot of blood. Finally, the ligature was made; the injured man fainted. I thought him dead, for he had lost 3lb of arterial blood; I had him carried away like a corpse, but the following day he was fine. I have rarely seen a thigh amputee as well as this man was the day after the operation: believing him dead, I dressed his wound very hastily and told the pharmacist, in the event that he were still alive in quarter of an

---

2. Longin: 11 June 1800.
3. Lower surgical grade equivalent to third class.
4. A Parisian military hospital.

hour, to have him take twenty-four drops of laudanum; he did it. He will heal and he will have an attractive stump.

This hospital contains, both in a rather beautiful room on the ground floor and in good outbuildings and barns, 350 patients. We have had another one prepared in the uninhabited house of a tax collector that had been turned into barracks: the building is superb; 300 wounded can be placed there very easily; there is a fountain in the courtyard.

Today, an order came for the citizen Réveilhas, my deputy, to go to the corps of the Bas-Rhin under the orders of General Sainte-Suzanne. I had already sent the citizens Cols, Dumoustier and Danvers, of the 1st class; Magnin and Vinay, of the 2nd, with ten surgeons of the 3rd class there.

Since the Prince of Lichtenstein had had his thigh fractured in its upper third during the passage of ... , citizen Lucas, *chirurgien-major* of the 11th Dragoons, applied the first dressings to him and citizen Henry, of the 3rd mobile corps, stayed close to him. He preferred French surgeons; the general-in-chief suggested that he have some sent from the Imperial army.

24th – I left Memmingen with citizens Simonet and Malapert, tasked by the general-in-chief with finishing the object of their previous mission, collecting 2,000 woollen blankets, 4,000 ells of cloth for dressings, etc. They did not want to let us go, believing the road to be unsafe.

We arrived in Mindesheim, and the commander offered us an escort of four *cuirassiers* as far as the other side of the wood that one encounters on leaving this town and that spans more than a league. We thanked him and did not meet anything on the way, although partisans had stopped and taken an artillery caisson two days previously; it is claimed that it was two squadrons of the regiment of Latour who, having found themselves between two of our divisions, were trying to escape and were looting on the way.

25th – Yesterday, I went to the hospital. I found the same surgeons whom I had left there ten days ago; they had lost twelve of their wounded. The left arm of a Wallachian was mortified and covered in blisters as a result of a wrist wound; it had to be amputated; it would have come back. The surgeon apologized for how little the Austrians had left him in the case. I found twenty-two Frenchmen, twelve of whom were wounded: a sabre blow that had cut open the joint of the arm where it meets the shoulder, a musket shot to the lower abdomen, a calf muscle torn away by a cannonball.

26th[5] – On the 27th, General Lecourbe left with his aides-de-camp Gauthier and Wadeleux[6] for Burgau. General Gudin has orders to seize the bridge at Donauwerth. Nearly all of the right wing is on this side. It is said that General de Kray is making his troops march to this point and that he is going down the Danube himself, along which all the bridges have been cut off.

The news, whether true or false, of the surrender of Gênes is gaining favour in Augsburg. This morning, *émigré* priests were circulating that we had been defeated on the left.

This morning, General Lecourbe dispatched the summary of Wadeleux's services to the Minister, certified to be consistent with the documents, with a letter in which he gave the most honourable praise to this young soldier; he is asking that he be made a captain.

It is very cold: the thermometer was at zero this morning at four o'clock; it snowed at seven, rained for part of the day, and I had to resort to an undershirt. The number with fever, rheumatism and sore throats is multiplying.

In the attack on the bridgehead of Donauwerth, Captain Cuenot threw himself in and began to swim, his sabre between his teeth. He untied a small boat and brought it back under enemy fire. The commandant of the Saint-Michel artillery was seriously wounded in the hand, which was pierced by a biscayan through its widest part. A cannonball that fell between Wadeleux and the general splashed them.

28th – I am leaving to see General Montroux, who has been seriously injured by a musket shot to the knee. The general is taking me to Burgau, from where I will go to Waldstetten, where the wounded man is.

The news of the surrender of Gênes has been announced.

---

5. There are two possibilities for the apparent confusion with the *Journal* having events from the 27th under an entry for the previous day: one is that Percy himself made an error, and the other is that Longin, the posthumous editor of the *Journal* in French, made an error when the handwritten notebooks were typeset.
6. Pierre-François Wadeleux was Percy's nephew. As well as sharing his first name, Wadeleux was also a surgeon, before being named aide-de-camp to General Lecourbe in the Army of the Rhine. Wadeleux repeatedly distinguished himself in the campaigns that followed, and became an Officer of the Legion of Honour in 1804. However, his career in the French Army ended abruptly; he joined the Russian Army following peace between the two empires in 1807 and he died four years later in a duel in Persia, while fighting against the Turks. Percy portrays him as brave but impulsive.

On my way to Burgau, I found the general-in-chief with the generals Dessolle, Decaen, Lahorie and Debilly, gathered to discuss the plan of attack that General Lecourbe has presented to them.

General Montroux is a young man with a handsome face, very well raised. On the 26th, he had his horse killed under him, and the same cannonball, having gone through the animal's stomach, met with the general's right knee, forcing his patella to the side and noticeably displacing it, chipping the bone of its internal side and tearing the joint capsules, teguments, etc. to shreds. Already there was considerable swelling in the thigh and in the wounded knee; the general was suffering greatly. He had hardly recovered from being shot at Engen a month previously, the musket ball from which had sunk the length of one side. The wound in his knee was not very reassuring to look at; it had spread to the size of the palm of the hand, and it seemed it had even been believed that the patella had been blown off; the excessive swelling of the knee supported this error, which I dispelled, having recognized the presence of this deformed and dislocated bone.

Such a case is one of the most awkward in surgery and it is necessary to have acquired a great deal of experience to manage the uncertainty that it creates. Should it be amputated? Can the limb be saved? It is hard to decide, let alone determine that a wounded person should undergo an amputation for a healthy and living leg, but on the other hand, by trying to preserve it one risks seeing the wounded person die. What decision should be taken? Sometimes the swelling of the thigh will soon leave only the cruel recourse of amputation, and if one dares to resort to it, one is accused of having done it too late. If the patella is shattered, all the fragments of it must be removed and the tendinous, aponeurotic parts must not be spared, and in particular one must use adductive bandages early to prevent muscle retraction, which often causes the onset of tetanus.

In the case of the general, I believed that I should state that amputation would be useless and that it was possible for the wound to heal while conserving the limb. Having inserted my finger into the wound, I found it cavernous, without adhesions or strips stretched across it; I would have destroyed them. The teguments of the inner face of the knee were detached, and I suggested that an abscess would form there that would have to be opened early. I advised warm oil, a lot of fomentations, poultices, etc. On the 29th, the report was good; on the 30th, and the 2nd of the following month, good news. I went to Dillingen on 1 *Messidor* to inform the generals Moreau and Dessolle of this good news.

Citizen Renauldin, of the 2nd class, is in charge of accompanying the wounded man, who will be evacuated by hand, on a large stretcher, to Memmingen in a few days.

After seeing the general, I returned to Wettenhausen Abbey, where I found the general-in-chief and General Dessolle, who, not without emotion, heard the account that I gave to them on the doubtful, perilous state of a brave young man whom they like a lot.

29 *Prairial* – I returned to Burgau, where citizen Desbureaux, head of a *wurst*, gave me somewhere to sleep. I left for Zusmarshausen at five o'clock in the morning without an escort and had reason to regret it, for in the middle of a wood that spanned 3 leagues that I had to cross, I found the bodies of two of our men still warm and a horse from the *carabiniers* also killed by the armed bandits who plague our rear. At Zusmarshausen, I took four dragoons with me to Augsburg, from where I made my way to Wertingen, where General Lecourbe had gone: it was so cold that one could hardly withstand it even in a carriage; the road is excellent.

I stayed in the castle that belongs to the elector. The general was on the banks of the Danube, bombarding Hochstett and trying to cross, which was impossible, since the enemy had cut off the bridges, removed the beams, the timbers, and cut them down as far as the tops of the piles. We bombarded various points for more than eight hours without success; it poured around six o'clock, and by nine o'clock the general had returned to the castle with his soaked aides-de-camp. At eleven o'clock, two of our gunners were brought in who had lost their left and right forearm respectively while cleaning the gun with a cannon swab, since the touch hole was badly clogged; the hand had remained on the ground with part of the ulna and the radius intact. The wounds were dry and shed not a drop of blood; this is what happens when part of a limb is torn away. I amputated each of their arms under the light of a lamp, without lint or cloth, with only oakum; one of them had a burned face. I have since learned that they were doing very well.

30th – The following day, the 30th, at five o'clock in the morning, we all left for the banks of the Danube, which the general still feared that he would not be able to cross. On the way, we saw the whole army in motion; we sank into a marsh, where we almost lost the four horses pulling the carriage. There, Captain Cuenot told the general that at four o'clock, the infantry had crossed opposite Blindheim. We went there on horseback. At three o'clock in the morning, ninety swimmers who had prepared for these expeditions had crossed the river naked, with a small raft beside them carrying their uniforms and weapons. When they arrived on the other bank, they had slung their cartridge boxes onto their backs, taken their muskets, and had chased away those who were guarding the bridgehead. While they were holding back the enemy, the sappers hastily mended the bridge with trees and fascines, so well that our infantry could cross within half an hour, not without some risks. Three pieces of cannon were taken, with which a quite considerable column was stopped for more than an hour; the bridge was re-established, so that it was possible to cross there, holding one's horse by the bridle; in this way, the hussars, cavalrymen of the 6th and a regiment of *carabiniers* marched across it.

However, the bridge a quarter of a league further up was worked on hard and after two hours, the artillery was able to pass. It was about time: our people had exhausted the ammunition of the three pieces taken from the enemy who, with eight of their own, were destroying us. General Lecourbe, whom I did not leave for a moment, made incredible efforts to hold on and give the pontoon workers time to finish the large bridge, because the other was too unstable, too weak even to carry the lightest wagon. The enemy was closing in on us; the cavalrymen of the 6th had suffered badly; the infantry, who were being showered with bullets incessantly, were losing heart. The general, seeing a column of infantry advancing supported by a fairly large number of cavalry, had the *carabiniers* charge. They halted these troops and took many prisoners.

I had found the *wursts* of Gouvion and Multon in front of the bridge all prepared to cross, but unable to do so until this bridge was re-established. I took citizen Gouvion (it was seven o'clock in the morning) with three surgeons in order to cross via the other bridge, which shook so much that it made us shudder. It was fortunate that I had this good idea, for the injured were arriving in droves to the village of … , which the peasants had abandoned. Sixteen horsemen from the 6th came with terrible sabre cuts. A *maréchal des logis*,[7] in charge of the 8th Hussars, had his thigh amputated. Several infantrymen had sustained leg fractures. All were dressed, given good beer found in the inhabitants' homes for refreshment, and then loaded on to wagons that crossed the Danube at eleven o'clock in order to go to Wertingen, where I had left five surgeons. It was around this time that Wadeleux, aide-

---

7. Marshal of Lodgings, equivalent to the rank of sergeant in the British Army. According to the celebrated military strategist Antoine-Henri Jomini, the term 'logistics' is derived from this grade.

de-camp to Lecourbe, at the head of some *carabiniers*, charged on an entire enemy battalion, disarmed their major and had them lower their weapons. The artillery was taken, with four flags and more than 2,000 prisoners. The few enemy soldiers who escaped withdrew to Donauwerth. This took place between this town and Hochstett.

The general took me to the left, where the enemy had also lost a lot of ground. We crossed next to Dillingen, which the enemy had been contesting with us for a long time; we passed through Lawingen, through which they had hastily made their retreat, and having arrived on the vast plain, we saw them rallied and with an imposing cavalry force. We had taken 1,470 prisoners, and it was now only a question of beating their cavalry. Klinglin had left with 1,200 horses from the area around Ulm. We fought for a long time; at four o'clock, the enemy no longer had a piece of cannon forward, and everything seemed to indicate that they were now thinking only of withdrawing; but at six o'clock, they manoeuvred skilfully with their cavalry. They presented the charge. Our cavalry's generals hesitated. Lecourbe spoke loudly; the two sides charged with equal ardour; they converged, then regrouped, and each side took up their ground again. Our men were going to yield without the 9th cavalry, which came to support them. What shouts! What tumult! I wanted to see this glorious and skilful carnage up close. Twenty-four *carabiniers* suffered very badly. Prisoners and horses were brought back.

Towards eight o'clock, the enemy had the cannon arrive. Yet our men held firm. Having left for Hochstett, we encountered General Moreau and all of his entourage near Dillingen: he made us return, having announced to us that he was bringing reinforcements in cavalry and that it was necessary to make a second charge to crush the enemy cavalry. We galloped onto the battlefield, a good half-league ahead of Lawingen. The enemy was firing from all sides: when they saw the gilded group in the middle of which I found myself, they fired on it fiercely and a ricocheting 13lb cannonball knocked Lecourbe's plume off; they fell close to us and, by showing that it was reckless to remain so grouped, we separated. The cavalry arrived; our infantry returned. The *wurst*, which was already at rest in Lawingen, also returned. We marched, we hurried; the enemy was waiting for us; but at the slightest clash, they fled more quickly and the battlefield was ours at ten o'clock in the evening. We then entered Gundelfingen. We did not have a single casualty.

1 *Messidor* – 1 *Messidor* will be remembered for the taking of a convoy of 150 wagons and more than 500 horses; it was the 6th *Chasseurs* who made this excellent capture; more than 1,500 sacks of oats, etc.

We entered Donauwerth this morning at six o'clock, and found large stores of wheat there.

# 1805 – The Austerlitz Campaign

I left Boulogne on 14 *Fructidor*. The roads were crowded; there were no horses at the posts, His Majesty having engaged everything.

I arrived in Paris on the 19th; I hurried to my house in the country; found my wife ill. She had an adynamic fever that had lasted twenty days.

I left Paris, or rather the hamlet,[1] on the 5th. I arrived in Strasbourg on the 8th; bought horses and baggage; I left for Rastadt on the 9th, for Pforzheim on the 10th, for Stuttgard on the 11th and rested on the 12th. The Emperor and the headquarters are at Louisbourg.

There are a hundred patients sleeping and treated miserably in Stuttgard. I wrote an urgent letter to the Intendant-general to have him establish two large hospitals for 1,500 and 2,000 patients respectively, one at the Solitude Palace, 1 league from the town, and the other in the barracks for the troops from this area who were leaving for the army.

I arrived in Schorndorf, a town surrounded by ditches and a wall, safe from a surprise attack; the large town hall is suitable for placing 200 patients; the superb church can hold 500. We stayed the night with a very drunk notary.

I called Chédieu to Stuttgard to be in charge. I left on the 13th for Gmünd, 10 full leagues from Stuttgard. I stayed in Stuttgard with *M.* Stockmeyer, Secretary of State, in a mansion; he is a good man.

I stayed in Gmünd, no. 142, near the gate to Aalen, with a very considerate baker. In this town, one may note the houses painted rather elegantly with frescos: that of an apothecary on the square depicts Moses, soldiers and prostitutes; it has the inscription: *Domus utilis et necessaria*.[2] The Calvar-Berg is the most beautiful mountain, dishonoured by the most disgusting sacred caricature: stations where Jesus, of such human greatness, is whipped, dragged

---
1. Longin: of Bordeaux, near Lagny. [Lagny-sur-Marne is now in the eastern suburbs of Paris.]
2. 'A useful and necessary house'.

by the most flamboyant-looking persecutors. There is a very old church, since it has a bishop's or canon's tomb from the year 1050 on display outside.

I arrived in Aalen at eight o'clock in the morning, 5 leagues from Gmünd: it is a poor place, without many resources. I left for Nordlingen, 8 leagues away. Three roads lead there. The best is that of Merckheim; there will be an evacuation line along this route, going to Spire. Nordlingen, famous for two battles, is an old, completely open town of little importance; it is surrounded by excellent plains. I lodged with the assessor[3] Valtz, near the church.

I spent the night of the 15th to the 16th in Marck-Zöbingen, a large, sprawling village.

Arrived on the 16th at Donauwerth, at ten o'clock in the evening; there are 14,000 men in this town; I had to sleep on straw with sixty *Gendarmes d'élite*. The weather is detestable. I arranged a hospital in the Bavarian veterans' barracks, a good building for 250 patients; we have requisitioned everything. I have placed Lejan, a *chirurgien-major*, there with four *sous-aides*. His Majesty has ordered that enough hospitals be established in Donauwerth for 4,000 patients, which is impossible.

I stayed on the 17th in Cokhaus with some conformist monks. The Emperor left at midday, on horseback, wearing a simple grey redingote.[4] Three thousand prisoners have been placed in the church of the abbey, all on top of each other, frozen from the cold. We are anticipating 200 injured. There are no amputation cases in the vanguard division, and Bancel and the physician Roussel have written a moving letter.

His Majesty has been to Wertingen, where 3,000 Austrians have been taken.

I wrote from Donauwerth to *M.* Dubos to dispatch the surgeons and the package of surgical instruments. I sent Benac and Deveyrines, from the 103rd, to Nordlingen on discharge, with an order to stay there and to retain some passing surgeons.

I left on the 19th, at seven o'clock in the morning, for Augsbourg, 8 leagues from Donauwerth. The weather is terrible, with rain, snow, cold and mud from which one would never emerge. I was with the colonel of the 1st Dragoons, a relative of His Majesty, who has been wounded by several sabre blows to the

---

3. A judicial position, less senior than a judge.
4. A redingote is a double-breasted coat adapted from the English riding coat. It is the famous overcoat that Napoleon is often depicted as wearing.

head, one of which cut a considerable flap from the occiput. I travelled in the war minister's carriage, to whom he is the senior aide-de-camp.

25 *Fructidor* – Arrived yesterday evening in Pfaffenhofen, where General Andréossy had placed us. This poor choice of position has prevented us from being useful for two days. We left an ambulance section there to recall it soon.

Yesterday, a bridge over the Danube collapsed and submerged beneath the waters two officers' wives who were passing over it in a cart, along with General Bailly's equipages, several other carriages and around forty people. This incident cut communication between the active army and us and delayed operations. As the conditions of the Emperor did not suit Mack, who was confined to Ulm, it will be necessary to fight today and gain the heights that overlook this city, which will cost a lot of lives. A few thousand Austrian foot soldiers still remain; it is said that the cavalry has left with Archduke Ferdinand.

Yesterday, I identified the hospitals, the one in the new barracks, where we had 300 wounded or sick five years ago, and the one established in the Capuchins' building: the greatest disorder reigned there; almost no straw, no *infirmiers*, little food and extreme uncleanliness. We have orders to separate the Austrians from the French and to gather 300 of them in the old barracks; I left Donat, the Austrian *chirurgien-major*, to care for them, with four subordinates from this army. The town is providing everything, and certainly the Austrians are much better treated by them than the French. It is true that the Austrians have behaved in a horrible way: Gunzbourg is devastated; everywhere they break, smash, steal, etc. No one represses the brigandage; we have no means of coercion. Under the pretext that no distributions are being made, the soldiers plunder and devastate everything; the foot dragoons are committing the most abominable crimes.

There was a fierce wind all night. The countryside has been swamped by the flash flood of the Danube, which slowed the operations more still. This morning the weather is fine, the sun is hot and everyone is drying out, but there is neither food nor fodder. The peasants' horses have all been stolen; everywhere horses are traded; people steal saddles; they are fighting and killing each other for a bridle.

Nearly 600 wounded have left Gunzbourg since the 22nd. Eugène, the *aide-major* is in Zusmarshausen with a *sous-aide* to receive them. How are they there? I have sent surgeons to Augsbourg: there is an order for my brother to retain those who arrive from Strasbourg there.

Vanderbach has sent 250 wounded to Dillingen, from where they were directed to Donauwerth: there were five amputees making the journey. The houses of Gunzbourg are full of wounded officers and soldiers whom the surgeons are going to dress.

Besson, *sous-aide* of the 15th Dragoons, has been killed by the enemy.

I conscripted and led twenty-five Austrian prisoners to the hospitals, chosen from a line of 500; I had a lot of trouble to get them to the hospitals, where they do not care to stay. No French workers or *infirmiers*; a sad service. I embraced my friend Gorcy; he was going to Augsbourg.

26th – I sent Bourdet, the *chirurgien-major*, and Bataille, a *sous-aide*, as close as possible to Ulm so that they are among the first to enter and can attend to the service there. They will only be able to do this in a few days, for the enemy, with a strength of 25,000 men, have obtained a respite, although they may yet surrender if help does not arrive.

We have a way in and we are waiting.

Most communications were cut when the Danube burst its banks and the bridges collapsed. The infantry can no longer join the army; the horses of the cavalry have water up to their shoulders; yesterday, a few badly guided cavalrymen drowned. The countryside around Leipheim and Gunzbourg is flooded: I have been unable to get surgical assistance through to Elchingen Abbey, where we have 400 wounded, to whom *M.* Larrey has been very useful; he has made some amputations, assisted by the surgeons of the Guard.

Gunzbourg is full of injured officers, who are staying there or cannot be transported: among them are some serious cases, shots through the chest, comminuted fractures, arm amputations; we are dressing them, and the townspeople do the rest. The Austrian unfortunates, who number 400, are delivered to their surgeons, from whom they receive pitiful assistance: these people are slow, burn through resources and are not very sensitive; the majority of those with serious injuries assigned to their care will die.

One sees only stolen horses; musicians, soldiers, workers, everyone is mounted on the same horses. They should be confiscated for the evacuation of the ambulances, but no order has been given.

The Emperor has been reduced to living on potatoes, as has General Murat. They are being sent at this very moment at Elchingen Abbey a baggage wagon loaded with food, which, because of the bridge collapse, has only been able to go 2 leagues from Gunzbourg; there, a raft will be found that will transport the items to the other side, from where they will be taken to Elchingen Abbey.

Ulm will only be ours in five days' time, it remains necessary that the enemy does not receive any support, for then we will likely fight again; it is said that they are holding 24,000 prisoners. Prince Murat is pursuing Archduke Ferdinand, who is fleeing at the head of 8,000 men, including 4,000 cavalrymen.

The dragoon division, under the orders of General Baraguey, is returning to Gunzbourg, then going to Donauwerth to pursue another column, or perhaps that of Archduke Ferdinand. The baggage train in Gunzbourg is diabolical. General Baraguey's ambulance division has lost four of its caissons and all of its instrument cases, which the enemy have taken from it; it was going to the aid of the hospital in Alpeck.

Good weather; wind from the south: we needed this change. There are few fevers, in spite of the previous fatigues, the marching and bivouacking in the mud, the snow and the rain. I do not know how the troops have survived. They have pillaged and lived on the spoils; the bread convoys were stolen along the way.

27th – There were nearly 600 wounded in Elchingen. Lejan, a *chirurgien-major*, with three surgeons and three pharmacists from Donauwerth, went there, leaving at the hospital in this town only a few people; the surgeons of the Guard, with *M.* Larrey at their head, have performed the service with few resources. The majority of the patients have been evacuated to Donauwerth, where they must have been very unhappy; from there, they were sent to Augsbourg. I was going to leave for Elchingen with five mounted surgeons. The whole region is still covered with water and the large bridge at Elchingen has not yet been repaired. The troops that passed back through Gunzbourg last night and tonight found it very difficult to find the path; a few people died in the waters. Yet they file past and are waiting for the Emperor. *M.* Paulet, from the Guard, told me that there would only be about sixty wounded left in Elchingen and that it was not necessary for me to go there, so I will spend the day in Gunzbourg. I had had the clothing bags filled with aid supplies and I had taken an amputation case.

The flooding from the Danube has disrupted our service considerably. In Pfaffenhofen, *M.* Andréossy, the assistant major-general, had sent to us the order to go to Elchingen. This order is dated the 24th; it was the response to our letter of the 23rd. It was only given to me by *M.* Lejeune, the lieutenant colonel, nephew of the chief justice, this morning; we may not have been able to comply with it so easily, but for my part, I would have left and that would have been useful and correct.

There is not a medicine chest anywhere. A few days ago, the enemy took cases weighing five hundred[5] that, because of their enormous weight, could not have been loaded onto other carts. No one has seen the cases of the subdivision.

The surrender is complete: the Prince of Lichtenstein (Louis) has been entrusted with it. General Mack had asked to take the 24,000 men to Austria, with a promise that they would not serve for a year; our Emperor refused it. It has been agreed that, since the rescue on which M. Mack seems to be relying is not arriving before the 3 *Brumaire*, we will enter that day, at noon, into Ulm, and that the Austrians, soldiers and non-commissioned officers, will go to France; the officers will return to their country on parole. I am keeping eight French and five German surgeons ready to enter Ulm on the 3rd, for there must be more than 1,500 sick and wounded Austrians there. M. Faschinck, the Austrian *aide-major* is going with them; he has been the secretary of M. de Mederer[6] for a long time.

There are, in Gunzbourg, nearly 500 Austrians, whom I returned to the surgeons of this nation.

28th (others say the 29th) – There was a white frost. The most beautiful sun appeared as early as eight o'clock; it is warm and the paths are drying out. The army has partly retaken the road to Donauwerth. The Emperor had to go to Augsbourg. Ney's army and that of Lannes remain for the evacuation of Ulm, which will start today at three o'clock. Mack has asked the Emperor if he can leave before the deadline expires; the officers are returning to Austria on their parole, and, since he is not on parole himself, he will be able to go wherever he wants, for which Napoleon reproached him; this humiliation is terrible. Ulm, it is claimed, contains 3,000 sick people; the Austrian army has ordered that each regiment should leave three or four surgeons to treat them. At nine o'clock, the French surgeons will leave Gunzbourg for this place.

It is said that there is an enormous number of wounded in Ulm.

---

5. Percy gives no unit of weight for these boxes. However, France introduced the metric system after the Revolution, implying that the weight of the cases was 500kg.
6. The Austrian surgeon Matthäus Mederer.

# 1806 – The Jena Campaign

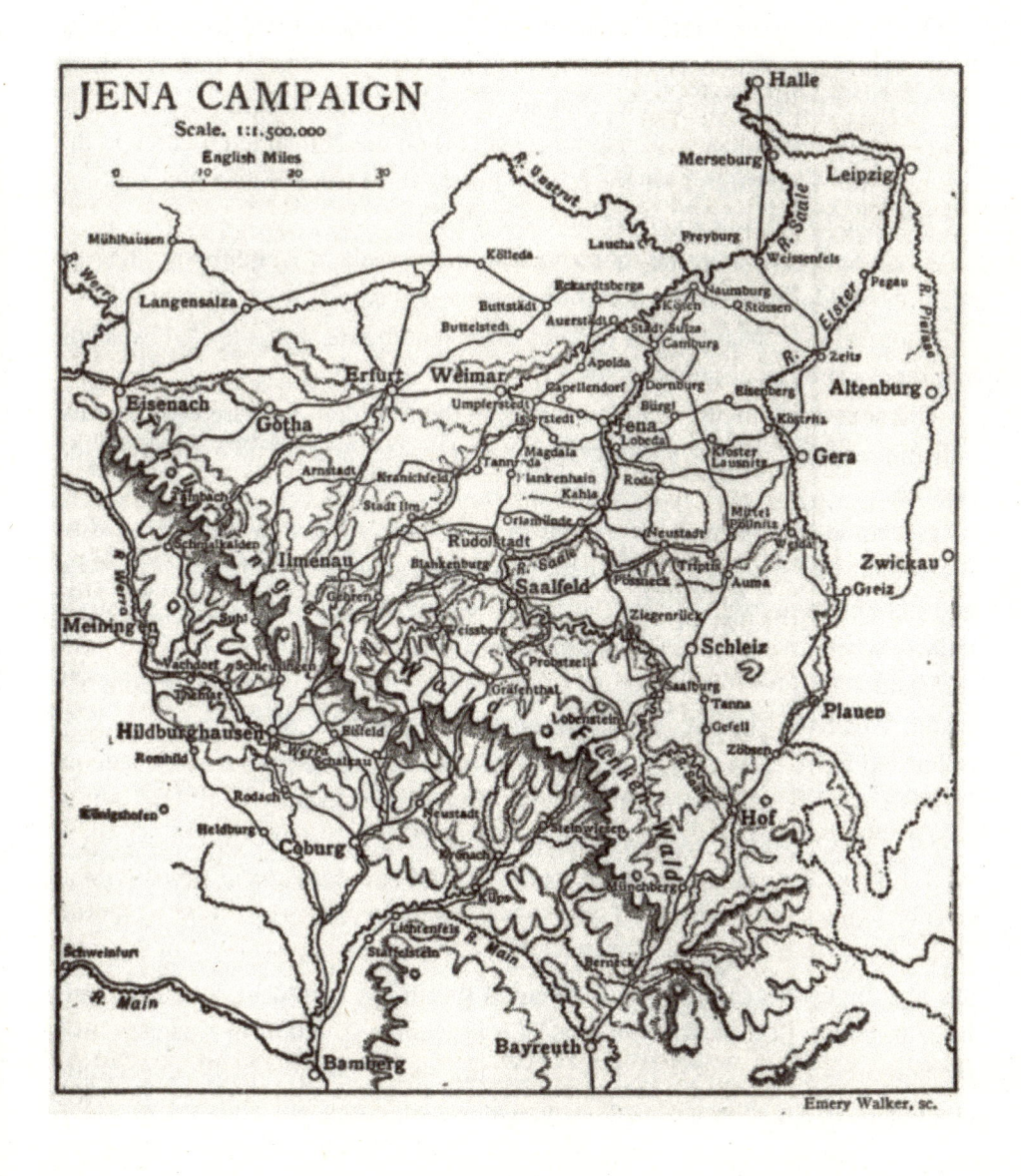

Everyone was preparing to pass back across the Mein and return to France; the official journals did not stop talking about the triumphant party at the camp of Meudon, of the public festivities. The two inspectors-general had been asked to go to Strasbourg to arrange the hospitals there and to receive the evacuations, which were going to be made very shortly. Suddenly we can hear cries of war: Russia has not ratified the peace treaty; Prussia is arming for war on all sides; all of Germany, all of the North, is stirring. The beautiful dream has vanished; we must go back on campaign.

On 25 September, I left Camstadt for Munich, where I was to spend a few hours with the Intendant-general to organize our service. He had left there on the night of the 27th to the 28th and I could not meet him. After sending many letters and orders to Augsbourg, I set off on the 28th at ten o'clock in the morning for Wurzbourg, where His Highness the Prince Major-General and the Intendant were due to arrive on the 29th.

At eleven o'clock in the morning, I found myself in Rottenbourg, having spent the coldest and mistiest night in a peasant's cart.

I stopped in Ochsenfurth, 4 leagues from Wurzbourg; I was tired, it was late and there were not enough horses.

The next day, the 30th, at ten o'clock in the morning, I entered Wurzbourg and immediately began to hurry to find premises and to take stock of the service.

My equipages have all remained in Camstadt. I am expecting it on 8 or 9 October; my wife will come here (Wurzbourg) with *M.* Chédieu, his wife and his children, and the three surgeons whom he has with him at Solitude Palace, where the establishment has been dismantled.

1 and 2 October were used to send service letters to several surgeons for whom I had the address, some already having served, and others who had requested to be called up to the army. I have asked Thomassin in Besançon, Ibreliste in Metz, Verdier in Mainz, Simonin in Nancy and Diebort in Strasbourg to send me as many surgeons as they could and to choose them well. I have persuaded the Intendant that I need ten more *chirurgiens-majors*, twenty *aides-majors*, and 160 *sous-aides*, and I have worked hard to recruit them. We will not be able to find everyone for this latter group, and yet they are absolutely necessary. It was decided that there would be 2,000 patients in Wurzbourg, 300 in Schweinfurt, 600 in Bamberg, 1,000 in Anspach, 600 in Nuremberg and 2,000 in Francfort, and that there would be evacuation staging posts in Offenheim, Closter-Oberbach, Langfeld and Seligenstadt.

The magnificent hospital, known as the Julius hospital, in Wurzbourg was charged with receiving 200 of our sick, and in the military hospital of the troops of Prince Ferdinand, we have placed seventy of them. The abandoned convent of the Carmélites will be converted into a hospital with 300 places; that of Unterzell, three-quarters of an hour from the town, will hold just as many. It will be possible to put the same number in the secularized abbey of the Benedictines of Saint-Étienne; which will still be far from the number we need.

The citadel of Wurzbourg, which has been placed in a state of siege,[1] will require a temporary service. I have already sent three surgeons to Kronach and the same number to Kœnigshoffen, other fortresses also in a state of siege. The surgeons have left for Nuremberg, Anspach and other destinations. Only Braunau now remains, where I have left six surgeons, and Augsbourg, where only three will stay.

His Majesty, expected in Wurzbourg for the past three days, arrived there on the 2nd at eight o'clock in the evening. The city is full of French people: I saw General Dupont's division pass through. The *chirurgiens-majors* in Mainz have received cloth, lint and instrument cases, and the regiments are equipped with hospital caissons. A case of instruments has been distributed to the other regiments of the army, which is improper: it would be better for the surgeons-major to have one of their own; that would cost significantly less and one would be sure at all times that there are enough instruments in the armies. Soldiers do not go to war without their weapons; surgeons must also have theirs, and it would suffice to give them some compensation to make it possible for them to obtain them. But as with each transfer and resignation of a *chirurgien-major* it would be necessary to start again, perhaps it would not be unreasonable to demand that everyone has their instruments. The distribution that is made to them from the cases in the magazine leaves us open to a shortage in the army's hospitals, for which at least 100 are necessary.

We have found in Wurzbourg, in order to set up hospitals there, in addition to the abandoned Carmélite convent, the abbey of Saint-Étienne, which is superb and completely new, but which is still full of households. Half a league from the town is the beautiful abbey of Oberzell, where a superb service can be established for 400 sick; the water is excellent there, abundant, and the building

---

1. A state of siege is declared when an authority decides to restrict movement of people and goods into and out of a city.

is on the Mein River, by which it would be possible to evacuate the patients. A quarter of a league further along, on the same road, is the old convent for women, which is called Unterzell. At one time the Austrians had their patients there; we have had them there as well. The building, although somewhat old, is vast and offers great resources; everywhere there are fountains gushing with water. The partition walls of the cells are being knocked down to create large rooms; it will be an excellent establishment. In three days the first patients will be placed there.

I saw in Wurzbourg the famous civil hospital founded by the elector Julius. It is a superb and very sizeable edifice, composed of two main buildings in parallel, separated by a narrow courtyard; behind it is a botanical garden with two greenhouses. A beautiful anatomical theatre and a conservatory are at one end of this garden; there are some beautiful items there, but nothing scholarly with regards to anatomy; the pathological objects are numerous there, especially concerning bone diseases. I saw there a calculus that had a musket ball at its base. The Siebolds, father and son, and celebrated surgeons, have given the Julius hospice in Wurzbourg a great reputation. The corridors stretch for as far as the eye can see; the wards consist of rooms, each with twelve or sixteen beds. The main building at the back is reserved for the elderly and the insane; the one at the front is the refuge for both medical and surgical patients. In each corridor there is a fountain; everything is well-kept, sweet-scented and swept. It is a shame that the rooms only have windows on one side, because of the corridor that leads to them; such is the style throughout Germany, in Vienna, etc., and in this beautiful town the hospitals are all flawed in this regard and because the casements are too high. It has been slightly remedied by small vents in the wall.

The troops of Prince Ferdinand, brother of the Austrian emperor, prince of Saltzbourg, formerly Grand Duke of Tuscany, where he was born, number only 400 or 500 men and have a small hospital that they share with us; yesterday we had there sixty-seven men. The Julius hospital has received or will receive a hundred of our sick; they will be there until the completion of our hospitals.

5 *Octobre* – Yesterday, the 4th, the fat king of Wurtemberg arrived here at eight o'clock in the evening. The Emperor went to see him; his only daughter is to marry Prince Jérôme, who accompanied his brother.[2]

---

2. Jérôme Bonaparte married Katharina Friederike of Württemberg in 1807 after the annulment of his first marriage by a French imperial decree two years earlier.

Our hospital equipment is gradually arriving, carried on miserable peasants' carts, where they are wet and nearly always spoiled. I saw one of them pass this morning and, through its slatted sideboards, one could see crutches and wooden legs, which made the troops laugh and mutter: they should be spared this spectacle, and why, for that matter, begin a campaign by bringing in these frightening implements, which can hardly be useful until the end?

6th – On 30 September, at seven in the evening, there was a terrible storm; rain fell by the bucketful and the majority of our troops were either on the move or bivouacking. Since this storm, the weather has been quite good. This region is superb. The town is surrounded by beautiful hills, where good wine is made; the grapes that are harvested in the northern part of the citadel are very highly regarded.

We received an order to leave for Bamberg and to be there by the 7th.

6th – We spent the night in Closter-Oberbach, halfway there, with a lady staying in the old lodge of the abbot of the beautiful abbey in this place, an abbey where it had been decided that we would set up a hospital, which is unnecessary, since the Mein River can be used to evacuate the sick from Bamberg to Wurzbourg. This means of evacuation renders the majority of the proposed establishments useless; Schweinfurt alone must be retained in order to receive the sick who are evacuated by the Mein there, as a staging post.

7th – Arriving in Bamberg on the 7th, at 11 o'clock in the morning, I found there in the Dominican convent a beautiful hospital started under the auspices and under the care of the physician Marcus, physician-administrator, an excellent hospital worker. The same evening, the Emperor sent Marshal Duroc there to see if the patients were well; he found the surgeons there who gave him a good report, and he went to make his own accordingly. The civil hospice, which is superb, has received 150 of our patients. Tomorrow there will be 200 places with the Dominicans and soon there will be 350 or 400. A second establishment will be set up: it is to be hoped that the French will not interfere with it and that the Bavarian administration alone will be responsible for it, as in Munich.

Nothing has arrived yet, not linen, nor lint, nor instrument cases; because there are not enough vehicles, everything is being held back. This evening, the *ordonnateur* Lombard was looking to borrow 2,000 *francs* to buy dressing cloth; the women of the town are making lint: what misfortune!

Bamberg is crowded with troops. I am lodged in the old abbey, known as Saint Catherine's Hospital. Tomorrow, His Majesty is leaving for Kronach. Many cases have been distributed to the regiments; it is to be feared that we are missing some.

8th – There is no fodder in Bamberg. The horses are dying of hunger there; it is twenty-four hours since mine have had hay. It will be even worse in Kronach, where we must go.

The order to leave for this fortress was brought to me at three o'clock in the morning on the 8th; it is said there that His Majesty wants us to go in a day to Lichtenfeld and the following day, the 9th, at six o'clock in the morning, to Kronach, taking (at his expense) supplies for eight days.

I was not able to leave until three o'clock in the afternoon; the whole morning was spent arranging a carriage and cow, which I had to leave in Bamberg at the lodgings of the *chirurgien-major* Philippe. I deliberated for a long time about whether I would make the campaign in a carriage or on horseback; in the end, to be more expeditious, I opted for the latter, undoubtedly the more arduous, but also the more flexible and more consistent with the swiftness that my service requires. I have six horses and three servants. Before leaving Bamberg, I visited the building that the Dominicans are said to run, where I found sixty French patients already lying, and a host of well-managed labourers who were preparing and furnishing the rooms for 300 others. In charge of this establishment is *M.* Marcus, a doctor of medicine and director-general of the hospices of Bamberg: he is the best hospital worker in Germany. It was on his advice and according to his plans that they built the large civil hospice in this place, which is beautiful, imposing, well-arranged, salubrious and admirably clean; he is its director and he commands everyone there. *M.* Marcus rendered great services to the French patients in the preceding campaigns, and particularly in those of the Sambre-et-Meuse army. I suggested to him that he should take sole charge of the administration of the military hospitals in Bamberg, and he agreed, provided that he was given one or two clerks at the entrances; he will have no other French workers. I have given him, in the name of the Intendant-general, a kind of certificate, the display of which will keep away the greedy clerks and directors who will come to meddle in the hospitals that this honest man is going to govern at the King of Bavaria's expense. From Bamberg, we will evacuate to Wurzbourg along the Mein River, stopping and staying the night in Schweinfurt, where I left Philippe and two *sous-aides*. The hospitals of Forcheim, Anspach and Nuremberg have become useless. In going to see the building of the Dominicans, I found the *ordonnateur* Lombard and the *régisseur* Mouron buying new cloth to make bandages and compresses while waiting for the arrival of the dressing cloth coming from France. We have no instrument cases.

I set off at last and it was already late. In less than five hours, we arrived in Lichtenfeld, a small town halfway along the route, having travelled along a generally good and beautiful road and through picturesque, mountainous, wooded and well-cultivated country; that is 7 leagues from Bamberg and from Kronach. I was losing hope of finding lodgings for my horses, my men and myself, but the headquarters had left at noon and I was given accommodation with a good woman, where we slept on the straw.

9th – This morning, at three o'clock, we left on a mild, but dark, night for Kronach, where I arrived at nine o'clock. I was lodged with the doctor Berner, a coarse man, to whom I made felt his dishonesty. I immediately went up to the Rosenberg Fort; I found there a small hospital with fifty places, where there were already twelve Frenchmen: it is a bad hospital, built against a wall of the fortress, which shelters it from the cannon. It will be possible to have another larger, more salubrious hospital, and there will only be casements to add in where they are missing. I have given an order of service to *M.* Charles-Guillaume Paul, doctor of the fort, a man of 55, a father to four children, and having a salary of only 30 florins from the King of Bavaria. The appearance of the surroundings of Kronach, seen from the top of the citadel, resembles that of some Swiss cantons. The garrison of the fort will be only 600 men: the Bavarian veterans and some recruits are leaving the post today. There is a lot to sweep and clear to make it clean up there; a pool of stagnant and foul water runs along the inside of one of the ramparts; the laundry room is dreadful. I will see if there is a way to find a building in the town for a staging post only, for it is a poor place.

I made amends with my host, the doctor Berner, who demonstrated to me that, not knowing me and seeing me arrive to stay with him with a large retinue, he had thought that I was going to take quarters that were intended for me and that he was protecting only for me. I gave him a written invitation to run the medical service of the hospital in Kronach, save suitable remuneration.

10th – I left at six o'clock in the morning. The weather is superb and warm; we stopped at the aforementioned town, where I took refreshment with the

Intendant-general, with whom I then travelled. We could hear the cannon to our left all evening. The dragoon division was marching with great haste and we found the three ambulance caissons from the VI Corps: I would certainly have liked to take linen, lint and instruments, which I am completely lacking, but they are awkward in this corps, and I returned by another way.

At last, we arrived in Lobenstein, a rather pretty little town in Saxony, built on a plain and surrounded by barren hills with an unpleasant appearance: a league away is the village of Ebersdorf, in the magnificent castle of which His Majesty has been staying. He left this morning for Schleitz, 4 leagues further on from there.

I have asked the magistrate of the town for linen and lint: they will be needed in the coming days, and *M.* Mouron, who has a lot of it, as well as instruments, is behind us, as is *M.* Lombard.

I found for a hospital of 225 places the Reuss mansion, at the end of the town: a beautiful building, where our soldiers have smashed everything. I have received the order to leave for Schleitz, where I must be tomorrow at eight o'clock; it is 5 full leagues from here.

11th – What a spectacle! Everything is pillaged, devastated; the inhabitants are fleeing; the houses are abandoned; in several villages the fire has consumed many of them. The road is narrow and dreadful; the region is barren and wild; it resembles Tyrol. In Saalburg, a large village situated on the height of a hill that is difficult to reach, I found twelve men in quite a good house. They were injured in the events of the 8th at the covered bridge by which one crosses a small river that runs at the bottom of this village; a surgeon called Zoeller was tasked with caring for them and was complaining a lot about this commission, not being able to obtain either cloth or food, and having been obliged to take the beds on which his patients were sleeping from the abandoned houses. The rest of the way is even worse than the part we have passed: the carriages break or tip; they move slowly in rutted tracks with steep edges, and which are always up or downhill. Having arrived at half a league from Schleitz and in a large village, entirely deserted, and which was being pillaged, I also considered looting and led my three servants to go to collect the linen and cloth that we could still find in the houses; in an hour we loaded a small peasant's cart with it. Tomorrow we will cut it into bandages and compresses.

Schleitz is a rather pretty town, with a well-built fortified castle. I found 150 wounded men there, who had been injured in the events of the 9th on the heights, a league away, by the gate to Leipzig; most of these wounded were lodged in the town. Sixty Saxons were gathered in a hospital established in the public school, all cut by sabre blows; three of our surgeons and two from the area were caring for them. The Intendant and I have found a spacious and clean building in which to set up a hospital of 250 places. The castle would have been still more suitable, but His Majesty had left a guard there to protect the town from pillaging.

Having hurried around, exhausted and in need, I ate something and risked buying an ironmonger's saw, in case of emergency and need; but, having remembered that there was a case of instruments at the hospital, I had it brought with 25lb of good lint, and I left at two o'clock with both of these aids for Auma, a little town 4 leagues further on. I thought I would meet His Majesty there, but he was 3 leagues ahead; all the lodgings are taken and the houses are crowded. General Roussel gave me refuge. A battle is expected tomorrow.

12th – Left on the 12th, at seven o'clock, in the morning, for Gera, 7 leagues away. A good road, a mountainous area, but better cultivated. The town is beautiful and quite large. At two o'clock, it was full; a large part of the army has passed through it. The houses are overflowing with soldiers; some of them have been looted. His Majesty spent last night there and will spend this one there again. It is terribly noisy.

The news of the success of Marshal Lannes has been confirmed; his corps, and in particular General Suchet's division, has taken a thousand prisoners, thirty pieces of cannon and killed Prince Louis-Ferdinand, uncle of the King of Prussia. On my way to Auma, 1 league from Schleitz, I crossed the battlefield of the I Corps: it was covered with Saxons and dead horses. The 4th Hussars were on the brink of yielding; they have some wounded.

The two bad little hospices of Gera have received sixty patients, including sixteen seriously wounded Saxons. Hospitals will be established for a thousand patients; there will be 200 of them in a small castle a quarter of an hour from the town. I made a request to the director of the orphanage to provide us, for tomorrow, the 13th, with 50lb of lint; we will go to look for all the linen we can gather from the houses, since the surgeon Bonjour abandoned the precious bundle that we had collected on the other side of Schleitz, despite my exhortations not to lose sight of it.

13th – I have organized a peasant's cart harnessed to two horses and loaded it with the linen that was supplied to us by the town and that our surgeons cut up in the morning. We had 40lb of lint; splints have been made for us; we have a case of instruments; our carriage, drawn by four oxen, carries ten surgeons, baggage and two barrels of good wine, the fruit of the pillage of Gera. Thus, we are quite well supplied. We are leaving on the 13th, at three o'clock in the afternoon; we must go to stay the night in Jena, and it is 9 punishing leagues away. We travelled for five long hours through the trains and the carriages, risking death with every step, and could only reach Roda, where the headquarters of several army corps were gathering. We had to sleep in a village and almost in a bivouac; I had a supper of potatoes without bread, but the horses have fared quite well.

14th and 15th – On the 14th, we left for Jena. Having made 2 leagues, we began to hear the sound of cannon; we crossed Roda, which is a very small town; further on, we heard the musket fire. Finally, having trotted for a long time among the troops who were forcing their march, we arrived in Jena. It was ten o'clock in the morning: they were fighting three-quarters of an hour from there, on the road to Weimar; the injured were arriving in droves. We dismounted our horses and I and the surgeons who accompanied me went to work in the large church at once. This was soon full; we made more than thirty amputations there; while I was sacrificing myself, the best of my horses was stolen, which a surgeon named Pissot was riding. Soon this building was insufficient: the sick were sent to the mental hospital, which contained 250 of them. It was necessary to fill the vast hall of the town council with them, and then the entire schoolhouse; the Black Bear inn was given over to forty-five officers; I put as many of them in another house on the main square. I amputated the leg of Marshal Ney's aide-de-camp and performed various other amputations or operations; each of my colleagues devoted himself with the same zeal. More than 2,000 wounded were dressed during the rest of the day and more than 1,200 during the night and the morning of the 15th. These unfortunates have been sleeping almost without straw, and the majority have had neither water nor food; we have hardly been able to find enough cloth. Beauquet, of the VII Corps, and Gallée, of the V, have helped us a lot with their instruments and their surgeons. There have been some terrible injuries. The Saxons and the Prussians have shown an astonishing vigour: they have sustained more than 800 injured, many deaths, and several thousand taken prisoner; among them were nine surgeons, whom I have retained. The town is full of Prussians and Saxons, who are streaming through. His Majesty will sleep there in order to go tomorrow to Weimar.

Along the length of a wood, there were still, on the battlefield, ninety wounded. We made a fire and tended to them; the surgeons of the Guard helped there. One hundred and fifty are still in the burned village three-quarters of a league from here; they will be brought this evening to our hospitals to undergo operations and treatment.

The colonel of the 9th Hussars has been killed. The colonel of the 8th was hit in the thigh by a musket ball; the *chirurgien-major* Charroy will stay with him and will be in charge of caring for between twelve and twenty other officers, including seven from this regiment. There are more than 400 wounded officers; I have amputated a great number of them. We are running back and forth to give treatment in the hospitals and to ensure that they do not lack the most necessary things. All the individuals who can walk will be evacuated; they will go through Lobenstein and Schleitz. I had proposed that we form a garrison for Jena, where the disorder is at its worst, with those who are still able-bodied. Everywhere we pass through, and here in particular, the houses are on fire, and the inhabitants are fleeing. Oh harrowing sight, am I condemned to see you for a long time yet?

Today, the 15th, I visited all the hospitals with *M.* Blin, colonel of the engineers, sent for this mission by His Highness Prince Alexander: we have found enough surgeons, but the wounded had spent the night without having had anything to eat or drink, at least in some establishments. Two hundred more of them were brought to us, all in the most unfortunate state; there will be sixty amputations to make. I am staying with the pharmacist on the square, to whom the greatest harm has been done and for whom I have already drawn my sabre five or six times.

I have had the order on the evacuations changed: 500 wounded who can walk will go to Gera, instead of Lobenstein. Tomorrow our hospitals in Jena will be completely empty; I am leaving two *chirurgiens-majors* two surgeons-lieutenant, ten Saxon surgeons, four students from the University and four Frenchmen there.

16th – Two hundred and seventy French and other wounded had been left 2 leagues from Jena, in a burnt village, near the first battlefield: we went to look for them and it was a *sous-aide* from the 32nd Infantry Regiment who led this evacuation; the surgeons of the Guard dressed them on the day of the battle. Lombard and Mouron are to stay in Jena, until the service is going well, which will take a long time and may be impossible, so badly treated has the town been, and so great is the number of wounded. This morning, all the unfortunates were still in the filth, in the middle of the excrement of those who could not stand up, legs and arms that have been cut off, corpses covered in blood, manure that the little straw on which they have been thrown has created. In some places they have been given a little broth and bread; it is hard to conceive how they have been able to survive until now. My amputees are faring quite well. While my servants were preparing my horses, I saw the church: it is in every way the most dreadful thing that one can see.

We left at seven o'clock in the morning. The surroundings of Jena are picturesque, but half a league away there is an aridity and barrenness that tire the eye and sadden the soul. In the middle of a rapidly ascending and spiralling path rises an ancient redoubt built in cut stone; it controls all the neighbouring mountains and, from this position, it is possible to halt anything that comes. The Prussians had wanted to hold it: with determination, courage and intelligence, 25,000 men would have crushed us, and although they had 100,000 of them, they were forced to abandon the most impregnable positions and to run away as fast as their legs could carry them, leaving many dead and wounded, as well as baggage. They had as many wounded as we had. We crossed the various battlefields. In one of their camps, I found some fine packsaddles and took one to carry my clothing bags, but I paid dearly for it, for, while I was having it placed on the horse, one of my servants forgot my hunting bag full of effects and provisions and lost it without return.

There are just 4 leagues from Jena to Weimar; only the first of them is bad, because of the almost-vertical climb to where the redoubt is situated; the rest are fine. On the approach to Weimar, we found camps with thousands of tents still erected; the paths and the fields were strewn with dead bodies, broken muskets, killed horses, etc. The Prince of Brunswick has been killed and Mollendorf injured. Weimar is a beautiful town; the residence is new. We found 100 wounded Prussians, the majority of whom will die. A hospital will be established in the pretty shooting house or in the redoubt, a quarter of a league from the town; nearly 300 patients will be placed there. In another building as many of them and more will be placed, which will suffice, I believe, for the current demand. I am leaving only a *chirurgien-major* and a German-speaking *sous-aide* in Weimar; the town will provide five surgeons from the area to treat the Prussians.

The King of Prussia almost died the day before yesterday from a fall from his horse, and he only just avoided being taken captive. He is asking for peace and this morning some envoys have arrived here, whom the Emperor has heard.

I saw the brother of *M.* Huffeland, a famous professor in Jena, from where he was called to Berlin. This brother is Hofmedicus[3] of the Weimar court. I forgot to say that a few years ago the University of Jena had lost eight of its most learned professors in all subjects and that in medicine and surgery Loder, Ackermann and Huffeland, paid badly by the duke, had left to go to Friedeberg, Halle and Berlin, such that in their time there were typically a thousand students in Jena and today there are hardly 300 of them.

Between Weimar and Jena is a superb, vast, well-cultivated plain: it is there that the Prussian troops were encamped; our men were able to attack them at will and they have been defeated, although the enemy had been keen to say that on the plain, if they could draw us there, they would destroy us.

17th – Today, the 17th, I am going to see the hospitals, although there is not much to see. I am staying with *M.* Muller, close advisor to the court, a young man with a handsome face, sensitive to the point of being gripped by spasms at the sight of what is happening in his country. Educated, he speaks French well; he has a kind wife and a good house, which no-one has dared to ransack, because the adjutant-major Dombrowski was lodging there.

I have retained for the Weimar hospitals seven Prussian surgeons of very good appearance and nearly all able to speak a little French. I had seven others leave for Jena, where they will be used. At my request, it was forbidden for the *commissaires des guerres* and the commanding officers of the towns to request any surgeon for the hospitals behind the lines, where enough have been provided for the service.

As I left, I gave to the *chirurgien-major* Damiens an old saw that cuts well, a large knife and some scalpels, to make the amputations that are absolutely necessary.

I wanted to have a horse with a packsaddle with hooks, but it is impossible to pass through the ranks and along the columns with this equipment; one can become stuck at any moment, and besides, the load turns too easily. I only need broad leather saddlebags and, for the ambulances, it would be suitable to have two flat cabinet-like boxes suspended by a spring that would be placed across the packsaddle or the large saddle.

I left on the 17th, at one o'clock. The fighting is terrible. The weather is superb, just as we have had without fail for the past twenty-five days. We again crossed some small battlefields to gain the road to Naumbourg: there

---

3. The chief physician of the court.

are so many broken weapons, scattered hats and bloody corpses! There are 10 leagues from Weimar to Naumbourg; the route is very beautiful. Having made 5 leagues, always travelling amidst the debris of broken weapons, dead horses and broken carts, we found the small town of Auerstædt, where we watered our horses.

It was all that we could do for them in this unhappy region, utterly pillaged and so ruined that Marshal Augereau, who would have liked to have rested in the castle and refreshed his entourage there, was obliged to continue his journey, for lack of provisions and hay.

A short distance from this town is a village reduced to ashes; the church has stayed standing. Thus, these unfortunate people will be without shelter, without livestock and without bread for the whole winter. As one advances, one finds, on the right and on the left, the excellent positions where the III Corps, with 26,000 men, fought 60,000 Prussians without respite across 2 leagues: the plain is immense, fertile, already sown; it is covered with corpses from both nations, broken gun carriages, abandoned cannon, muskets, stakes and cartridge boxes. In some places there are twenty-five corpses in the space of a few *toises*; both sides of the road are littered with them; most of those of the French are still there and the sight of them is even more deeply distressing. The III Corps wanted to stop the Prussian army from fleeing with all haste. The fury was matched on both sides; they fought (on the 14th) with a frightening fierceness. The Prussians could not be stopped; many of them were taken prisoner; they passed and continued to Magdebourg, where they are preparing for a final battle. Two leagues from Naumbourg we met convoys of caissons, on which were being loaded the last of the 1,800 French and Prussian wounded, who had spent the two preceding nights in a bad village; these unfortunate people spent the night of the 17th to the 18th in these caissons, crying out from thirst and splitting the air with their screams.

We arrived in Naumbourg at eight o'clock. The shouting that I heard as I passed in front of the large church, near the square, made me immediately dismount from my horse: it was an injured man who was being amputated. In this church were nearly a thousand unfortunates sprawled on a bit of straw and to whom fifteen surgeons were making an effort to offer assistance; I saw them handing out broth, bread, meat and wine. In the church, which is called the cathedral (everything is Lutheran), there are more than 900 wounded, including eighty-five amputees. In a small church named after St Thomas, I counted 250 of them; in the shooting house, a charming place, but devastated, there are 380 of them. Indeed, the whole town is filled with wounded. General Debilly has been killed; a number of colonels and officers staying in Naumbourg are out of action; this battle has been one of the most terrible. I am leaving around thirty surgeons for all these wounded. The head surgeons of the III Corps will stay for a few days to organize the service. I have two cases of instruments.

19th – We are going to go to Mersebourg; it is midday, the weather is magnificent. A part of the army is heading for Leipzig. I have just seen the eighty-five pieces of cannon and the thirty bronze pontoons that have been taken from the enemy. The town is rich in stores of flour and oats. His Majesty had the Elector of Saxony told to expect him in Dresden and to receive him there as a friend, otherwise he would have imposed himself.

We left at three o'clock, and had only just arrived by nine: there are 6 fatal leagues and from time to time bad country roads. There are more than 9,000 men and countless baggage trains passing through Mersebourg; never have so many wagons, carriages and trains been seen in armies. I lodged at no. 410, in the *faubourg*: a large house in which there were twenty-five *grenadiers* of the Guard and four officers, which has not prevented me from being quite well, despite the racket from the caissons and carts, which filed past my windows throughout the night. The town is beautiful and pleasant. The weather continues to be superb. His Majesty is reviewing his Guard: I saw the surgeons of this guard, with Larrey at their head, all of them in full dress, and the *infirmiers*, in uniform and commanded by a decorated officer, take to the parade ground.

20th – We are leaving at midday for Halle. I am leaving here a *aide-major* for the sick who will remain there.

The road is blocked with vehicles; they collide with each other, one risks one's life twenty times an hour while passing along the length of the trains, among bayonets, horses, caissons, etc. The weather is magnificent. At half past five, we entered Halle, an old town, but beautiful, big and rich; its church steeples can be seen from afar because of their green colour or the malachite in which the copper that covers them is coated. One must cross the Saale River to reach Halle. The enemy, with 20,000 men, tried on the 17th to contest the access to a small stone bridge a quarter of an hour from the town with our men; they fought tirelessly. It is the I Corps of our army and the division of General Dupont that withstood this fighting, in which the Prussians lost a lot of men. I found the hospitals full of their wounded, among whom were some of our own, but in small number. The *chirurgien-major* of the 9th Light Infantry has made some operations; since he left, it is the surgeons from the town who have been in charge of the service. A great insalubrity reigns in the hospital in this place; the poor wounded sleep on little straw there, all dressed, and nearly heaped one on top of the other. The fighting continued as far as the town itself, and the roads were still strewn with corpses.

All of the Imperial Guard and the dragoon reserve have gone to Halle; around the town, more than 50,000 men are bivouacking this evening.

I am bringing with me ten surgeons on horseback and twelve on foot, marching with a wagon drawn by four oxen: I will need these assistants in a few days. I have not been able to see *M.* Loder, nor *M.* Spinger, both famous professors in Halle: the former is in Russia to perform a waist operation on an important lord; the other was so afraid of the arrival of the French army that there was no way to meet him. Eighteen hundred students who stayed in the town and who cried out on Monday, during the battle between the Prussians and the French 'Long live the king! Die Napoleon!', have been driven from the town; I retained some for our hospital and they are the most honest young men in the world. This hospital was established in the catholic residence, which contains the anatomical theatre and the natural history conservatory: the French who are spread among the houses and mixed up in the hospitals will be brought together in this establishment. This evening, Marshal Duroc and *M.* Daru, whom I accompanied, visited all our wounded and distributed 20 *francs* to each of them; a soldier from the 32nd Regiment who had had both arms amputated received 60.

Today, *M.* Villemanzy ceased his functions as Intendant-general and handed them over to *M.* Daru.

I am leaving eight surgeons in Halle for the 300 wounded who find themselves there, as many in the houses as in the hospitals. We leave tomorrow, the 21st, for Dessau, 10 leagues from here. The order of the day reports that His Majesty blames the generals Klein and Lasalle greatly for having allowed two Prussian columns to escape and for having unwisely believed their general Kurgel,[4] who assured them that there was a six-week truce.

21st – I have been well lodged at no. 230, on the square, with a Jewish man called Salomon Herz, who has treated me well. We are leaving at six o'clock in the morning for Dessau; on nearing the Elbe River and following the Mursa, it is very foggy. More than 30,000 men left during the night.

---

4. Longin: The general that Percy calls Kurgel is none other than the famous Blücher.

The route is sporadically very beautiful. The countryside is vast: there are plains as far as the eye can see; there is a lot of fallow land. The villages are few and far between: the soil is mixed with sand; it is more suited to growing rye than to wheat. The inhabitants make good use of tobacco, which grows very well here; turnips, cabbages and beetroot fill the countryside at the moment. The houses are built from rammed earth, quite neatly kept and inhabited by gentle and patient men. We stopped halfway through the journey in a fairly good village, where excesses had already been committed. In the house that we entered were two horses that the peasant had had the idea of unshoeing to deter any admirers; there was also a very well-made caisson from the region. We spared the horses and the cart, but will they have escaped the rapacity of the others?

We arrived very early in Dessau, capital of the States of the Prince of Anhalt-Dessau. This prince, with his son and a small entourage, went to meet our Emperor, who received him well and was treated well by them in turn.

Three leagues from Dessau there is a vast park, full of big game animals: the road that crosses it is planted with large poplar trees that create a very beautiful effect. Everywhere it is as if one is seeing a garden, or rather groves in the English style; towers built in brick in the twelfth-century style; statues dotted here and there; the view of a village church, a romantic farm. Indeed, everything contributes to the beauty of this place. The town is modern; its houses are beautiful, with wide roads and a considerable surrounding wall; the residence is not particularly remarkable. I have been very well lodged. In general, the whole army has had to rent from the good inhabitants of Dessau, whom heaven wants to preserve from all harm. One sees long plumes there, as in Prussia; my good host, who does much to flatter, has one that is 42 inches long sitting atop a large cockade.

As one enters the town, one sees an orphanage that serves also as a house of correction; above the door is this inscription: *Pro miseris et malis*.[5] Further and on the same road is the *lazaretto*[6], where I left forty Frenchmen with a *aide-major*.

22nd – I left Dessau on the 22nd, at eight o'clock in the morning. The way leading out from the town is quite beautiful; in addition, several well-placed windmills suggest industry and affluence. English-style *bocage* is

---

5. 'For the wretched and the bad.'
6. A hospital for infectious diseases.

still in fashion and one travels a league along a magnificent drive lined with large poplars. However, the good road soon disappears; the track that leads to Wittenberg is terrible in some places; nearly everywhere, it is made of a sand in which one can sink 10 inches and, from time to time, there are deadly ravines. One travels in the middle of the woods, without a road; we saw countless hares, roe deer, hinds and stags. The forest reverberated with musket shots fired by our men and though perhaps no beast was killed, they passed by us while fleeing. After making our way for four hours, we stopped in a village, where our horses drank and ate, and so did we. I even gave the children of the peasant a meal; they laughed and frolicked, these poor children, while their parents, whose misfortunes they did not sense, were stricken with suffering. Someone tried to steal their geese while we were there; I had the *grenadiers* of the Guard give up their catch, having taken three of them, and I showed the peasant a hiding place in which to conceal them from the greed of the soldiers.

We arrived at five o'clock in the evening in Wittenberg, which was already full to overflowing with Frenchmen. We saw the Elbe and crossed this beautiful tributary, or rather this beautiful river, over a bridge to which the Prussians, while withdrawing, had set fire; but the inhabitants, fortunately for us, had extinguished it with pumps and care, such that it has remained passable. Work is taking place near this bridge to establish batteries: 500 peasants were engaged there. We are going to put the town of Wittenberg into a state of defence. It is quite beautiful, and there is a large university there, which I have taken in order to establish a hospital. This town has contained and fed, during the day from the 22nd to the 23rd, 60,000 Frenchmen: our poor host has gone without bread and has treated us miserably, albeit with the willingness to do better.

23rd – I am leaving a division of surgeons in Wittenberg. We are leaving this morning, the 23rd, and taking the road to Potsdam. After 3 leagues I encountered the surgeons who had left in advance to prepare lodgings; they told me that the headquarters is staying there and that it is necessary for everyone to bivouac. It was raining and very cold; we all readied ourselves to spend the rest of the day and night in the meadow, near ten or twelve huts already filled with *chasseurs* of the Guard. Our young men had killed a pig and found plenty of straw and hay for themselves. His Majesty was staying in a bad castle a quarter of a league from there; dinner was prepared for him in the bivouac. I did not want these bad lodgings and I pushed on further in search of a refuge; after half an hour I saw a secluded house where we would do better than in the meadow from which I had moved away. I sent one of my companions to announce this news to our men bivouacking, and they came to settle as well as possible in this house and in the neighbouring windmill; I heard from them that they had not been uncomfortable there. As for me, I reached a village, then another, then a third: everywhere was full; on all sides, poultry, pigs and calves were being killed. There was not even a small corner free from horses and men. Having entered the courtyard of a house, six officers of the Mounted Guard thought at that moment that they had spotted an enemy; but, having seen that it was me, they made me feel very welcome, providing me with a barn for my horses and allowing me to enter the *stouff*.[7]

25th – Yesterday, the 24th, I left early. Having met a cart on the road, I climbed into it next to the deputy *aide-major* Verner, the best man in the world and the most industrious on campaign; *M.* Fillod took my horse. We stopped for refreshment at Treuenbriezen, quite a pretty small town 7 leagues from Wittenberg. On the door of the townhouse is this inscription:

'*Hæc urbs promcruit quæ briccia fida vocetur
Principibus belli tempore fida fuit.*'[8]

We went further and after four hours on the road, we again gave the horses hay and oats because I wanted to reach Potsdam.

It is impossible to imagine the roads of this country: they are made of moving sand in which one sinks 10 or 15 inches; the horses, especially draft horses, suffer a lot. The road is not marked; one goes through fields, choosing the best areas and finding sand everywhere. The countryside is all sand too; the fields near the villages are extremely productive. There, they harvest rye, buckwheat and excellent oats; cabbages, turnips, etc. also grow there; elsewhere, there are enormous pastures, or fallow land that lasts for ten years. To reach Potsdam, one must cross vast pine forests and barren countryside; 2 leagues before this town starts the beautiful avenue of the king; it was time that we joined it. Our horses, who had travelled 11 leagues in the sand, could not take any more of it. Finally, having cut through numerous columns of cavalry and equipages, we arrived at nine o'clock in the evening in Potsdam.

---

7. Longin: *Stube* [establishment serving alcoholic beverages, especially beer], *chambre à feu* [a room in traditional houses containing the fireplace], stove.
8. Approximately, 'This city, which is called Briccia, can be trusted. It was loyal to the leaders of the war at the time.'

Today, the 25th, having rested well in quite good lodgings, I wandered the town. Just as I left my accommodation, I met the *commissaire* ... of the Imperial Guard, who, as we embraced, told me that he had taken my wife to Wurzbourg, where he has left her in good health, although afraid of the partisans: this good news gave me the greatest pleasure.

I have seen the castle, which is nothing spectacular. The surroundings are badly maintained; the water is stagnant in the neglected ponds; the lawns are covered with mutilated statues, as if our patriots,[9] in the time of their vandalism, had travelled through this otherwise imposing place. The tomb of the first two kings is insignificant: there is a large and beautiful pulpit, all in white marble with four large columns of grey marble.

The public buildings are magnificent. The townhouses are equally beautiful and elegant; but the people are poor and everything there implies destitution. I visited the Orphanage, for the children of soldiers who died in service: it is a superb establishment, well run, well administered. The boys, numbering 400, are fresh, in good health, without scabies or lice, dressed as soldiers, with good lederhosen, good shoes, white linen and wearing a copper badge on their left arm. The girls, numbering 150, are just as well dressed and give an impression of gaiety and health. The refectory is vast: it is a beautiful vault supported by fine stone columns; its appearance is truly beautiful. The dormitories are very clean; each child has their own bed; there are one hundred of them in each room and one cannot smell any bad odours there. This institution, started by William the Great, was completed by his descendant.[10] It is a model of its type. Sixty officers' sons, also orphans, are looked after in this house at the expense of the king, who provides 5 Prussian Crowns (20 *francs*) every month for each of them; as they grow up, they move to the school for cadets in Berlin.

I have seen the five *lazarettos* intended for the service battalions of the king: very poor condition; in total, they offer only 189 places. I have retained the vast teaching room for the troops during the winter, which can contain 300 beds: it is an unparalleled place; and also the barracks of the bodyguard, with the stables, which are as beautiful as any; we will put 800 sick there. It is likely to be necessary to keep 2,000 patients here instead of evacuating them behind the lines, where they are lost and die of hardship. Besides, how can we send these

---

9. 'Patriot' was a term given to citizens with republican or revolutionary ideas during the French Revolution. They opposed the *Ancien Régime* and aristocratic values, often with violence.
10. The orphanage was built between 1722 and 1724, during the reign of Frederick William I.

unfortunate people back to Wittenberg, where there is nothing, along impassable paths of sand and through countryside and villages that are utterly devastated?

After eating, I went to Sanssouci, very close to Potsdam. Its castle is quite pretty: on display are Voltaire's room, that of Frederick the Great, the tables on which they wrote, etc. The Sanssouci mill is there, which brings back interesting memories. There are groves, beautiful avenues of greenery, Chinese-style pavilions, a superb view and a hall where the foreigners of distinction stayed when they attended the great review, which was never more than 14,000 men; they were made to manoeuvre on the flat land in front of Sanssouci. I saw all this without much emotion. The furnishings of the castle where the great man lived are pitiable; the paintings are mostly by Watteau and there is a gallery of restored antiques. In general, the statues and paintings of the region are Germanic in style and are in bad taste, but they build well and elegantly there.

26th – Left on the 26th, at seven o'clock in the morning, for Berlin. The road, which is 3 miles (6 leagues) long,[11] is the most beautiful that I have ever encountered; it is lined with trees and cuts a path through pine forests or past beautiful lakes. To the right and to the left, as one approaches the capital, one finds beautiful villages and charming country houses, tasteful, with English gardens, greenhouses and well-chosen ornaments. The Germans take pleasure in embellishing their rustic manors; inclined to melancholic ideas, they like everything that can feed and satisfy this penchant.

What an imposing sight, what a spectacle is Berlin! The gate and the road by which one enters it are superb; the buildings of this vast city are majestic; the roads are for the most part drawn in perfectly straight lines. The only criticism is that they are paved with uneven stones; pavements are installed along them. The protestant churches, old residence, arsenal, barracks and a thousand town houses prove by the beauty of their design, by the elegance of their architecture, by the boldness of their dimensions, that in Berlin, just as much as in Paris, there is ingenuity, taste and talent. Learned societies abound in this town. The arts largely take pride of place there. We found there that the citizens were full of confidence and felt safe, coming out to meet us, but with a brazen, cynical and superior air;

---

11. This conversion is hard to reconcile; a league is generally considered longer than a mile, although the length of both measures varied before the adoption of the metric system. It is 30km from Potsdam to Berlin, similar to a distance of 7½ leagues (of approximately 4km each), but much greater than 3 miles.

it is said that the Prussians are the Gascons[12] of Germany; those in Berlin merit the application of this proverb. It has been recommended by His Majesty to exercise moderation and respect around them; we will obey him, although with each step one is tempted to strike or to expose a crowd of braggarts who come to look down on you. The Emperor will only leave one squadron here, which is ordered to fall back as soon as it sees the enemy return in force. However, he has given the order to have a hospital there of 400 beds. The Austrians are more worthy than these people here; Vienna is less beautiful than Berlin, but the Viennese are much more honest than the inhabitants of Berlin.

Around the equestrian statue of Frederick I are the four nations in chains; France can be seen raising its suppliant hands towards the Prussian hero. This monument will not stay as it is, but the moment has not yet arrived.

The headquarters of the Emperor is in Charlottenbourg, 1 league from Berlin. I have been ordered to go to establish two hospitals in Spandau, each for 300 places. I am completely alone; *M.* Legendre, the only agent who was still with me, thought to kill himself this morning by falling off a horse. It seems that His Majesty has taken Spandau, Wittenberg and Erfurt as fixed defence points. Spandau was taken yesterday with eighty cannon and 1,200 men, and without even having to light a fuse; Marshal Lannes, under the pretext of negotiating, presented himself there and had a battalion of *grenadiers* file past, in the face of which they lowered their weapons.

I am well lodged, on the Road of the Horses, at number 3: it would be hard for me to be better.

I am returning from the theatre: they staged *Iphigénie en Tauride*. I am delighted, I am still in admiration. The enemy is in Berlin; Prussia is conquered; the king is on the run with a terrified army, and yet the opera house was full and nobody appeared to be thinking of their homeland, nor sympathizing with the court, nor worrying about the future. Everyone applauded the singing of Iphigenia, and especially the ballets, which were charming. I doubt that it would have been done better in Paris; the decorations are at least as good as ours and some of the dancers would be applauded back in our country.

I am going to hold back 400 places in the hospitals of Berlin and will not establish a hospital there; I will leave next for Spandau, in passing through

---

12. 'Gascon', the name given to a person from the portion of south-western France that borders Spain and the Atlantic Ocean, is sometimes taken in French to mean 'conceited' or 'boastful'. Natives from this region supposedly lived up to that trait.

Charlottenbourg. I have saved the horses of my host from requisition for this commission.

27th – I left for Spandau at eleven o'clock. The road to Charlottenbourg is superb: it is a mile long and one passes through a beautiful forest as pleasant as the *Champs-Élysées*; the town and the castle are small, but pretty. The road to Spandau is unpleasant and made only of sand. The town of Spandau is quite modest; the fort is on the same level as the town, surrounded by fortified walls and a moat, without any outside works. I saw the former prison where Frederick II learned to play the flute. The Baron von Trenck had been imprisoned at Magdebourg, and not at Spandau, as far as I know. The order of His Majesty was that I should form a hospital for 1,200 patients there and that I make two more of them for 300 places each in the town. To do so is completely impossible, short of taking all of the barracks and recesses of the fortress, which, incidentally, has nothing more to offer.

On my return, I saw the Emperor mount his horse and make his way, followed by a glittering escort, towards Berlin, where he entered triumphantly at five o'clock.

I reached an agreement with the administrators of the hospices of Berlin for them to see to feeding and caring for the 400 patients that His Majesty has ordered me to keep in Berlin. In this way we will not have a French administration in this town, and the service will only run better for it; I will leave some surgeons with the patients in order to arrange their service.

28th – The 400 places retained in the house of charity[13] are already almost entirely filled. The sick are arriving from all sides; they are fatigued men, with a slight fever or lesions on their feet, or light injuries, or some kind of rash; there are some also who are afflicted with scabies, with plaques such that they cannot go any further. It has also been necessary to receive those with venereal diseases, but only those with an open and ulcerated swelling, painful chancres or symptoms that mean that they are unfit to continue marching. All of them are too well fed; the Prussian administration is making big sacrifices to please us. Tomorrow I will have the payment supervised and everyone will receive that which will have been prescribed to them. This hospice does serious harm to our service.

(Longin: The workbook in which Percy had consigned his impressions of his stay in Berlin is missing.)

---

13. A form of religious hospital or hospice.

# 1806 (continued) – The Polish Campaign

24th *Novembre* – I was quite at ease at the headquarters in Berlin. I had sent surgeons everywhere, and as far as each staging post; my service was perfectly assured. Suddenly, I received a letter from Kustrin stating that there were no medical officers at the hospital established in this town; this news reached His Majesty, who ordered us to go to the site ourselves. After some hesitation, we climbed into a carriage, on the 24th, at six o'clock in the morning, in a terrible fog and complete darkness, taking absolutely nothing with us. There was no talk at all of the Emperor's departure. Having travelled a good 5 leagues, we refreshed the horses in a vast farmhouse that had been completely devastated; many troops were passing by. At four o'clock, we arrived in Muncheberg, 10 good leagues from Berlin. The town is small, situated in the middle of the sands, poor, and yet we found rather good lodgings there, which we had to share with seven infantry officers and six *chasseurs* of the Guard, who entered through the window.

25th – On the 25th, at eight o'clock, our spare horses, which I had sent the day before yesterday to Muncheberg, believing that we could make the journey to Kustrin in one day, led us in eight hours to this stronghold along dreadful paths and across sands and marshes. The day before, the weather had been quite fine. The next day it rained, and it was an upsetting sight to see our men soaked, holding their shoes in their hands and marching barefoot through the peaty marshes that we could hardly cross with our horses. What a sad country!

The sight of Kustrin is imposing. The Oder is superb; in front of this site, this river is four times the width of the Rhine. The fortifications are good; the bulk of the settlement is well built; it consists of a few hundred houses and there are 3,000 inhabitants. The public buildings are beautiful. Vast magazine stores were found there. The hospital is on the square; we were satisfied with its cleanliness and its good condition. I wanted to know if it was true that there had been no surgeons at the beginning. There were some there on the 17th; I had sent a division and a sub-division of them on the 3rd and 9th November, and it is the fault of the *commissaire* and the director if on the 14th, the day that the hospital opened, they were not called upon, for it was not possible to be ignorant of their presence, since they had their coupons signed every day. Be that as it may, they had their reasons for shouting; everyone was involved in it; even Prince Murat wrote to His Majesty that there were no medical officers in Kustrin, and all this noise meant nothing, unless, envious of the gracious and favourable reception that we had received from the Emperor a few days previously, they sought to counterbalance its effect through some kind of complaint, which cannot be attributed to the Prince, but to some subordinate instigators. A certain *commandant*, an important man in small matters, also spoke out. I made a scene at the hospital to the director and to the parties involved; I threatened, I gave a refutation to the persecutors and proved for my part that there were surgeons; that Waghette, Wadrot, Lévêque and Kuhn were there before the 17th. They kept quiet and shuddered when they saw me writing a report for His Majesty. I took advantage of this event to ask the Intendant-general to call us and have us called surgeons, and not medical officers, a vague and generic designation in which we are loath to be included and that, moreover, causes frustrating misunderstandings for us. On the 23rd, there was neither a physician nor a pharmacist at the hospital in Kustrin: there you have the medical officers with whom ours, who were at their post, were confused.

26th – His Majesty, who seemed so at ease in Berlin, left on the night of the 24th to the 25th. We were very surprised in Muncheberg to learn on the morning of the 25th that he had just passed through there: he arrived at Kustrin the same day at noon and we at four o'clock. He visited the fortifications and this morning (26th) at two o'clock, in terrible weather, he left for Posen. I must also go there: happy would I be if I were not to go any further! I was unable to return to Berlin for my equipages; *M.* Coste left at noon to return and stay there; he will send me all my horses, my luggage wagon and my colleagues.

Today, the 26th, it rained all day and all night; a south-easterly constitution. There are many fluxions, catarrhs, diarrhoea. The soldiers are exhausted, badly fed and badly housed; they march at night and are always sodden.

I am leaving tomorrow with *M.* Maugras for Landsberg and then for Driesen, halfway to Posen, where I will arrive on the 29th or 30th. My equipages will not be there until 2 December. What a season, what a country in which to make war! One must take food for five or six days at a time, which kills everyone.

I have had a terrible cold for the last fortnight and I am coughing somewhat. It makes no difference, it is necessary to march: I have only that which is on my body, nothing but my shirt, my pair of boots, my handkerchief. It makes no difference, it is necessary to march; where I fall, they will bury me.

27th – Left at half past seven from Kustrin. Bad weather, bad path: we could only go at walking pace with three strong horses, yet there are some good stretches of track and even of road. It seems that the sea once covered all these lands: the mountains of sand similar to the cliffs on the shores of the ocean; the countryside entirely covered with sand; the enormous polished and rounded stones scattered here and there; the blocks of quartz, of granite, also softened by traction and collision. Everything suggests that the Baltic covered this country, which, in spite of its harshness and its infertility, is quite well populated. Most of the villages are built of wood and mortar: we have found them all deserted, looted and devastated. Halfway along the road, or rather, after we had travelled 6 leagues, we dismounted in front of a house of quite good appearance to warm ourselves and to feed the horses: everything there was upside down; we could hardly find a bad earthenware pot in which to cook some potatoes.

We arrived in Landsberg at six o'clock. Our accommodation was prepared there. It is a rather beautiful town: we have been treated well there; we have seen only very good people, obliging, trusting and familiar. I found some sick there in a house serving as a hospice and left the *aide-major* Sabet to care for them, as well as those who would arrive there, but warning him to be wary of the soldiers who would present themselves at this hospice, because almost always some arrive who, having done something foolish behind the lines, seek a note of hospital release to legitimize too long an absence once back in their regiment. Tomorrow, the 28th, we are leaving for Friedberg.

28th – There are 6 leagues to travel: the road is good and the weather superb; it has frozen; the sand is firm; there is no mud and the sun is shining. We pass through fairly good villages and pine woods. The territory of Landsberg, one league in radius, is good, well cultivated and has a beautiful appearance, which explains the beauty and cleanliness of the town, as well as the air of health, cheerfulness, trust and civility of the inhabitants.

The little town of Friedberg, situated on a large plateau, is quite pretty; its inhabitants are good, well housed and well dressed; the men especially are richly clothed and almost in our style. We are lodged with the Jew Moyse, whose manor is clean and with whom we found a good table and very good beds. In this town, there is an Israélite physician of good appearance from Francfort-sur-Oder, who speaks our language fairly well, is an astute, intellectual man and has given us good information about Poland.

The wind is to the north-east. The frost is increasing: this is a great fortune for the army, a sixth of which has been put in the hospitals by the southern constitution of the last few days.

29th – I was mistaken about the frost: during the night the wind turned to the north-west; it snowed, and it is snowing and raining this morning; there is some black ice; the weather is not cold, but the roads are dreadful.

We left Friedberg at eight o'clock, very content with our Jewish host and our Jewish host very content with us. Nothing is cleaner than the house of this brave Israélite, father to five children, widower of a woman who died of a gangrenous hernia, and with Miss Migna, of the same sect, to help him in his widowhood.

There are 5 leagues from Friedberg to Driesen: sandy road, poor country, sad villages. We arrived at one o'clock and stayed in a very good house. This town is quite pleasant; it suggests affluence. I found the commander there to be an officer of the 7th Mounted *Chasseurs*, who had been shot in the back of his neck, the musket ball having hit the occipital buns: *M.* Hermann, *aide-major* to this regiment, has stayed to care for him and to keep an eye on the service of the civil hospice. The sick are evacuated in groups of twelve to fifteen (per boat) on the Netze River, which flows into the Oder near Kustrin; they are on good boats that are enclosed and heated. The *commissaire* is the amiable Catuellan, a charming young man from Rennes, who has had us given good white bread and mutton for three days, with a suspended carriage waiting that will take me to Posen, for tomorrow I will leave my colleague Maugras, who, since Kustrin, has given me a place in his cabriolet; he is going to Bromberg or Thorn, and I am heading right to go towards Posen, where His Majesty is. We have not yet crossed the Vistula. The Prussians, who are on the right bank, facing Thorn, have fired a few cannon shots at our men; but we silenced them by threatening to burn down the town where they are with incendiary shells.

The weather is extremely bad; it rains, snows and is freezing; there is not much black ice. Tomorrow, the 30th, we are leaving, five of my surgeons and I. I will only see my equipages on 3 December. Everybody makes us fear Poland. We are in the best part of this country; beyond Posen, it will be nothing but misery and dirt. The Poles are very dirty; the old Prussians have a poor opinion of them and they all speak of Poland with disdain.

30th – We travelled our 6 miles quite swiftly; *M.* Catuellan found a good suspended carriage for me harnessed to four horses that took me quickly.

We arrived at one o'clock in Zirke, a small Polish town on the Warta River. The IV Corps was passing through it; everywhere was full. The commanding officer would certainly have liked that I go to find accommodation in a village 1 league further on: I insisted on staying in the town, and I have received fairly good lodgings there with a Polish man who speaks Latin well, who is honest, an important farmer and the owner of a former Dominican convent; it will be difficult for me to keep hold of my farmers and their horses, even though I keep them under lock and key without leaving them to want for anything. The countryside resembles the surroundings of Ambleteuse; everything is sand, and sand as pure and as fresh as if the sea had passed just yesterday through these sad regions, which it surely covered. Stanislas Leczinski[1] was heir apparent to the three most considerable estates in Zirke when he was dispossessed. Already in this country one sees only men with moustaches or thick beards, with a kind of long coat or habit and a belt; they all wear boots and have a fur cap. There are many Catholics in Zirke.

Having had some difficulty in retaining our lodgings, which two generals were coveting, we thought about our dinner. Our host always replied to us: '*Curabo ut sitis bene.*'[2] To everything we asked, he replied: '*Curabo.*'[3] This man speaks Latin perfectly. We had a really excellent supper and perfect Hungarian wine; that is the kind that they drink in this country. In Prussia, it is the red or white wine from Médoc;[4] in Poland, it is wine from Hungary. It is fortifying, slightly warm and very pleasant. We had game, vegetables, pastries and fish; pike is very common in Prussia and Poland; it is good there and it is eaten both salted and fresh.

We had a fine and generous meal and I was able to make quite a good bed on an old wing chair. My companions had good straw.

---

1. Stanisław I Leszczyński (1677–1766) was King of Poland from 1704–1709 and again from 1733 until 1736. Stanisław's daughter married Louis XV of France, and he became Duke of Lorraine, living at the palace in Lunéville. Percy was familiar with Lunéville as, at the start of his career, he was garrisoned there as part of the Scottish company of the *Gendarmerie de France*.
2. 'I will make sure that you are well.'
3. 'I will make sure of it.'
4. A French wine-growing region just north of Bordeaux.

1 *Decembre* – The wind was terrible all night. I slept and this morning, after drinking a coffee and thanking our host in Latin, who came to apologize for having done so little for me and who had put on a Polish habit with a superb belt, we left for Samter, 8 leagues from Zirke. The weather was quite good; little wind, no rain; our troops have not suffered today. The road is still in the sand; there are many bad little bridges. Sandy landscapes, some completely barren, others cultivated; woods of sparse birch trees; miserable hamlets; houses, or rather the huts of very poor people: this is all that we encountered for 4 leagues. Then one comes across an immense plain, sown, interspersed with a few villages where one sees awful houses of mud and straw and some pretty dwellings. I saw a very beautiful castle, brand new, built in brick and with a peristyle of eight columns in very good taste. Everywhere the roofs are made of straw placed in tiers and very badly arranged; they do not know how to make a continuous roof in this country. Not a single house has a floor on the ground floor; it is earth, or rather sand, and few have a first floor. Saint John of Nepomuk[5] and the Virgin Mary are starting to appear on the bridges and along the roads.

We have passed through Ostoroch, a miserable town consisting of forty earth huts inhabited by people with moustaches, wearing long sheepskin habits with wool inside and Polish caps on their heads. Rye, oats and many *catouffles*[6] are grown; it is these that we call potatoes; there are some fruit trees. The small town of Ostoroch is surrounded by slats and has wooden gates, which form its outer wall. That of Samter is a little more elegant; there are some fairly reasonable houses, but they are still made of veneer and wood. We are lodged with the schoolmaster and in a single room; fortunately, we have bread, wine and meat. Our hosts speak German. The weather is not cold; the wind is towards the south-west. Tomorrow, 2 November,[7] we will arrive in Posen. The part of Poland through which we are travelling at present is what is called the first division.

2nd – The picture of the most absolute barrenness: sandy plains as far as the eye can see; a few shacks scattered over the area or gathered to make a sort of hamlet; a few woods of birch trees, withered fir trees; a lot of small streams and bridges on the brink of collapse. There are a few women who do not have a bad appearance; some men resemble devils. Such are the things that one encounters from Samter to Posen.

---

5. The saint of Bohemia. He was drowned in the Vltava River in 1393 and canonized in 1729.
6. Longin: *Catoffeln*, potatoes.
7. Longin: Percy inadvertently wrote 'November' instead of 'December'.

I should not forget the pleasant evening that we spent with our *schulmestre*,[8] whose wife, sister Éléonora and children are interesting and tender; they all joined in. I wanted to pay the expenses and we lacked nothing, because we had wine, bread, meat, sugar, etc. These good people were cheerful and ate very well with us; we even procured for them some wood, which we went to steal. The night was noisy, because of the wind and rain; I slept in a bed; our six surgeons, the two carters and a young servant slept around me on good straw, the stove being quite warm.

At eight o'clock we left; it was not cold. I found that the time passed quickly. At two o'clock, we arrived at the first triumphal arch, a quarter of an hour from Posen: it is made of wood painted with distemper, which means that the wind and rain have damaged it considerably. On the pediment is written: 'To the victor of Marengo.' Further on is another arch with marbled columns, which has also suffered from the rain; one can read this inscription there: 'To the victor of Austerlitz.' The third is the most considerable; at the top and to the left is a painting of a Pole, with a sabre in his hand, and to the right a phoenix with these words: '*Resurget ex suis cineribus*';[9] in the middle is written: 'To the restorer of the Polish nation.'

What mud there is in Posen! How difficult it is to find accommodation there! Everywhere is full. They are decorating everywhere with lights; the concert hall, which is at the entrance to the city and brand new, is surrounded by festoons and greenery, as are the houses in this quarter. Today is the anniversary of the victory of Austerlitz, but the weather is terrible and the rain will extinguish the paper lanterns.

The display of lights took place as best it could.

There was a proclamation today that His Majesty will not lay down arms until he has forced peace on his continental enemies and had England return the possessions she has seized.

3rd – Having slept fairly well, despite a terrible coughing fit, I mounted my horse and saw the three hospitals that have already been established, namely one in the seminary, quite far from the town, the other at Saint Joseph, a beautiful new convent, and the third with the ladies of the Bernadines. The latter is as miserable as the convent and the unfortunate women who live there;

---

8. Longin: *Schulmeister*, schoolmaster.
9. 'He will rise from the ashes.'

the others are fine and well kept. They can hold only 500 patients in total, and we are likely to need 2,000 places here.

The chill wind is very harsh and stings one's face. It has frozen; there is a thick, stinking mud, in which one can sink up to the calves.

I saw the Intendant-general, who informed me that His Majesty wanted a fourth hospital in Posen; two hospitals, one for a thousand wounded and the other for a thousand fever patients at Leczyca, 45 leagues away, on the road to Warsaw; a very large hospital for 2,000 venereal and scabies patients at the gates of Kustrin; and a hospice in the castle of *M.* de Lucchesini,[10] at Miseritz. His Majesty does not want us to evacuate beyond the Oder. The surgeons have left for all these new establishments.

The people of this region live more or less as they do in Holland: a lot of butter, which is of good quality; coffee, beer and white wine from Hungary. The apartments of the rich are clean and well decorated, but what people! The Jews are ugly-looking and repulsively dirty.

4th – It snowed a little last night; the weather has become milder. When I rose, I read the beautiful proclamation of His Majesty, as well as his decree on the monument in the *Place de la Magdeleine*. Everyone is complaining about the weather, the buildings, the accommodation, the food. The Poles are arming themselves in large numbers and are already paying dearly for the plan they formed; soon there will be no more food in this country.

The hospitals are hardly able to support themselves; everyone is living there from day to day. The sick are flocking there; space is being made for them by sending the venereal and scabies patients back to Kustrin.

My nephew, with all of my entourage, arrived this evening, with a carriage, caisson, etc.; he killed some stray pigs on the way, which we will salt tomorrow for our use. We will pull through.

5th – It has frozen and snowed heavily; the wind is north-easterly; it is difficult to travel on horseback. In the evening, the weather became milder; a little snow is falling.

6th – The night was mild; the north-westerly wind is prevailing; it is raining a little. The coughs, catarrhs and fluxions are multiplying.

I have received a letter from *M.* Danbe, one of the Prussian surgeons-general; he was in Magdebourg, from where he has returned to Berlin. He

---

10. The diplomat Girolamo Lucchesini, who served Prussia.

implores me to ensure that his pension of 1,000 *Friedrichs d'or*[11] continues to be paid to him. He has served under three kings; Frederick the Great is still dear to him.

*M.* Goercke, the most senior surgeon-general, has written to me via Grand Marshal Duroc, who was with the King of Prussia on 22 November; he recommends his Institute to me; I will reply to him by way of diplomacy.

7th, 8th and 9th – Superb weather, beautiful sunshine, autumn days, a known phenomenon in this region, where at this time of year the barometer shows 12 or 15 degrees. Today, the 9th, it is 3 degrees; the sun is warm; it is the most beautiful weather in the world.

I met with His Majesty to discuss our service; he welcomed me well. I recommended my colleagues to him; he granted them each 5 ells of fabric, saying that they were officers and that they should have been included in his decree on 12 November. The Emperor has taken a great interest in medicines; he spoke of quinine, emetic and camphor, and was surprised that there were so few supplies in the army. I told him of the towns of Dantzig, Stettin and Hambourg, where they can be found for a price.

Tomorrow, the 10th, we are leaving for Warsaw. I have obtained some food for myself for this miserable journey; my cold has improved, but I am no better for it. My colleague Coste had his trunk stolen from the back of his carriage as he re-entered Berlin on his return from Kustrin; he lost 1,600 *francs*, his papers and all his effects. This incident, together with a certain brusqueness on the part of the Intendant-general, whom he met on the way, has left him very upset.

10th – Left at eleven o'clock, content and calm. My service in the three hospitals is assured, although I have left few surgeons there. *M.* Kurtz has received a long instruction to retain the surgeons who are likely to be needed not only at Saint Joseph, where he is in charge, but also with the ladies and at the seminary. The weather is mild and beautiful; the road is bad and full of ruts. We arrived at Kostrzyn at three o'clock; it is only 4 leagues away; since our caisson had taken a left turn, it was necessary to have it travel 6 fatal leagues to reach us; I found that very difficult. A poor little town, made entirely of wood, as in the rest of the country. We went to the castle, *M.* Mouron and I: now, this castle is a wooden house, with only a ground floor and large stables. We made an excellent

---

11. A Prussian gold coin used between 1741 and 1855. It was first minted by Frederick II (the Great) of Prussia, from whom it took its name.

dinner there; the lord with his family remained hidden in his chambers. We slept on straw, eight of us in the same room; our men were next door.

11th – Left at seven o'clock, for Wreschen, 3½ miles further along. Mild weather; no frost; the sun appeared very bright from ten o'clock until noon; the mist has eclipsed it. Same road; sand, ruts that could have consumed us; fields as far as the eye can see; miserable wooden huts; many windmills; some woods with a mixture of fir, birch and oak; well-defined road, lined with sparse willows. We took refreshment in Nekla, around halfway, in the inn of the local lord, for here one is a serf and everything belongs to the lord. The lord of Nekla has eighty villages.[12]

There are churches built of wood; the statues of saints outside, on the bridges and in the squares, are miserable effigies made of pinewood. In these houses, one finds poultry, cattle and pigs. The latter are small, stocky, short and have a crest on their backs, which is made from those fine bristles that cobblers seek and which are so expensive to buy. The hens resemble ours. The cattle are small, as are the horses; the carts are much the same; the wheels are not iron-rimmed.

At four o'clock, we arrived in Wreschen, a large village entirely made of wood, although with a castle and a church made of stone. We are lodged with a Jew with a bushy beard, wearing a big fur cap, a belt and a long gown; such are the typical clothes. He wanted to kiss my clothes, presented his wife to us, who was fine, and his daughters, who, although almost dirty, are pretty. We were given quite a lot of dinner; we provided half of it, as there is no wine here, and the bread is black and made of rye. We slept on straw, but warm and comfortably, because we have our blankets and sheets. Several times in the night, we were woken by troops arriving in a very bad mood.

12th – At seven o'clock, I rose, had breakfast and left. A beautiful cold, heavy frost, sunshine in intervals; paths sometimes passable but more often dreadful; miserable huts, few and far between; a rather fine castle on the right.

I arrived at Slupca at two o'clock, although it was only 3¼ miles. What a poor place! Houses made entirely of wood; ragged inhabitants who are already ruined. We are lodged with a widow in the town; we will be fine given the weather and the country; we have food of all kinds.

His Majesty has ordered that there be a hospital of 500 places in Slupca: an impossible thing. A small hospice of twenty or twenty-five pallet beds will be

---

12. The abolition of serfdom in Poland was a gradual and non-linear process. Indeed, as Percy notes, serfdom persisted in parts of Poland into the nineteenth century.

made there, above the townhouse, and that is all. *M.* Lagarde, the *chirurgien-major*, with Hormois and Sauvage as *sous-aides*, will remain there until they receive a new order.

13th – I spent an excellent night in the small bed of a nun, without a fire, but with my good blankets; we were all perfectly well.

Left at eight o'clock. The weather is very mild: never has a day in April been more beautiful or warmer. The roads are terrible. We killed larks along the way; they are large, fatty, with lots of feathers, have long, strong beaks and have a crest of two small feathers on their heads; they are more grey than tawny and their species is the strongest that I have seen; they are only found around houses. The route is only 6 leagues; but the horses cannot go further, so tiring do they find it. I handed over two letters on the cheery topic of fistulas to a messenger and to a lieutenant-colonel of the engineers going to Posen.

Arrived at three o'clock, in Kleczewo, an average town made of wood; lodged with a bailiff or similar, with a kind and very obliging young wife. General Guyot was lodged with us, which disturbed him and me both. During the night, there came a crowd of Frenchmen seeking somewhere to take shelter; the poor lady (she had eleven children) was losing her head because of it. We provided everything, even the money for two bottles of porter, for which they had the dishonour to make us pay 24 *sous* each. I found it repulsive; it was, I think, ordinary beer into which they had melted liquorice sap and added a small amount of colocynth or essence of absinthe.

14th – We slept all together; by misfortune, there was a mouse in my straw that disturbed me all night. The wind was tumultuous; it rained; this morning the weather is mild and it is drizzling slightly.

We left on the 14th early in the morning, animals and people, being well rested. The road is as ever; we crossed a superb forest 20 leagues in circumference, so they say; it is certainly 3 leagues long following our path; its pine trees are magnificent and densely packed. After passing through this wood, one finds marshes, in the middle of which a path has been made out of large pine trees; this kind of causeway, 4ft high, is several hundred *toises* long. Beyond the marshes and from time to time in the wood, one comes across houses surrounded by a little arable land.

Sempolno, where we arrived at one o'clock, is a poor little town like the previous ones, but where there are already a few earthen houses covered with sand and lime plaster, with tiled roofs. The church is made of wood. We are staying with an apothecary who speaks excellent Latin and also practices medicine and surgery, which he hardly understands; there has never been anyone from either of these professions in this place, except for a physician who could only stay there for a few months.

Tomorrow we will have 16 leagues to make.

I found an Elzevir edition of *Tacitus* at the home of the pharmacist, which the foul man wanted neither to hand over nor to sell to me. He is a Harpagon,[13] and I will take this opportunity to note that this word comes from *harpago*, meaning hook, fang, and that never have I seen more claw-like fingers than those of our host. I slept on a pallet bed 18 inches wide and 5½ft long; hence, I was very uncomfortable there.

15th – Left at seven o'clock, in a twilight full of fire, the weather being superb, mild and spring-like. We encountered bad roads. The small town of Babiak, through which we passed, resembles an American dwelling; it is composed of wooden houses or huts arranged in a circle around a beautiful, dry and clean lawn, which is rare in this country; in the middle is the church, made of wood.

The girls and women of this colony-like settlement are very fine and dress with elegance. In general, the sex is beautiful, and as much as the Jews are unsightly, their women have, in their uncleanliness, grace, freshness and good features; some are very well dressed. The children and women of these people go barefoot in the mud up to the backs of their knees.

We found in a rather simple house, built of wood, several very well-mannered women, elegantly dressed and who spoke French; we spent an hour with them.

In Klodawa, a rather pretty small town in comparison with the others, we stayed with the landowning count of the place, which is to say that I slept on the straw in a large room that had been abandoned for fifty years and was full of mice. Behind this room is a beautiful garden, with covered walkways and a lot of fruit trees. There is a poor little abbey in Klodawa, from which we have made a hospital where the patients will only stay the night before being evacuated to that of Leczyca. One sees roofs of beautiful minium-coloured[14] tiles and rather pretty brickwork houses in Klodawa. Alsatian *émigrés* had

---

13. Harpagon is a character from Molière's comedy *L'Avare*. *L'Avare* translates literally to 'The Miser', and Harpagon is the story's Scrooge-like character.
14. Minium is a colour similar to vermilion.

them built; there are twenty of them in a single row, separated by a few hundred *toises* of land that was granted to these *émigrés*.

16th – Left at seven o'clock on the 16th. Weather still mild and beautifully sunny, but awful roads; our horses were worn out by midday. Arrived late at Kutno, a large village or town like most of the previous ones: fortunately, I was lodged in a very pretty castle by a count and three women, one of whom was young, pretty, too fat and spoke our language perfectly. The generals Marulaz and Wathier gave me a place there. It is raining this evening; tomorrow it will be very bad.

The lady of the castle, who has had amaurosis for four years, wanted to consult me. She told me that, having taken warm baths during the summer, she wanted to go for a ride in a carriage and that, her eyes having been struck by excessively fresh air coming in through the windows of the vehicle, she returned home blind. A certain *M.* Wolff, a physician from Posen, helped her to see again for some time; but, having died without passing on his secret, she lost her sight again, which no doctor, neither from Vienna nor from Warsaw, has since been able to restore. I limited myself to giving her a little hope and some empty words of advice, being quite certain that it is an illness without a cure. Galvanism has been very harmful to her.[15]

17th – Left on the 17th at nine o'clock. It is the kind of road where one risks dying a thousand times: we could only manage 4 leagues and had to stop in a village on the route. Our servants stayed with the horses and the local priest, and we stayed with the lord, a father to nine children, with Jewish tailors busy dressing the fifteen soldiers that he is obliged to provide; that is, five for himself and ten for his peasants. He told me that he gave these peasants somewhere to live, livestock, marriage, etc. in return for three days' work that they give him each week with his own farm tools and his cattle; it is reminiscent of the servitude of the negroes.

It is not yet cold; it is raining a bit. We will sleep on straw and will eat a cockerel that we have bought for our supper. Tomorrow, the 18th, we will go to Lowicz, a fairly good town 6 leagues from here; it is necessary to establish a hospital there and to leave some surgeons.

---

15. Medical galvanism was the therapeutic use of electrical currents to relieve certain symptoms. The Italian physician Giovanni Aldini (1762–1834) is associated with this medical application of electricity, which would have been a very new treatment at the time of Percy's writing.

## 1806 (continued) – The Polish Campaign

18th – Instead of taking the road to Lowicz, we followed the route to Sochaczew, through the woods and along unimaginable paths, and thus our carriage had an accident. With a belt at the back having broken, the body of the carriage fell sideways until it was in the mud and I found myself with my companion Mayot lying on the left side in the middle of a dreadful mess, without getting wet or even dirty. We got out of trouble as best we could and, since our caisson had arrived, we corrected the body of the carriage and suspended it with chains, which worked well. But as our horses could take no more and as the sun was beginning to set, without seeing any sign of a town along the vast horizon, we began to fear that we had made some unfortunate mistake and a German-speaking Jew convinced us that Lowicz was on our right, that we were 4 leagues away from it, and that we were just as far from Sochaczew. As a result, I immediately took my leave and went straight to a village off the track, half a league from the road. There we found an excellent castle, where we dismounted and were received by a young Pole, who spoke French, and his niece, who spoke only her native language; our horses and servants were led to a house in the village. We will all be perfectly well: the house is pretty, neat and tidy, with a beautiful garden, a large farm and countless livestock. The lord is in Warsaw to form a company there, which he will captain. I am worried about my friend Le Vert, who is in Lowicz and who is undoubtedly just as concerned for me; I hope to find him tomorrow in the next town.

The weather, which was windy and rainy last night, has been lovely all day. The sunset, red and gleaming, forecasts a charming day for us tomorrow too.

The fire, the meals and the beds will make our stay here marvellously comfortable.

19th – Left in the fog, having coughed horribly all night and having been unable to sleep.

I still have a bad, dry cough; the mist only irritates this cough and I am really quite ill.

I arrived early in Sochaczew, an insignificant little town inhabited by hideous monkeys from the forest, who are called Jews here: these wretched people, all horrible, have spread their communal metal-work and other goods in every direction; they are covered with lice and shake them off by the handful when they bite too fiercely. By special grace, I was lodged in the house of the burgomaster, where the honest clerks in charge of the food, meat and drink supplies received me well and gave me some good soup; my horses were also well stabled, but without fodder. In the evening, my friend Le Vert arrived;

immediately the cooking was underway and at eight o'clock I had a good supper, which my cough prevented me from enjoying.

20th – We all slept in the same room with two *gendarmes* and a prisoner dragoon. I slept a little.

We left at seven o'clock on the 20th in mild weather. The way from Sochaczew to Blonie is only 6 short leagues and the road, often very bad, is generally the best we have had. In this poor market town, where there is absolutely nothing, they were not able to find us lodgings. We were pointed to the castle of Musenheim, 3 leagues further on; despite the bad track, we arrived there in good time. We found a young surgeon of the mounted artillery there with three officers from this corps, who showed us much consideration. We placed the cooking pot on the fire, arranged the straw, put away the horses, and everything suggests that we will be well.

His Majesty, arriving by carriage at Lowicz, left there on horseback and, at the risk of killing himself, has travelled a long way in a few hours. *M.* Duroc dislocated his arm near Kutno; *M.* Caulaincourt has also been wounded, both their carriages having overturned on the way.

22nd – Arrived in Warsaw yesterday at one o'clock, frozen, penetrated by the cold and damp, coughing like a wretch. This city is not worth its reputation: it is very extensive, but generally badly built, and the Jews, who constitute more than half of the inhabitants, make it loathsome because of their ugliness, their dirtiness, their horrible appearance. I am staying at the Prussian trading post, a beautiful and grand building where I would be treated wonderfully if I could only eat.

As soon as I arrived yesterday, I had to hurry to see the Intendant-general and spent three hours with him making my reports. This morning, at ten o'clock, we went to see His Majesty, who was in a very bad mood. He protested about the pitiful state of the administrative service and went so far as to say that the nation had become the most barbaric in Europe in relation to the hospital service; that the army was, in this respect, inferior to those of all our neighbours and that the Cossacks acted better than us towards their wounded. Having asked where the chief physician was, he lost patience again and said that he no longer needed such people; that this old fellow should long since have returned to *Les Invalides*; that he had served his purpose and that it would have been better to send Desgenettes to the army than a homesick septuagenarian who was afraid of dying in Poland: 'No,' he added, 'these are not the men I need; I want them to be young, active, somewhat sharp and lively and having ... '[16] He asked me question after question and, having made the Intendant-general take the quill, he dictated more or less the following:

> 'A chief physician in an army corps is an absurd and useless being. All the physicians will leave the corps and divisions to which they are assigned and will remain either in the hospitals or with the main headquarters. The physician must only appear when the army has a territory and, in reality, this only exists when it is stationed or has conquered a lot of land. The *chirurgien-major* must also serve as a physician for the army. There will only be surgeons in the active army.
> 
> 'Four types of ambulances:
> 
> 'First type: ambulance of the regiments managed by the *chirurgien-major* and one or two *sous-aides*; it must have a caisson, since it has been paid for in advance.
> 
> 'Second type: ambulance of the divisions; it will be managed by a *chirurgien-major* behind the army's lines and under no circumstances can it be directed by a regimental *chirurgien-major*; the *aides-majors* and *sous-aides* will be drawn from the regiments; this ambulance will have caissons supplied by the hospital administration.
> 
> 'Third type: ambulance of the army corps marching with the headquarters; it will be served by the surgeons following in the army's wake; the administration will provide it with caissons and other necessary resources.
> 
> 'Fourth type: ambulance of the main headquarters.'

His Majesty, indignant about everything that is happening with regard to the equipment of the hospitals, the multitude of workers who are paid but not present, the means of transport, etc., said again that it would be desirable that the surgeons be charged with the care, upkeep and supply of the caissons assigned to their ambulance division; that they would take an interest in it and be meticulous, instead of always being promised much and given nothing.

---

16. Longin omits the final word. The Physician-in-Chief of the Grande Armée at the time was Jean-François Coste (1741–1819). It is believed by some scholars that Percy played a part in turning Napoleon against Coste, and he lost his position in 1807.

After a moment of silence and reflection, he delivered these memorable words: 'They have lost me my surgery by burdening it and by giving it over to their foolish plans.'

'Is it really true,' the Emperor asked me, showing me the register that I had just handed to him, 'that you have all these surgeons here?'

'Yes, Sire,' I replied, 'and you cannot do me the injustice of doubting it; but your Majesty should know that almost all of them have returned to the army only for him; that not one has been supplied to me from Paris, and that I have personally called nearly 200 of them to me.'

'You have done well,' said the Emperor, in whose eyes and gestures I thought I noticed a great discontent against the primary source of the disturbances that cause his complaints, and against the authority that maintains and increases them through meanness and unjust conduct towards the most honest people.

His Majesty ended by announcing to us that there would be a great battle on the 24th or 25th of this month. Consequently, as soon as we left him, it was necessary to hurry about the city to find new premises. Six are already filled with 1,700 sick; we need space for 6,000 wounded; I proposed having the 350 scabies sufferers who are filling one of them leave and rejoin the army, and that we send to Lowicz 350 venereal patients who are in another, and evacuate all those with fever who can be transported to the same city, so that we can find seven or eight hundred ready-made places in the hospitals already established.

I have an order to leave tomorrow for Jablona with all my available surgeons.

I requested that earthernware pots be bought for soup, candles, rice, lard, etc.; we have sugar, *eau-de-vie*, white and brown bread, in short, everything that we need to survive for eight days. I am taking five divisions of mounted surgeons, each of which has been given a caisson on two wheels carrying some aid supplies.

23rd – After quite a poor night, having coughed with more ease than during the previous ones, I saw that the service was assured for the 1,900 sick who remain in Warsaw. I agreed with the physicians Duval, Brassier, principals; Jusserandot, Rampon and Mourge, ordinary, that everyone would make an effort to support this service until our surgeons returned. I have only left six *sous-aides* to help with the visits and distributions; the physicians and pharmacists will do the rest. *M.* Magnin, a Comtois physician who has been living in Poland for twenty-five years, will take charge of a hospital with six Polish surgeons. With His Majesty having forbidden evacuation, this statement was interpreted to the letter and the Intendant-general did not want the 300 venereal patients to be sent to Lowicz; as for the 400 scabies sufferers, *M.* Duval has promised me that they will be given their *billet de sortie*[17] to go to fight the enemy with the others.

At two o'clock, I left on horseback with my young friend Le Vert and a single servant. My post wagon, despite having fallen to pieces, is harnessed to two good horses and loaded with good supplies, pots, cooking pans, raw mutton, candles, linen for dressings, lint, blankets for bivouacking, oats, etc. What a majestic river this Vistula is! It is eight times wider than the Seine. However, one must cross it via a dilapidated bridge, built half on boats and half on trestles. On this fragile bridge, so unworthy of the magnificence of the river, but so useful and so beneficial to His Majesty's plans, a hundred thousand men have passed or are going to pass, the cavalry on foot, one-by-one, and the infantry in threes. The carriages are waiting their turn; ours is unlikely to cross before five or six o'clock in the evening.

And so we crossed and remounted our horses, but what roads! The rustic carts disappear in the middle of thin, wet mud and are swallowed by ruts several feet deep. No one wants nor dares to help them out of them; it would be necessary to enter up to the middle of one's thigh. Yet I pity the poor peasants and their livestock, and more than anyone I am interested in their wagons, on which I am counting for tomorrow.

We could hear the cannon. At first, I thought that they were firing on a reconnaissance party or a vanguard, but the frequency of the shots increased and became mixed with the sound of gunfire: it is a position that we want to take and defend. On arriving at Jablona, one of our surgeons, a Gascon and very loquacious, told me that the Emperor left there at six o'clock in the morning (he had passed through the village of Praga at four); he added that everyone has orders to advance, that we have been fighting since three o'clock, etc. Instead of staying the night in this place, as His Majesty had ordered me to do, I am pushing further on, entirely set on bivouacking and waiting where God wills for the dusk that will surely signal the death and pain of some and the glory and honours of others. We travelled 2½ leagues in a cold rain and through thick forests that our men were working to clear to use for their bivouacs. As we advanced, I thought about what my babbling Gascon had said, and remembered that he had not told me anything about our ambulance carts,

---

17. An order of discharge from hospital.

nor about the *ordonnateur*, nor about the principal director. What am I going to do so close to the battlefield, I told myself, if I arrive empty-handed with no aid supplies? So, turning the horse, I returned to Jablona, having travelled 5 long leagues entirely unnecessarily. This morning the aforementioned Gascon had left Warsaw with orders to find me a certain isolated cave in the woods behind the castle and to have straw carried and a fire lit for me there. On my return from the ill-fated duty, I found my man, who only obtained his reprieve at the sight of this charming cave, where a good stove, a good open fire, mattresses and straw spread out on the ground soothed my anger. I dried my clothes and fur cap and immediately sent a letter to the *ordonnateur* to find out what had become of the carts and workers. At the same time I was given the order from the hand of the Prince Major-General to spend the night at Jablona with all my companions and to leave before daybreak to go to the bridge over the Narew River; the aide-de-camp carrying this order was himself ordered to go as far as Warsaw. I will be well tonight and until three o'clock tomorrow morning. What a day it will be! Everyone thinks it will be terrible and bloodier than any that preceded it. However, let us leave it to our great man: he knows how to master fate and slay his enemies.

24th. – From ten o'clock in the evening until three o'clock in the morning we were firing; we have continued to hear the cannon and musketry. I did not sleep at all and my cough has fatigued me horribly. It was too hot in our cave and my arduous, as well as useless, errand in the evening had in no small way contributed to this bout; moreover, we were disturbed by some people seeking lodgings and by the frustrating news that our light ambulance carts, which we were counting on finding in Jablona, had not appeared anywhere, which exposed those in charge of the administration to all His Majesty's animadversion, to whom they had vouched for their existence and their arrival.

At two o'clock, I rose. On the way, my friend advised me to get into a carriage, which suited me well; I slept there for at least two hours in the middle of our baggage. Arriving at the break of day at Nowy Dwor, a recently built village in place of another that a terrible flood had wiped out a few years ago, I learned that the Emperor was a quarter of a league further ahead, in a bad village, where a bridge had been built over the Narew River, which the people in this area also call the Bug, because this river flows into it a short distance away. I also learned that there had been about 300 wounded, of whom seventy were seriously affected and the rest had only minor injuries. Only three amputations have been made, two of which were to the arm and one to the leg. *M.* Bousquet, *chirurgien-major* of the ... infantry, in charge of the ambulance from a division of the III Corps, ran the service: I replaced him with *M.* Douche and his four *sous-aides.* His Majesty having mounted his horse at eight o'clock, I found myself in his path; he had me summoned to ask me how many wounded we had. I told him about 300, three-quarters of whom had only light wounds. A little earlier I had seen His Highness the Prince Major-General, to whom I had given the same account. I attended to some dressings and showed the young men how to pinch and raise the skin in order to cut a fold over a musket ball that they wanted to extract from a Russian hussar, near the armpit. During another operation, a purse of 40 *louis* was stolen from the side pocket of *M.* Bousquet's uniform, which was all of his means since the fire that ruined his entire regiment by reducing to ashes the caissons locked in a barn near Posen.

The Emperor lodged in a small wooden hovel; Prince Alexander was in one still worse. The Imperial Guard has bivouacked, officers and soldiers. Large numbers of men are filing over the bridge, and it continually breaks apart, which delays the passage over the Bug. The Russians have abandoned the position that we had so contested with them last night; they are gathered in their entrenchments 2 leagues further ahead; it is there that we will have to attack them.

This evening we have 250 wounded at Nowy Dwor, where we have returned to seek refuge until two o'clock in the morning, the moment fixed for our departure. The service is extremely difficult, the means of transport are useless and the roads are dreadful. This country has been devoured by the Prussians, the Russians and the French: what a desperate situation! I am coughing a lot, have no appetite, and still keep going: where I fall, I will be buried. We made a big bivouac fire in the little village; we prepared our dinner there, a good bacon soup and mutton with chicken. All this was eaten standing up, a large tree serving as a table. It rained all evening; the wind is to the west, without frost.

25th – Lodged with a poor priest with twenty other people: I coughed a lot and, without having slept more than two hours, we left at three o'clock in a dreadful wind. It was necessary to pass over three pontoon bridges, cross the peninsula where the Russians had defended themselves, follow an awful path through the marshes and woods, then continue for two hours through a beautiful forest and finally arrive at Nasielsk, a town occupied entirely by Jews, built in wood, full of mud and ruined by the Russians, who turned all the rooms of these unfortunate people into stables. We saw the debris, the waste, the traces of barbarity of the Muscovite savages; our people chose to imitate them. At the cries of a group of Jews who were pointing to a dragoon running away with a package in his hand, I rushed over and stopped this man, who showed me a large loaf of bread that he was carrying in a handkerchief. A loaf of bread! Was it necessary to shout so much for that? However, the cries redoubled when they saw that I was letting him go. I stopped him again; I opened the package and under the bread was the golden tablet of the Decalogue and a large silver crown that the scoundrel had flattened to better conceal.

Having only just arrived, I had to enter the mud up to my ankles to go to see some of the wounded men scattered around the houses, including one whose thigh required amputation: he was a mounted *chasseur*. Major Simonin has just communicated to me a letter written in the name of His Highness Prince Alexander, in which he is charged with telling me that His Majesty is unhappy not to see me at the outposts, and yesterday he spoke to me there! At my age, to be at the outposts! The Emperor could not explain himself in a way so far from his spirit of justice and reason. Nonetheless, we set out to go further.

Having crossed the muddy square and the awful streets of the town of … with difficulty, we joined a fairly good path, which led us to the battlefield of the previous day. This field of pain and of death was covered with the corpses of men and horses; that of Réal, the son of a well-known judge, was in the ditch on the left; this young captain was serving in a regiment of mounted *chasseurs*, and the skirmish had taken place between some French regiments of this force and Russian hussars undoubtedly forming the rearguard. One resents the curiosity with which one contemplates the victims of war, but one cannot help it; it is a sad pleasure, the charm of which is in that secret feeling that makes us enjoy the happiness of not suffering the same fate. The road passes through woods of fir and oak; I did not find it long; in the villages, it is barely passable.

We arrived at Nowemiasto, believing that we would find His Majesty there; but how can he stay long in one place, when the enemy is so close to him? He had left for Sochoczyn, 3 leagues further to the left; we had to continue to there, but the horses needed to rest and we spent two hours in this small town, the streets of which are paved; this is all that is remarkable about it. We had to follow a winding path, because of the ponds and marshes; one must go through the woods and we had no guides. Having continued on for three long hours, we arrived at the headquarters, where nearly everyone was bivouacking: it was raining and the weather was cold. We were given a small corner in the room of the local marshal, where twenty-five people were already lying on the straw. I found *M.* Ribes, of the Imperial Household, there, as well as four of our surgeons; they had tended to the wounded from the combat that had taken place in the village that very evening, a combat in which a mamluk had his nose cut off, but it was still partly connected; it was reattached to him. Several *chasseurs* of the Guard had been cut; *M.* Bockenheimer stayed to look after them. Fortunately, I was given two glasses of broth and a good bundle of hay, on which I slept reasonably well. I arrived at half past eleven. My poor friend Le Vert chose to sleep in the carriage, where he was very cold. Our horses, all wet with sweat, were like an icy rain for him during the night. What a job! The Cossacks had left us part of an ox at the marshal's house; this stroke of good luck served us well! I wanted a soup to be made, believing that His Majesty would not leave until late; but no sooner had the pot been placed on the fire than our departure was sounded, and it was necessary to remove the meat and leave.

26th – It is cold and very windy. There we were in the cart: we were on our way; but, after advancing half a league, we came across the regiment of heavy cavalry, which we had to watch pass by slowly and often in single file, because it was bad underfoot. We tried to avoid them by going across the countryside: several carriages remained there; ours barely managed and still the path continued to worsen. I then took the decision to ride on horseback and send the poor crew back to the village from which we came, proposing to come and find them the next day with permission from the Major-General to return to Warsaw. I rode in a wind mixed with hail and snow, which I could not tolerate; on all sides, one sees debris from carriages, horses buried in the mud and unable to get out, oxen dying while sunken into the earth up to their stomachs. Here was a battlefield from the previous day: luckily, there were only a few corpses. The houses there are burning, and we passed behind them so as not to be suffocated by the smoke. All that could be heard were cries to incite the beasts and men to redouble their efforts in this unfortunate terrain where what one calls the road has disappeared underwater and in the mud. His Majesty's six-horse carriages suffered the same fate; the wheels fell into colossal ruts and the white and superb team of horses falling and rolling round in the mud was soon no longer recognizable. The artillery train left behind several caissons. Some auditors dismounted from their beautiful sleeper to push at the wheel and their cries mingled with those of the coachmen and postilion riders; but, just as the carriage was about to get out of its predicament, the trace broke and my poor travellers were thus condemned to spend the night in the bivouac. Alas! Everyone has their own sorrows; mine are to cough with pain, to be horribly fatigued and unwell.

We arrived at Ciechanow, a small town with a rather poor abbey, which the Cossacks had already mistreated as they withdrew yesterday. At five o'clock in the morning they were still with their horses in the room that we had the good fortune to take as ours; we removed the manure; we made a large fire there to dry our clothes and to cook the hens and geese that *M.* d'Albavie, my colleague, had managed to procure. We had to let sixty soldiers of the IV Corps enter; these poor people were soaked and dejected; they wished to die and fight rather than to lead such a life for more than two days more. General Kirgener of the engineers, with his two aides-de-camp, asked us for lodgings, which we hastened to give him.

27th – We did not lack hay: I slept on four good bales spread out and, apart from a few coughing fits, I slept well enough; but this morning my head and chest were suffering. I ate some honeycomb that one of our surgeons had discovered for me in a forest yesterday: it is known that it was the Poles and Russians who taught us how to keep bees.

Having considered that the Major-General had told me yesterday that the Russians were on the run and that there would be only small skirmishes there, I decided to turn back and to write to him that I was going to the rear to collect the large number of sick people who were languishing without help in the abandoned hamlets and huts and to bring them together at a hospital that I would establish as best I am able in Sochoczyn or Nowemiasto. My letter was carried by the *chirurgien-major* Godefroy to the headquarters and, without waiting for an answer, I am going to leave to find my crew and return to Warsaw, being entirely sure that if I persist foolishly in marching with the headquarters, I will die of a fluxion of the chest. My great sorrow is to know that my friend Le Vert left yesterday on horseback to join me; that we did not see each other on the way; that he pushed on to the headquarters, 3 leagues further than Ciechanow, where we had intended to find him, and that the poor child is going to suffer death and passion for me.

I mounted my horse at nine o'clock and rode towards Sochoczyn, following the same route that I had taken yesterday. I met Marshal Lefebvre, who pulled a face and told me that he would speak to His Majesty about all this. The

Guard came after him, very tired, very muddy, having travelled up to 18 or 20 leagues in mud that one can scarcely imagine, murmuring softly and without an ounce of bread. This is the state of the army: it lives on meat, when one has the time to cook it; and on potatoes, *catouffles*, when one can get hold of them, for the peasants bury them in the fields and often one does not know where. I will spend the night in Sochoczyn, at the risk of having to engage with the Russians, who plague the rear and steal or kill everything they find: the peasants brought me one of five who were looting what the French had left; they had disarmed him and tied him up with ropes. I sent them back to the burgomaster.

My friend Le Vert has just arrived, frozen and starving. I am delighted to see this young friend, who has just proved his tender attachment to me so markedly again. We are in a bad room; the wind is blowing from all sides. Tomorrow we leave for Nowemiasto.

28th – I coughed all night and my body is broken, so cramped was my straw bed, or rather my litter. Here I am in a carriage like a poor dying man. My coachman found two good horses on the battlefield; he hitched them to our carriage and they are going well. We no longer recognize the roads by which we passed a few days ago; they have been destroyed as a result of the vehicles that were moving to join the army, and, at each step, we risk tipping over or dying. Several caissons and wagons will spend the winter in the holes where they fell. The drivers turn back, terrified at the sight of these unfathomable ruts. Shoes, uniforms and regimental effects are held back for fear of accident, and yet the soldiers have great need of their relief.

We arrived at Nowemiasto, which means 'new town', at five o'clock in the evening. On the way, I saw Major Simonin travelling to the main headquarters. I asked him to give *M.* Larrey a letter in which I warned him that I have established staging posts after a fashion in Ciechanow, Sochoczyn, Nowemiasto, Nasielsk, etc.; that I am leaving surgeons there but that there is no bread, nor any means of subsistence in these unfortunate places. I have requested that he take charge of my service, to go to inform His Highness the Major-General and to do for me what I would do for him in a similar situation. My letter will not reach him until 1 January, for His Majesty is marching every day, which leaves everyone to despair and pushes our shared misery to its furthest limits. But the Emperor has grand plans; we must wait until he has fulfilled them before passing any judgement, before uttering any grievance.

Never has the French army been so unhappy. The soldiers, always marching, bivouacking every night and spending their days in mud up to their ankles, have not an ounce of bread or a drop of brandy. They do not have time to dry their uniform and they faint from fatigue and starvation. Some are found dying on the side of ditches: a cup of wine or of brandy would save them. His Majesty's heart must be torn apart by all this, but he is marching towards his goal and fulfilling the grand destinies that he is preparing for Europe: if he had had the misfortune to fail or obtain only mediocre results, the army would be discouraged and would protest. It is presumed that his intention is to cut off the Russians' retreat and to corner them between the Vistula and the Baltic Sea so as not to let any of them escape. So be it. Yet the Russians are withdrawing in good order; their army, 70,000 men strong, is well led; it has sustained a small number of casualties so far. It seems that they are finding something to eat and that it will be difficult for us to throw them into the trap that we are preparing for them. The roads are full with our troops who are trying to regroup. The Guard has left many of them behind; these men have no bread; they live on meat and potatoes, when they have somewhere to cook them.

We have returned to our lodgings in Nowemiasto, but what a difference! It was full of soldiers who had filled it with rubbish; we had to use shovels and brooms to clean it. The pots were immediately put on the fire and the supper occupied my whole escort. It was good: not being able to eat my share of it, I claimed it for the people of the house, to whom I gave a quarter of a goose, a piece of ham, oily rice and Russian bread, which made them cry with joy. My coughing has grown worse; it has not let me rest tonight on my straw and in the midst of my companions and two officers, including an artillery captain of the Guard, whom I must have tired horribly with my dry and resounding coughing fits. Misfortune had it that at midnight the fire took to the house; the gunners of the Guard and the soldiers lodged under the same roof as us succeeded in extinguishing it. If it had not been noticed, in half an hour the house, made entirely of pine wood, would have been in cinders and we would perhaps have died there.

29th – Left at half past seven. We were afraid of the bad roads; however, we managed well. We found the battlefields of the 24th still covered with corpses and dead horses; the unfortunate Réal, stark naked, was lying along a ditch, inside the field. What reflections are not made at the sight of all these victims of a war of which they knew neither the motive nor the pretext! Yet, one must do one's duty, and should our mutilated bodies remain unburied, if the master has ordered us to die, we must suffer our fate and die in obedience. The crows only attack human bodies as a last resort; the dogs dare not touch them and the wolves tend to favour horses.

I stopped a league beyond Nowemiasto to feed our horses a little buckwheat in the form of oats. The miserable hospital of this sad town has received more than 300 wounded or sick, which it evacuated as best it could having fed and cared for them according to the time and premises. I gave orders to four surgeons, namely the *aides-majors* Baltz and d'Albavie and the *sous-aides* Bordenave and Wolhert, to march towards the main headquarters, leaving one of them in each of the staging posts where there will be a commanding officer for the town: it is a terrible fatigue that I am having them undertake. I crossed the three pontoon bridges without accident and found, at Nowy Dwor, *M. Gay, aide-major*, who lodged us well. There were 300 wounded in the small hospital of this village, five of whom required amputation: this evening I lent one of my cases to carry out these operations, and tomorrow we will make a decision on the means of evacuating to Warsaw, from where we are no more than 8 leagues away.

30th – My night was very bad. It is mild and there is a lot of fog. One of the *grenadiers*, who, having withstood the amputation of his thigh with so much courage last night, was found ill and unconscious, could not be shaken from this weakness and died.

We left happy and delighted to return to Warsaw. In three hours we arrived at Jablona and I had the satisfaction of warming myself well in my beautiful cave, where no one since us had entered; my good old lady made us a good fire there; she also had half a loaf of *kommißbrot*[18] and more than a pound of excellent ham, not to mention a few coins that we only gave her when we left. At five o'clock, we had crossed the Vistula, and at six I was already well warmed in my lodgings, which had fortunately been kept for us. There are more than 1,200 wounded in Warsaw and twice as many ill with fever. His Majesty is returning with his Guard. Thank heavens! I trembled with fear that he would persevere in prolonging his stay in this country cursed by nature and where there is nothing to drink but swamp water and nothing to eat but *catouffles* and lean beef.

---

18. Percy's original term is '*pain de munition*' ('Munitions bread'), which described a type of standard bread given to soldiers on campaign. It is sometimes known by the German name *kommißbrot*, a loaf made from rye and wheat. The German term means 'soldier bread'.

If I have ever known happiness in my life, it is certainly here, in a warm room and a good bed, where I have already eaten a broth. My cough is extremely bad and I am starting to frighten all those who come to see me. I found M. Poussielgue and M. Gallée, my principals, in mule slippers and nightcaps, quietly warming themselves; they have been back for three days. M. Delacoste has not left: what servants! The latter will do whatever he wants with his *ordonnateur*-in-chief, an unfrocked priest, nervous and cowardly like an abbot, running away at the first cannon shot and not having the right to think badly of others who do the same.

31st – Having coughed terribly, having had only short intervals of sleep, I took at day break two grains of antimony potassium tartrate.[19] I want to attack this cough with purgatives; it is purely gastric, I am sure of it. The physicians suggest potions of oxymel, red antimony oxide, incisives and delayants:[20] all that is real nonsense.

I spent the day coughing, working, giving orders; in the end, I fatigued myself excessively, for I was assailed by everyone. The sick arrived by the hundreds and were truly worthy of pity; covered in mud, haggard, thin, frozen, cut to shreds, dying of hunger, hardly able to drag themselves, they filled the streets, asked where the hospitals were and flocked to them. It is not freezing, but there is an icy mist that penetrates more than the frost. The army is returning little by little, sometimes a regiment, and what a regiment! Sometimes a platoon.

---

19. A strong emetic tartar.
20. *Incisifs* ('incisives') were remedies that were believed to break down thick and coagulated humours to aid circulation. *Délayants* ('delayants') were remedies designed to thin the blood.

# 1807 – The Campaign of Eylau

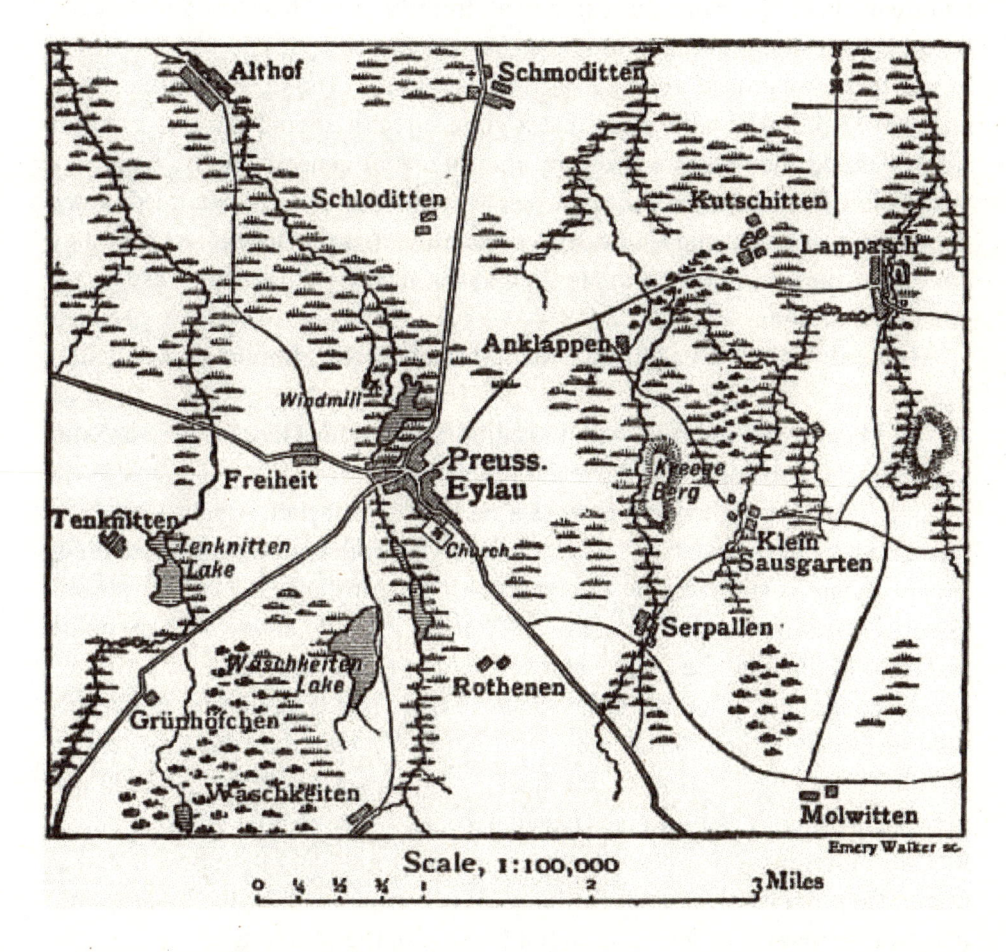

1 *Janvier* – I think I coughed less last night. As soon as it was morning, I took twenty-four jalap pastilles in a glass of tepid water saturated with sugar. I am overwhelmed with requests; I must work constantly. I have few surgeons and the number of patients is incalculable. For some time to come we will make

use of Polish surgeons; one of them, *M.* Magnin, who is Comtois and a very kind man, has taken charge of the service of the Radziwill hospital. The town is making great sacrifices: the bread is good; there is wine that has been bought and paid for at a high price. The hospital service has been given a lot of money; but a slowness of procedure and a heaviness of action still prevails, leaving the service to languish and the poor patients to suffer. The Intendant-general has assigned a *commissaire des guerres* to each hospital, and there are fourteen of them: he rebukes them, takes all the complaints he receives out on them and treats them like mercenaries; they all tremble under his cane and they are on their feet, night and day, to make the service work. It is a pleasing thing to see them breathless, running, asking, shouting, bending over backwards, and why? To do the hard work that a good director should do. But I am far from blaming the measure taken by the Intendant-general: firstly, there is a multitude of *commissaires des guerres* who should be kept occupied, since they were made to come to the army; secondly, it is due to the fact that they have more time and more resources to make things work than a simple director could find of both.

My head is much clearer and I feel infinitely better. Tomorrow I will start again.

His Majesty has returned with his entourage and his Guard. There are still troops on the other side and powerful bridgeheads.

2nd – I have coughed less and, as a result, I slept better. Again, I used my jalap, with which I have been very satisfied. This purgative works wonders for me; everyone is surprised by the way that I treat myself, and the physicians especially seem to be chuckling inwardly about it, but I know what I am doing and most of the time the same cannot be said of these gentlemen.

My cough leaves me for quite long intervals and is becoming noticeably less severe. It is not like a cough produced by catarrhal engorgement or inflammatory engorgement of the lungs; nor does it resemble the cough of peri-pneumonia. It is of a particular nature, and here is how one recognizes that it is foreign, so to speak, to the lungs: it is loud and the noise it makes comes from the whole area of the lungs. It is hard to see how the lungs do not tear and the vessels of the head do not burst with the coughing.

28th – For three weeks we have been working according to a state of organization that conforms to the decision of His Majesty dated 22 December: it was presented twice without being approved, because the surgeons designated for the light ambulance divisions and others of the corps of the armies were not found present in Warsaw or at the posts for which they were announced, being for the most part behind the lines. On the 27th, I submitted a new statement and gave my word that all the surgeons named therein were ready to leave at the first signal, or were already at their destination; but I asked that, because I am unable to pay them the salaries that they are due, I be given a few thousand *francs* to distribute to them before setting out, and today, the 28th, I received 2,000 *francs*, which I shared with them in 50 and 100 *francs* to immediately cross the Vistula and return on campaign. The order was given to sleep in Jablona and to be in Pultusk tomorrow. We were wrong not to go to Seiroch, which would save us 2 leagues.

I am leading thirty-six mounted surgeons and twenty-four on foot, with twelve carts loaded with aid supplies. I have left eight *chirurgiens-majors*, eight *aides-majors* and only sixteen *sous-aides* for the Warsaw hospitals; however, sixty-four Polish surgeons will be distributed among these hospitals after my departure.

*M.* Delacoste, principal of the III Corps, who remained ill in Warsaw, received a very detailed instruction on what was to be done, in my absence, to ensure that the curative service was taken care of; he is in charge of placing the arriving surgeons and of sending me those who have orders to join me. I am leaving my best equipage and two servants in Warsaw to take care of it. I am taking only four horses, a poor carriage and saddlery of little value, because the ground is freezing hard at present; but, if the thaw comes, all is lost and only the good horses will get through the mud.

It is one o'clock: I am leaving; the paths are splendid.

29th – We found ourselves alone at the beautiful castle of Jablona. All our surgeons have left. Such is the order of His Majesty, to whom I have promised, under my personal responsibility, that I would always have about forty of them at the headquarters.

There is a heavy frost. It took us five hours to arrive at the bridge at Bruck, still travelling through the woods and encountering, from time to time, a flurry of snow that bothered us greatly. When we arrived at the bridge, we found 100 carriages and 500 horses awaiting their turn to cross. My companions went to beg the major of the pontoon builders and an officer of the artillery of the Guard to let us go, and we crossed the river and its two tributaries on the most miserable and rickety bridge that has ever existed. Beyond it is a large castle with outbuildings that we could use as a hospital, or at least a staging post. We pressed on to Schlirock. There we stopped to feed the horses and to eat ourselves: a fire still burning in the middle of a barn warmed us up. Near this covered bivouac was a little boy of 10, almost naked, as beautiful as an angel, with Russian boots on his feet, and on his body a female corset in pieces: we treated him to a meal and everyone gave him some coins. If we were to return just as we came, I would have taken this poor child with me, who told us in Polish that he no longer had either a father or a mother. All these villages are devastated, absolutely drained of resources and almost deserted.

We arrived in Pultusk at half past five. The town is quite beautiful in the winter and in the frost: when it thaws, the square will be covered with 2ft of mud and perhaps 4ft of water. There is a bishop's palace, a seminary, a hospital for the sisters of charity and a Benedictine abbey in this small place. After the skirmish on the 26th, we had nearly 200 wounded piled on top of each other; there were 100 of them with the sisters and 225 in the house of the curacy. The latter was evacuated, and in the others I found fifty-two complicated fractures and twenty amputations. The beds in the sisters' hospital are only 5ft long; the poor wounded are very badly off there, and those who have a fractured leg will not be able to avoid being shortened by several inches; besides that, the place is quite clean for the country. Here, as elsewhere, the nuns are stern, miserly, selfish and full of vices or imperfections; it is only among the young, still in the fervour of their vocation, that one finds humanity. No one is more stubborn and more unkind than old women, and in Warsaw, in the Infant Jesus Hospital, where we have 150 sick or wounded, it is the same as in Pultusk and everywhere else where such women live, who nonetheless remain better at caring for the sick than the men.

In the Benedictine abbey, eighty wounded men are lying on a bit of straw and have no supplies of any kind. Their comrades have procured for them a few old blankets, some bad feather mattresses and other effects, which, already dirty and disgusting in themselves, have become even more so because of the grease, pus, blood and sputum with which they are soiled. Some amputees, despite this miserable state, have healed. There are a few fractures that are faring well. When the civil commission supplied the food, it was quite good; the undertaking was handed over to the French, and from then on, everything was spoiled, contaminated. Well might one cry out: this continued until the news of His Majesty's arrival in Pultusk. Then better wine was given out; the straw was changed and linen was procured for dressings, etc.

On my arrival, General Baville, the commanding officer in the town, informed me of a letter from Marshal Davout, ordering the chief medical officers of the Pultusk hospitals to go to the civil commission, and from there to the villages where, according to the report of the physicians of the country, there was an epidemic. I wanted to entrust this care to *M.* Micaleff and *M.* Boudet, of the III Corps, commanded by the same marshal, all the more so as they had already made a report on this over-accredited rumour; but they were about to leave, and that would have interfered with their plans! After a few errands and enquiries, I learned that the epidemic in question was merely hunger and a scarcity of food and that the remedy and antidote would be foodstuffs, of which the army had left no supply. Moreover, a Polish physician, who had distributed thousands of flasks full of a preservative liquor to the inhabitants, was seeking only to charge the Pultusk apothecary who supplied them, and with whom he undoubtedly had to share. That is all there was to it.

I saw at the sisters' hospital, among the complicated fractures, a dragoon who, having sustained a complete fracture after he fell from a horse, and hospital gangrene having destroyed part of his muscles, was in the most unfortunate state. The fractured bones were showing with their ends exposed; an awful empty space appeared around them, and the thigh scarcely left the sad recourse of amputation. The hospital stinks: as one enters it, one is hit by the smell of rotten cheese, a sign of the great amount of suppuration. The pharmacy is run by the sisters. No fumigations are performed.

30th – His Majesty arrived at noon, and everything suggests that we will leave this evening. Indeed, at three o'clock, the order was given to assemble in the square to observe the marching order drawn up by the Major-General, who must surely not have believed that it could ever be complied with in such difficult circumstances. At three o'clock, the square was covered with two dishevelled regiments, whose leaders believed that the Emperor would inspect them. His Majesty contented himself with saluting them as they passed; he was in his small open carriage, with Prince Alexander beside him and his faithful mamluk in front. I followed his carriage fairly closely, but a hold-up on the bridge having delayed me and the convoy having begun to file out, I was forced to follow in his wake, and so slowly that, with only 4 leagues still to travel before arriving in Marcow, I was not able to reach it until half past eleven in the evening. Two of my companions had found me bad accommodation in a barn. Having waited for them for an hour at the place without seeing them arrive, I decided to lay siege to a house whose shutters and doors were carefully closed. I shouted, knocked, threatened; at last they opened to me, and I was very surprised to find stretched out on a pallet bed *M.* Boyer, my colleague, and his two workers.

31st – Left for Prasnitz in six-degree cold and a superb frost, where I arrived at one o'clock: it is a good 6 leagues. The IV Corps left a hospital in this city, rather well built, but more or less unavailable: 120 sick remained there, and more than 400 must have arrived there the following day, so many filled the road! We are evacuating to Plotz, where I sent some surgeons over the last few days. It was necessary to leave three of the surgeons of the IV Corps in Prasnitz, one of whom is sick: another has lost all his effects, and a third is asking for nothing more than not to have to march.

At three o'clock, having found the general of the artillery of the Guard ready to leave by carriage for Colchiren, 5 leagues further on, I took advantage of the opportunity and made my way there very comfortably. We arrived at half past six; we were sent to a castle, a quarter of a league from the town, where General Lariboisière, my friend, with his aides-de-camp, those of General Couen and fifteen officers of the artillery of the Guard were gathered and, indeed, at the table.

1 *Février* – On 1 February we left, but not without having lunch. I obtained a sack of oats and a good bale of hay for my horses, which were to arrive, and having climbed into General Couen's carriage, I descended in front of the first house of the village, to wait there for my equipages and my men, who had remained in Prasnitz. *M.* Thérin, *chirurgien-major* of the artillery of the Guard, who procured the hay and oats for me, had them deposited near the aforementioned house. There I warmed myself well, shaved my beard and saw, after three-quarters of an hour, all my company and my entourage arrive. His Majesty had ordered that a hospital be set up at Marcow; but, apart from the fact that it is impossible to find a site suitable for holding a hundred patients, the distance from this place to Prasnitz is only 5 or 6 leagues and consequently very short. We left for Wittenberg,[1] 3 leagues further on. At three o'clock, we had already arrived and found accommodation, which is to say a shelter from the cold, in a room where there must have been eight or ten of us on the straw. I cleaned myself up a bit and paid a few visits. His Grace the Major-General appeared pleased to see me and to find that I had forty-eight

---

1. Longin transcribes this town as 'Wittenberg', but it is more likely to be Willenberg or Willenburg, now called Wielbark. Wittenberg is instead in eastern Germany, and Percy had passed through this town before travelling to Potsdam.

surgeons with me and a large quantity of aid supplies. *M.* Larrey and I, while walking around, visited the Lutheran church and identified that 300 patients could be put there, if a huge stove were placed there. In the two neighbouring houses and in the huge stable where His Majesty's horses were being kept, it would be possible, if necessary, to put another 300 patients, who would be sufficiently warm there.

Wittenberg is a pretty town that offers many resources. It is the first town in Old Prussia, where we have finally arrived. No more Poland, no more Polish: German is spoken in the country. The frost is heavy and the very starry sky promises one that is even heavier; there is not much snow. The Major-General is constantly consulting his thermometer, which is shaped like a watch and the effect of which, being very exact, depends on the expansion and contraction of a metal rod. Everyone is asking for frost, because if, by misfortune, the thaw should come, we would be very troubled; however, the earth would still remain firm enough for eight days to put us within reach of our destination, which depends on events to come. There are some magnificent mills in Wittenberg and a reasonably clean building, which is known as the castle: His Majesty was staying there.

2nd – We were quite well yesterday. Today, at eight o'clock, in extremely cold weather and a north-easterly wind, we set off for Passenheim, a small town 8 long leagues from Wittenberg. The road is detestable; it is the most direct route and the country is very mountainous. Having been preceded by the vehicle train of the Guard, we had to travel slowly in its wake and through the high furrows of the countryside, which so shook the carriage that, this morning, the 3rd, we realized that it was in no condition to go further. Having made half of the journey, we let the train go and entered an unfortunate village that had been abandoned and looted. We had a little hay there and found a very warm room that fifteen or twenty soldiers evacuated at the sight of us; they were removing the rest of the peas, broad beans and potatoes from it. We thought we were alone in this hovel when the sighs of an old woman, lying in a secluded bed, struck and saddened us. She is 80 years old. This unfortunate woman, having been unable to follow her children into the forests to which they have withdrawn, was abandoned by them. She was wrapped in disgusting rags; her eyes told of a fatal hunger. I gave her some white bread and a piece of cooked beef, which she ate well, although she no longer has a single tooth. She drank a glass of white wine that I presented to her very well; but, when she saw me give her a piece of sugar dipped in the wine, she hesitated and was afraid. However, when she took it to her lips, its taste pleased her and all that has properly restored her. We left her, asking Providence to save her and being very satisfied with our good deed.

At six o'clock, we arrived at Passenheim, where our surgeons charged with our accommodation had found us a corner with thirteen officers of the Guard. The horses were better than we were; they did not want for anything. Our officers were all occupied with their supper, on which they were making a head start, when I entered the room that I was to share with them; they showered me with respect and consideration. Everyone dined well. The room was filled with fresh straw; I laid my sheets, blankets and fur overcoat in a corner and by ten o'clock, everyone was snoring. At three o'clock in the morning, they came to give the signal to the officers to leave, then there was a counter-order and they did not leave until eight o'clock. His Majesty ordered us to be ready at all hours and to stay until an order had been sent to us to go quickly to wherever we were to be led. Thus, our staff and our equipment are waiting and, from one moment to the next, we expect to march. The Emperor and all the headquarters, equipages of all sizes, have left for Allenstein. It is said that 15,000 Russians are surrounded; a great assault is expected; His Majesty has announced it.

Our carriage is broken beyond repair. We have discovered another, but this one is bad too. We will have a good sleigh for our baggage; my nephew has taken a crazy, wild horse, which he hopes to break in; *M.* Le Vert has obtained another that is muzzled, which will not prevent it from pulling the sledge. We have saddlery; all in all, our business is going quite well.

3rd – You have never seen a spectacle of devastation such as that presented by the poor town of Passenheim: our people, and especially the Russians, must have eaten 200 cattle there; everywhere is covered with the heads of cows still with their skin, the stomachs and internal organs of calves, oxen, etc. We are promised a little bread, which the *ordonnateur* has had made for our small headquarters. It snowed a lot last night; the weather is cold, a little foggy; we are on the alert.

We have an order to remain in Passenheim and to wait there for the promised order. We can hear the cannon. It is said that the Russians are holding. The III Corps is arriving so as to move slightly to the right tomorrow. We have renewed our equipages, changed our carriages and kept our horses ready.

4th – We have slept well on good straw. The weather is superb; it snowed slightly at ten o'clock, but the sun is showing and easing the cold. At half past eleven, we received orders to leave. We are going to Allenstein, along 4 leagues of track and 4 of road. I climbed onto a rather pretty sledge, pulled by quite a good horse; I had to leave my carriage in Passenheim, since it was absolutely worn out from travelling so frequently; I am taking a small rural cart in its place.

I arrived at Allenstein at half past four, having trotted the whole way, in spite of the very hilly path and the 8 leagues, as much of track as of road. The little town is in a valley; its appearance is not unpleasant: its houses are quite well built. It is cluttered with equipages, carriages, caissons, etc.; the VI and VII Corps have theirs there; those of His Majesty and his entourage left at four o'clock, shortly before my arrival. I found the surgeons of the VII Corps wandering through the streets with a case of instruments, which at first made me fear that there were many wounded, but they told me that they had only about 200 of them, of which very few were serious cases. These are mostly those of yesterday, for there was a fierce battle 2 leagues from here. Today again, the battlefield was a similar distance away until noon; then the Russians lost 4 leagues of ground, having defended themselves fiercely and having caused us much harm. The 4th and 28th Line Infantry of the IV Corps suffered greatly. The VI Corps charged. Gilbert and Tissot are on an assignment in Thorn and the service is going as well as it can. Tomorrow we will have five or six hundred wounded at Allenstein: I am leaving four surgeons there with an order for four others who will pass through tomorrow. There is no way to evacuate: everything is ruined along the route, everywhere is deserted; even the Vandals never did so much harm. I am sure, from the countless number of heads of cows, oxen and sheep, which one meets at every step, that there is not a soldier who does not consume 4lb of meat each day. It is true that they rarely have bread and that they live on hardly anything other than meat and potatoes. The fire and the smoke of the bivouacs make them yellow, gaunt, unrecognizable; they have red eyes; their clothes are thick with filth and smoke. They are thin, sad, deep in thought; they are too often affected by maledictions, imprecations that despair and impatience draw from them.

We are lodged in a large house that, like all the others, has been pillaged and stripped. I went to bed at eight o'clock and slept until midnight. The snoring of twenty people lying in the same room, the excessive heat from the stove, the bugs and fleas woke me up. My tongue was as dry as wood: I drank water and, unable to fall back to sleep, I rose to write these miserable lines by the light of a small tallow candle from the fields of our homeland. I looked around at our crowd of sleepers: on the right, nine surgeons on the straw, and on the left twelve people of the house lying on the floorboards and snoring very well there.

At four o'clock in the morning, we will all leave; I have given the order. Three hundred sledges have preceded us. *M.* Larrey and his six aides have tended to the day's wounded. Without the inconceivable order given to us by the Major-General, we would have been at yesterday's and today's events: His Majesty will be informed of this order and its results. It is said that 2,000 Swedes and 10,000 English soldiers have docked and are joining forces with the Russians and Prussians.

5th – The night was cold; it was still snowing and at four o'clock we could not see a thing. We took a guide with a lantern; I climbed into the Russian sledge of the *chirurgien-major* Thomas, and we all left together. I had with me around twenty-four surgeons on horseback and ten on foot. We travelled almost blindly until half past five: the road is quite good up to the first village. Here we found thirty wounded spread over several houses, and I had been told that I would find 400 of them there. In the second, we found the same number and saw the colonel of the 4th Line Infantry with a simple contusion on his arm. At half past seven, we met the equipages of the VI and VII Corps in a large village; we had to follow in their wake, which delayed us severely. It was bitterly cold; the snow was falling in heavy flakes; the entire route was strewn with the corpses of men and horses, splintered muskets, broken carriages, dismantled Russian artillery caissons and cannon, two of which were still in position, loaded and primed. The cartridge boxes, the finest leatherwork, powder bags and cartridges were scattered all over the place. The beautiful white carpet of snow was stained with blood and had been trampled by the men and horses who had manoeuvred there. The Russians lost many people there and left behind a lot of baggage on the 3rd of the month; in other words, the day before yesterday.

We intended to go to Guttstadt, but we were told that His Majesty was at Liebstadt and we continued on our path, after resting the horses in a desolate and ravaged village. We had entered a house owned by some poor people, who had deserted it; two wounded Frenchmen had withdrawn there, and it was cold in the room that had been turned into a stable. One of our surgeons, who wanted to make a fire in the stove, saw two human feet sticking out of its opening. He told me about them. I found these feet hot; I pinched them, and immediately a plaintive voice was heard from the bottom of this sort of cave. It was a Russian who had climbed into this stove to seek a bit of warmth there; we pulled him out of it. This unfortunate man had received several blows from a sabre, among them one that cut his skin and the muscles covering his occipital and another that had made in his vertex an '*apokeparismos*'[2] as wide as 6 *francs*; we bandaged him as best we could and left him to the care of Providence, while waiting for the surgeons, whom I had ordered to collect these unfortunate people, to pass through.

Before arriving at this village, we had seen a short distance from the road, near a dismantled carriage, a Russian with terrible cuts to his head, who was naked and had spent the night on the ground, sheltered only by a shred of rug. He was barely 18 years old. He said to us: '*Nix braute for Rousse*' (the Russian has no bread). Alas! None of us had any on us, and none of our surgeons could put a head-covering on him, for lack of compresses, with which their pockets should have been filled.

This caused me great sorrow and drew from me bitter reproaches to my colleagues, who have not forgotten the small supply of lint and linen since.

The army had pursued the Russians through woods and uneven country, where it would be impossible to pass if it were to thaw. On all sides are lakes, ponds, pools and streams, now frozen, covered with snow and over which one passes without realizing. However, we were twice forced to make a considerable diversion to avoid dangerous passages, already worn down by the columns that had preceded us. It was on these routes that we were able to note the traces of the manoeuvres of the two armies. Here and there, there were a few corpses and some Russians still alive, who, having resisted the cold of the first night, would have perished from that of the second without us being able to help them: it is a misfortune and a terrible fate.

Having travelled for a long time, still following His Majesty's equipages, and having been obliged to ride on horseback, so slow and uncomfortable was the sledge, because of the furrows through which it was necessary to pass, we arrived on a height where all the carriages of the entourage were stopped. By then, they were fighting vigorously on the left, near Liebstadt; the cannon and musketry were going strong, and quite close to us. I saw the coach of my colleague Boyer, who had given a seat there to General Gardanne (of the pages),[3] who had been hit by a dead musket ball.[4] I continued and arrived

---

2. A Greek word meaning 'decapitation' or 'detachment'.
3. Gaspard Amédée Gardanne was a French general in the Grande Armée in 1807; however, Percy's reference to 'the pages' suggests that he meant Claude Mathieu de Gardane, who in 1805 was named 'governor of the pages', a title given to a senior aide-de-camp in Napoleon's entourage (and previously under the *Ancien Régime*).
4. In French, a '*balle morte*', or 'dead musketball', is one that has reached the end of its trajectory and is not travelling fast enough to cause any harm.

in a large village called Wolfsdorf. Throughout Old Prussia, the villages are beautiful, though most of the houses are still built mostly of wood; there are beautiful plantations of lime trees and fruit trees; in summer, the houses are cool and pleasantly shaded. In Wolfsdorf were 150 French and fifty Russian wounded, near whom I left *M.* Boyer's division, with orders to join me, when it had evacuated these wounded to Allenstein.

It was late: the VII Corps, bivouacking within cannon range in a small wood, and already making soup, had just beaten the drums and sounded the call to leave. It was said that His Majesty was in Landsberg; others assured us that he had slept on this side, in a village beyond which he had not been able to go. I wrote to the Major-General that I would stay the night at Wolfsdorf for the wounded who had been directed there and among whom there were more than eighty dragoons, including two officers who had lost their legs. The day before, 6,000 dragoons had charged against 1,000 Cossacks, who, constantly darting around and among them in dispersed order, while they were doing their manoeuvres, had slashed and stabbed them with their lances. These Cossacks were supported by two pieces of cannon, which had done much worse still, so that the 16th and 4th Regiments had been almost entirely defeated.

I believed the Major-General to be in Liebstadt and I had charged the *aide-major* Baltz with carrying my letter to him, but the latter was afraid of the Cossacks and learned moreover that His Highness was not in the small town in question. I found in my village the adjutant-major Vuilleminot, the topographer, who was kind enough to have a sentry guard a large and beautiful house for me, which, although looted and devastated, provided me with a good refuge and gave me a good night's sleep. *M.* Chappe came to share this stroke of fortune with us.

6th – Having given the orders to the surgeons who remained in Wolfsdorf, I set off at eight o'clock, believing that I would go to Landsberg and find the main headquarters there. After 2 leagues, on uneven country roads that made my sledge jump and shook me horribly, we arrived in a village where His Majesty had spent the night, before leaving in the morning; *M.* Lombard had bivouacked there. We learned from this *ordonnateur* that the Major-General had reproached him for having left Allenstein without any orders, and that His Majesty had not intended that we should be exposed to spending nights in the bivouac. What should one make of the situation of a headquarters as large as that of the Emperor, when it is necessary to establish it in a village such as Hermendorf (that is, I believe, the name of the commune in question)! This village was empty and more or less deserted; nothing had been left there, and the streets, the surrounding area, the front and back of the houses were covered with straw shelters, if not bivouacs still smoking. In each of them a cow, a pig, etc. had been eaten and their skin, entrails and head were still there. The meat from these animals had been cooked, as was our custom, using doors, furniture, carriage wheels, winnowing baskets and farming equipment, in the absence of other dry wood, such that the poor inhabitants, when they return to the houses from which they were driven by fear and violence, would find neither livestock, nor ploughs, nor food, nor resources of any kind.

I lodged at random and was fortunate. I helped my host and his wife to remove four cartloads of bedding straw and manure that filled the room where twenty-eight *grenadiers* of the Guard had spent the night and left all their waste. We took over this room and immediately looked in the bivouacs for something to live off. Here we found good meat, pots made of earth and iron, and firewood. A freshly killed pig was lying in the street; it was only missing a thigh: we took advantage of the good find, and our servants, directed by me, set out to remove the other leg. Soon our cooking was under way. We went to kill the rest of the local priest's pigeons; we took six of them. Wanting to see if there were any oats in the barn, I noticed a hen there, the only one to have escaped the previous day's captors; *M.* d'Albavie had soon wrung its neck without making it squawk. What a feast we have, but I have little appetite and my *rôtie au vin*[5] mixed with sugared hot water gives me more pleasure than anything else.

The village is full of wounded; there are 180 of them. I am ordering the *chirurgien-major* Mornac to see to them with his division. Three hundred Russian prisoners are gathered in the church (which is splendid and which these barbarians will have soon devastated); I sent *M.* Mayot there to bring me back an altar candle, an essential thing while on campaign. We have shaved; my breeches, which were torn, are being mended for me. Everything is going well: I have brought back some iron wagon parts found in the bivouacs for our host; my nephew has had our host take the hides of the livestock that our men have eaten; we have given him some of our bread, which his wife and children ate voraciously, so starving are they. We have had an excellent night.

---

5. A medicinal tonic made by toasting and then garnishing bread with lemon zest, sugar, cinnamon, wine and water.

7th – I am ordering two *sous-aides* both of whom have a sore foot, to remain in the village to continue caring for the wounded, but to join me as soon as they can without adversely affecting this duty. We are all leaving for the village of Gross-Claudow, where we were called by the Major-General during the night. The aide-de-camp, or rather the deputy who was to bring us the order, lost it and has, reportedly, been dismissed, given the harm that our delayed arrival has caused.

On bad roads, we travelled the 8 leagues quite swiftly from the village of Hermendorf to that of Gross-Claudow. What a season! What cold! What a country! We passed through extremely dense woods, where one could lose one's way a thousand times without an assured and faithful guide; but in large armies there is almost always an uninterrupted stream of soldiers and carriages that direct the traveller from their departure to the stopping point. I travelled very quickly in my little sledge. It was four o'clock when we arrived. His Majesty, with all his Guard and the entire main headquarters, had spent the night in this indescribably desolate village. The colonel of the 75th Infantry Regiment, who had been wounded in the arm and was accompanied by his *chirurgien-major* Lejan and four officers, was staying in the Emperor's room; otherwise, I would have lodged there.

As soon as I had arrived, I had put twenty of my surgeons to work throughout the village, where there were still a hundred wounded who had not been bandaged; the corps surgeons and those of the Guard had dressed just as many of them the previous evening and in the morning. They had fought with unparalleled doggedness 1 league from the village. The Emperor who, on the 6th thought he was going to spend the night peacefully in Preuss-Eylau, 7 leagues from here, was stopped by a very large Russian line, which appeared suddenly, took up good positions and readied itself to fight. The cavalry, and particularly the *cuirassiers*, charged with fury; the 75th Infantry Regiment, among others, fought valiantly. Both sides attacked and defended themselves with an almost barbaric obstinacy, and this unexpected encounter yielded around 300 wounded, who were taken to Gross-Claudow. His Majesty asked for me several times: it was the failing of the general staff and its deputies sent to find me that I was not present. The Emperor's chief surgeon, *M.* Boyer, saw some of the wounded; *M.* Larrey saw some others; in any case, they conducted the surgical service reasonably well. I slept on a pallet bed, which I had well cleaned, and I arranged my feather quilt, my sheets and blankets over it. Never have I slept better. Having arrived outside this house, which was then full of soldiers, and while looking for the leftovers of those who had preceded them there, I saw the owner and four women, each with a child latched to her breast, who did not dare to enter and who, without me, would have spent the night at the door. I showed them in and gave them some scraps of bread and meat. Our surgeons put themselves in a tiny room that I had great difficulty obtaining for them, since it was full of soldiers who did not want to leave it; they killed a sheep, from which they cooked a leg of mutton that they could hardly tear up; the majority bivouacked.

8th – As soon as day broke, we received the order to go in all haste to Eylau. Soon everyone was on his horse. I am leaving *M.* d'Albavie and *M.* Fizelbrand in the village to continue their care of the wounded for a few days and to evacuate them. I climbed into my sledge and left swiftly. The night was extremely cold; it snowed and is snowing still. The path is mountainous; the country is wild and wooded; we are always climbing and descending.

Having travelled three-quarters of a league at most, we found the battlefield from the day before yesterday. Oh, what damage the killing frenzy has done! Never had so many corpses covered such a small area. Everywhere the snow was stained with blood; the snow that had fallen and was falling still was beginning to conceal the bodies from the distressed looks of the passers-by. The corpses were piled up wherever there were a few clusters of fir trees, behind which the Russians had fought. Thousands of muskets, caps and cuirasses were scattered on the road or in the fields. On descending a mountain, the reverse of which the enemy had undoubtedly chosen to defend themselves better, there were clusters of a hundred bloodied bodies; horses, maimed but alive, were waiting for starvation to topple them in turn on these heaps of corpses. Scarcely had we crossed one battlefield before we encountered another, and all were strewn with bodies, among them Frenchmen too.

At nine o'clock, we arrived in Landsberg, a small town where the retreating Russians, and our men pursuing them, had wreaked every kind of devastation imaginable; everywhere was full of carriages; the artillery trains passed through in succession; we had great difficulty entering the town with the sledge and our little cart. I found the principal surgeon Poussielgue there with his division and the surgeons of the vanguard of the cavalry reserve; he had just performed his last amputation and was leaving immediately. I left behind *M.* Pla, *aide-major*, as well as four *sous-aides*. At ten o'clock, we went back on our way: it was cold and a heavy frost of snow and ice was forming. At eleven o'clock, we met some wounded soldiers, some bandaged, others not, and all of them making their way towards Landsberg, forming a column that was growing increasingly long as we advanced. We could hear the frightening sound of the cannon; on all sides, the bombs and artillery shells were exploding; the musket fire was unrelenting. His Majesty had stayed the night a quarter of an hour from Eylau, which we had seized the previous day, and since early in the morning the fighting had been underway on the plain on the other side of this small town, previously so pretty and so prosperous. Having arrived half a league or even less from the battlefield, we saw the whole wagon train of the Emperor's headquarters stationed on the high ground. Continuing for a quarter of a league, I was warned that, in a large house near the road, there was a crowd of wounded men, and that more were flocking there constantly. I entered and was reassured to find the principal Chappe, surrounded by twelve good surgeons competing in their zeal and effort to assist this respected leader and to withstand such a difficult service. Through great effort, the operations were performed; only the fractures and amputations were held back; all the other wounded were sent to Landsberg. Around this sanctuary from misery and pain were countless carriages, several regiments waiting for the signal to leave and a crowd of wounded unfortunates who could neither enter nor find a place to be dressed. I neglected to say that on the way I had seen my friend General Levasseur, going to Landsberg in a good covered sledge, with a fracture to the upper third of his left arm.

Beyond the ambulance building, I saw several *grenadiers* of the Guard, as many on foot as on horseback, returning from the battlefield bloodied and more or less seriously wounded. This greatly affected me, for the Guard is a reserve corps that His Majesty risks only as a last resort, and to see it return covered in wounds and in retreat is a bad omen. The mounted *chasseurs* had been felled. The infantry of the Guard had not charged; the grapeshot and the Russian artillery, so well-served, had wrecked them where they stood. The mounted *grenadiers* had charged very ill-fatedly. The gunners of the Guard had suffered greatly, such that *M.* Larrey, *M.* Bockenheimer, *M.* Thérin and other surgeons-in-chief and their subordinates were very busy and had only dilapidated sheds for a ambulance. I had to share this place with them in order to treat, dress and operate on the wounded of the line, whose number was continuing to grow constantly.

The senator and general d'Hautpoul arrived in a sledge with a comminuted fracture a few fingerbreadths above the knee. *M.* Larrey was finishing dressing him when I learned of this cruel accident. As he clasped my hand, the general wanted the bandage untied so that I could see his wound; *M.* Larrey was prepared to make this gesture of deference, but I did not agree to it and repeated several times to the wounded man that my colleague was worthy of all his trust. Marshal Augereau had already seen us, having been shot in the leg, General Leval had a musket ball in his arm and General Ricard had a wound that I can no longer remember. General Heudelet had been hit in the lower abdomen by part of the musket ball. My poor good friend General Gudin had been killed, as well as the colonels Lemarrois, Lacuée and others of whom I was also very fond. The brave and kind Corbineau, general aide-de-camp to His Majesty, had just died, after a cannonball tore through his thigh. General d'Allemagne,[6] colonel of the Emperor's mounted *chasseurs*, had been riddled with lance blows by the Cossacks and was in a state of anxiety and spasm that worried me greatly for his life. A large number of corps commanders and distinguished officers had died. The massacre was terrible, and our surgeons could not cope with the throng of wounded. Fire had broken out in several houses in the small town of Eylau, below which we found ourselves. The noise of the artillery, the smoke from the blaze, the smell of the gunpowder and the cries of the wounded on whom we were operating, nothing that I saw and heard will ever leave my memory. Our men had spent the night in the town; *M.* Poussielgue had dressed the wounded there until ten o'clock in the morning; but the enemy was launching so many shells and cannonballs towards it that it had been necessary to abandon this position. Yet our soldiers continued to go there to steal food, or rather to find some way of surviving.

Around one o'clock, Marshal Augereau crossed the town, followed and preceded by a large escort that was moving quickly, because of the cannon fire. This small company was taken for a Russian corps, and everyone fled as fast as they could as far as our sheds and even further still, which gave rise to a general alarm and caused a real rout. It was merely a question of who could get away most quickly: officers, soldiers, cavalrymen, servants, everyone ran away. My coach driver Paul, who is very cowardly by nature, brought me my horse quickly, which I mounted as a precaution, not knowing what this movement might become. He had unharnessed the best of my horses from the carriage and he had already started his retreat on it when I cut him off and sent him back to my wagons, making fun of him. However, I must confess

---

6. Longin: The general that Percy calls d'Allemagne ['of Germany'] is General Dahlmann.

that, still not having been able to find spurs large enough to fit my huge riding boots, I counted myself lucky in such circumstances to notice a very large and open one on the ground. I hastened to fit it to my right heel, in case of need, since I was riding a horse that does not move quickly without being stirred. I let the deserters run; finally, my nephew and I, shouting that it was only a panicked terror, just a false alarm, succeeded in rallying an infantry regiment and holding back most of those who were following the bad example. An *ordonnateur* and his secretary left their horses and ran on foot; another took the time to mount a horse and fled very far; only one of our surgeons (Charpentier, *aide-major*) allowed himself to be swept along and travelled nearly 2 leagues in less than three-quarters of an hour; all the others remained firmly at their post. However, out of an excess of precaution, I chose to move my carriage and my horses away and make them ready to make off before the others, if it became necessary. As a result, we led them close to *M*. Chappe's ambulance and against the gable of a badly damaged little house, already half-exposed, and in which Colonel Henriot of the 14th Line Infantry, who had been wounded in the hand, had withdrawn with his *chirurgien-major* Courtois and seven or eight officers from the same corps. More than 300 wounded from the same regiment had been dressed in this building. Since Courtois and the colonel promised me a portion of soup and a small corner in this derelict lodging, I had a good fire lit for our servants, had the wagon train covered and guarded, because of the snow that continues to fall in large flakes, and saved a place in this bivouac for some of our surgeons. Then I returned to our sheds, where *M*. Laurenchet, *chirurgien-major*, and his division were busily dressing the wounded. We had not been able to make ourselves useful earlier, because the ambulance carriages had not yet arrived; once they came, we opened one, and there was no shortage of linen, lint and instruments. We made a large fire a short distance from the first shed, to spend the night around, for the cold is becoming more and more biting and the snow continues to fall.

We went, *M*. Le Vert, *M*. Mayot and I, to the highest part of the cemetery to see the end of the battle and to appreciate the spectacle of the two formidable armies that were present. The artillery of the Guard had taken this position. The reverse of this hill was covered with the corpses of the brave gunners killed at their cannon in the morning; one cannot fix one's gaze anywhere without seeing twenty and fifty corpses at a time; the slaughter is terrible. To me, the enemy seemed very strong in number; only their skirmishers, arranged in a line and spread out from each other by 7 or 8ft, were still shooting, and only a few cannon shots were now being fired. The cavalry of the Guard had withdrawn; the rest were in battle. The plain is vast, and against its snowy backdrop one can easily observe the fighting corps, the infantry in their lines and the cavalry always ready to charge. The movements of the troops, the glint of the weapons, the manoeuvres and the fire of the artillery, the men marching, the countless corpses of those who have perished, etc. – what a sight, so curious and so harrowing all at once! On the other side of the cemetery, the side of the plain, blood had flowed terribly; it was that of the Russians. Around the church, in the town, in the farmyards, the houses – in a word, everywhere – we saw only corpses and dead horses. The carriages pass over them; the artillery trains tear them apart and crush their skulls and their limbs. The enemy has launched many hollowed cannonballs and shells on the town, which have not succeeded in driving away our pillaging, starving soldiers who, for a fistful of potatoes and a pot for soup, lay themselves perilously open to being killed.

Returning from the battlefield, where more than 300 wounded Frenchmen were still lying without it being possible to reach them, I went back to our sheds. On the way, I saw His Majesty observing the movements of the Russians from the top of a hillock and on horseback; several times during the day he was the target for more than one battery, and five or six shells fell near him, the fragments from which flew around him. I found the surgical service in our sheds in full operation, but what a service! Legs, thighs and arms cut off, thrown with the dead bodies in front of the door; surgeons covered in blood; unfortunates with hardly any straw and shivering with cold! There was not a glass of water to give them; nothing to cover them; from all sides the wind was blowing under the sheds, the doors from which the soldiers were removing to establish their bivouac a few feet away. I had a few bundles of straw, already broken up, brought in to cover these brave people slightly. The barn doors were set back in place on the side where the cold wind was blowing most fiercely, and having exhorted my colleagues, arranged around me on all sides, to hold firm to their work for as long as they could, I returned to my wagons a quarter of a league away. I made sure, as I passed before the bivouac of the ambulance carts, that the majority of the wounded would receive broth; I had candles carried to the surgeons, as well as a fresh supply of linen and some more cases of instruments.

Having reached our carriage, we provided for the supper of our men and arranged the horses to get through the icy night that threatens us. I saw five or six officers of the general staff coming, who, seeking refuge for the night, thought they would find it in our shack; I told them that it was full of wounded, showed them Colonel Henriot, Major Dupuy and seven or eight other wounded officers, which immediately drove them away. Then we each took a small corner; a *cantinière*[7] made us soup; I spread out my feather bedding and lay down under my fur overcoat.

9th – This morning, at six o'clock, some men came on behalf of the Major-General to ask for me. At seven, I took the rest of yesterday's bad broth and drank a mouthful of white wine that a wounded lieutenant-colonel furtively gave me. I was going out to see my men in the bivouac when I noticed the Grand Duke of Berg[8] returning from answering the call of nature behind our hut. I greeted him; I spoke with him for a moment and my nephew thanked him for having offered him a place on his staff yesterday. This proud and gallant nephew, seeing or believing that he saw the army in full flight, had run to His Majesty and asked him if he had the honour of being recognized by him. The Emperor answered 'yes'. 'In that case deign to give me a sabre, a horse and a command, and Your Majesty will see if I am worthy of his esteem.' The Emperor smiled, and the prince told our *chevalier* to join his staff, which my nephew did not deserve. Having taken my turn in the place from where the prince was returning, I found a superb sabre, which I believed to be his, and which I was taking back to him when General Bertrand, its true owner, claimed it, having left it behind in the place where the three of us had all gone. His Majesty's aides-de-camp saw me and informed me that the Major-General was waiting for me with *M.* Lombard, whom they had gone to fetch. I made the short journey from my hut to the Emperor's, which is only 200 paces away, and no less miserable and destitute than my own; I put my embroidered redingote on outside and came running to the Palace, where *M.* Lombard was arriving. The Major-General showed us into His Majesty's room, where he was lying fully clothed on his mattress with a face that signalled serenity and safety. He welcomed us with consideration and kindness. 'Do you have many wounded?' he asked me.

---

7. A woman attached to the French army as a sutler. They would sell food and alcohol to the soldiers.
8. Joachim Murat, who, from 1804, was also a *prince français*. Murat had married Napoleon's sister Caroline in 1800.

'Sire, I think we dressed about 4,000 of them.'

'Are the wounds serious?'

'One thousand are of the greatest severity.'

'How many of this number of wounded will you lose?'

'A third, because the grapeshot and shell fragments have wreaked the greatest havoc.'

'Have you also had wounds from blades?'

'Many, Sire. The lance, the sabre and the bayonet have caused much damage; one of your Guards had the full blade of a Russian bayonet pushed to the top of his thigh and into his buttock, and its socket had been broken by the blow; we removed it from him without effort and this wounded man will recover.'

'Have you seen our wounded generals?'

'I met General Levasseur, who has a fracture to the upper third of his left arm; General Leval was shot under his Achilles tendon; General Heudelet was hit in the lower abdomen; General d'Hautpoul had his left thigh fractured by a biscayan musket ball; General Augereau was hit in the leg; General d'Allemagne was struck by ten lance blows, one of which was to the lower abdomen and emerged from the omentum.'[9]

'Do you think you can save General d'Allemagne?'

'No, Sire: the blood-streaked urine that he has passed, the convulsive vomiting, the hiccups, his faint pulse, the insurmountable cold in his extremities, his anxiety, everything indicates an imminent and unhappy end.'

'And will General d'Hautpoul pull through?'

'I like to think so, Sire; he is in a castle 2 leagues from here and is expecting me this morning.'

---

9. A layer of fatty tissue sitting in front of the stomach and intestine.

'You will not be able to go there; you have a duty to all and not to one. Why did you not amputate his thigh?'

'It was my colleague Larrey who saw and dressed it, and he told me that there was a good chance of preserving the limb.'

He asked *M.* Lombard if he had anyone to assist him. He was told that he did not; that there were no bookkeepers, no workers, no *infirmiers*, but that we were not short of linen, lint, instruments, etc. 'What organisation!' said the Emperor. 'What inhumanity!'

'Sire,' added *M.* Lombard, 'when one is sure, in peacetime, of being cast aside, whatever good conduct one has demonstrated during the most gruelling and perilous war, it is difficult for one to have zeal and to decide to follow an army as an employee or as an *infirmier*. Even this title, on our return to France, will be a loathsome reference.'

'That is true,' said the Emperor, 'because indeed hardly anyone other than rogues and vagrants throws themselves into the profession of the hospitals, which they abandon very quickly if they do not find any business to do there.'

'Your Majesty,' I felt I should say, 'would never confuse your surgeons with such men, but even so their outlook is no more reassuring.'

'I am pleased with their efforts, their devotion, their good conduct, and I want all this to be better arranged in future; everyone can be sure of keeping his job and there will be a sustainable and military organization.'

'Sire,' I said, 'the evidence of the necessity of this organization is incontestable, and its advantages are no less so. If in your Guard a fairly good ambulance service was provided, despite the weather and setting, it is because you have given it workers, *infirmiers*, some of whom are officers and others soldiers: we require the same, and it is particularly essential that our surgeons constitute a corps, as I had the honour of proposing to Your Majesty.'

'Very well. What has become of your wounded?'

'Sire, the false alarm that took place at one o'clock caused more than 1,500 of them to leave suddenly; they were bothering us to be dressed all at the same time and had only minor wounds. I know of no better secret for clearing an overcrowded ambulance.' The Emperor and the Major-General smiled.

Someone knocked at the door and His Majesty said, 'Enter!' It was an aide-de-camp of Marshal Davout. We withdrew after receiving permission from His Majesty.

I went to put back on my ordinary redingote and placed my *vitchoura*[10] over it, tied simply at my shoulders. Dressed like this, I mounted my horse. I met Marshal Bessières; he asked me for news of General d'Allemagne, whom I spoke to him about as if speaking of a lost man. I went to the bivouac of His Majesty's aides-de-camp; *M.* Larrey was warming himself there with them, and in front of *M.* Boyer. The latter said to me: 'Ah good! You have arrived.'

'As you can see, colleague,' I replied. 'And you, colleague, how do you find it? A few campaigns like this will end up making you quite the hussar like me,' I continued, 'for you will notice, gentlemen,' addressing my words to the whole bivouac, 'that in my old age I have become a sort of pandour.'[11] General Caulaincourt began to laugh and congratulated me on my cheerfulness and good health. 'What a pity, colleague,' I said again to Boyer, 'that we do not have our red and black doctoral gowns here! They would keep us warm.' My colleague turned his back on me, and I spurred on my horse, causing it to stamp to better resemble a hussar, of which my lambskin helmet and wolf-fur *vitchoura* give me quite the appearance.

I saw General d'Allemagne again and persisted with my unpleasant prognosis; he is leaving for the castle of Vrinec, where General d'Hautpoul is. There are more than thirty officers in *M.* Chappe's ambulance, most of them maimed; one cannot get close to them, so tightly packed are they on the floor that serves as their bed. I went to our sheds and found our poor wounded there shivering with cold; the neighbouring buildings were being dismantled and exposed to find wood and straw. The Guard bivouacked. Our surgeons, frozen, with hardly a bit of black bread with potatoes for their supper and having spent the night in front of a fire in the bivouac, had already set to doing dressings and amputations. While they sacrifice themselves, their horses, belongings, swords and even their hats are stolen from them. Nothing matches the selfishness, the rapacious fury and the inhumanity of the soldiers: they walk on the corpses; trample severed limbs underfoot; they hear the screams of the wounded, whose arms and legs are painfully amputated, and do not pause for a moment. Occupied by their own interests, everyone searches for some means of survival, runs to gather a little fodder, something to live off. They even dare to take the straw that we have obtained for the poor wounded, and we

---

10. A fur-lined coat, from the Polish *wilczura*, meaning wolfskin.
11. Eighteenth-century Hungarian soldiers reputedly known for their pillaging and brutality.

have to stand watch to prevent horses being placed among them and to avoid them being crushed under the feet of these animals. There is no sympathy in the armies; no sensitivity, and one finds only soldiers roused by combat, valiant and brave, if you like; only courageous and intrepid officers; one must not expect to find a man there. Compassion, philanthropy and a love of one's fellow beings reside only among the surgeons; everything is cold-bloodedly barbaric, and, if I dared to say so, I know well the name that I should give to the mass of individuals who constitute an army. It is true that once distanced from the bloody theatre of all the horrors that war spawns, French soldiers regain their natural gentleness and kindness.

I went around nine o'clock to the town, the houses of which, mostly spared from the fire and the shells of the Russians, have been terribly ruined by our people and perhaps by the enemy; I found a lot of wounded there. Having learned that the main headquarters may well be established there, I hurried to take up lodgings and had to chase away the soldiers eating potatoes, looking for pans and cooking pots, etc.; then I removed two cartloads of waste that were filling the room that I was to occupy. While we were working, the town became crowded with troops, generals, and fortunate were those who had had time to find accommodation. Although it had been intended for eight surgeons, I shared our room with *M.* Lombard and his entourage; we wrote, ate and slept there. Our surgeons divided the labour among themselves: sixteen divisions are spread around the town, going from house to house to tend to the wounded, for there is not a building where fifty of them could be placed together. We were supplied with 828 rations of bread from the IV Corps and of brandy; a few crumbs were given to the wounded, with a cup of broth for most of them; the surgeons each had a loaf of bread, and what bread! At home, one would not give such bread to even the most savage animals; but, when one is hungry, anything seems good. We performed sixty amputations in the evening. I had the corpses that had been crushed in the streets by the artillery trains removed; those in the houses and ambulances were similarly taken away; the Russian prisoners were charged with this task. We went to scour the battlefield, half a league from the town, for any seriously wounded Frenchmen, whom we could not bring back the day before and who had spent the night on the ground; there were hardly any of them under these circumstances; my nephew had discovered them and called attention to them during the day. Several wounded Russians, lying on the corpses of their comrades, were looking for the vestiges of warmth in them or using them as a mattress to avoid lying on the snow;

many of them were collected on sledges. I saw the officers who had been tasked with collecting the bodies of the generals, colonels and notable officers: those of my closest friends were heaped on top of each other and most of them were horribly disfigured.

Having visited some of the houses to witness the operations and to judge their necessity, I was struck by the singularity of many of the wounds. I saw a 3lb cannonball in the thickest part of the calf of a skirmisher, whose bones it had fractured. I saw a young conscript who, having been shot in one of the malleoli,[12] with a fracture at the head of the fibula, had the musket ball in his scrotum, which made me think that he had been wounded while fleeing as fast as he could. A thin, frail young man had more than sixty Cossack lance blows to his body and none of them had penetrated. A gunner had both legs blown off and had not lost any blood: it is known that, given the appalling attrition caused by cannonballs, blood rarely flows, and, in the cold, there is even less haemorrhaging. Our *chirurgiens-majors* like to take advantage of my refractor when amputating the thigh: nothing, in fact, is more convenient than this instrument. I will have a fairly good bed: I would to heaven that all our wounded were as fortunate as I am!

10th – I slept quite well, and I needed it, for I was extremely tired. Last night, at eight o'clock, my nephew and I were still roaming the streets to find sheds for our wounded and feather quilts to prevent them from dying from the cold. Having found forty, which we had taken to them on a sledge, we went to visit them and to have the large doors of these sheds put back on, after the soldiers had again seized them for their bivouacs. I ordered a surgeon on guard to stay not far from them during the night; they had had broth and some bread; but there was nobody and no utensils to give them a little water until the following day. Our servants poisoned themselves with potatoes cooked in a cauldron full of copper oxide: they undoubtedly saw the verdigris, but hunger, or rather gluttony, prevailed; they vomited and had salutary diarrhoea. I have obtained a good little covered carriage that will be very useful to me, for it is going to thaw; the wind is to the south-west and the weather is mild. Our service was beginning to take control of the situation: we had recalled the inhabitants to their homes; everywhere broth was being made for the wounded; straw was arriving; the surgeons had more time to operate and bandage, when suddenly His Majesty's foot-

---

12. The bony protrusions on the sides of the ankle.

guard swept into the town with permission to occupy it militarily. Since then the poor wounded fell back into their deep misery; the pot in which their broth was being made, and the broth itself, were taken away. They seized the fireplaces; they took the straw; they filled the houses; the lodgings of the surgeons were forcibly occupied in their absence. When they returned from dressing the wounded, they found no more room, and some of them no more belongings; the horses were driven from the stables so that those of the generals and officers of the Guard could be placed there. They quarrelled; they fought, and each one had to complain about his lodgings and his lot. As for me, having gone to see the wounded in the pastor's house, I found a room there that was still undiscovered and vacant. The pastor had reserved it for himself: he needed it to withdraw there with four women who appeared to be his sisters; but, at the sight of the Guard tearing down the doors, breaking everything and making a diabolical racket, these five unfortunates fled. Thus here I am, the master of the place, ready to defend myself here from the attacks and the plans to usurp it. I have arranged myself well there with my four companions; we have gathered cooking utensils, an axe to chop wood and food to sustain us there for several days. Twenty-five foot-guards are lodged near us, and the ground floor of the house is occupied by sixty wounded, among whom there is one whose gangrenous right leg emanates an unbearable cadaverous stench. I am going to have it cut off, which is the only means of saving the life of this unfortunate man, who is appealing determinedly for this sad recourse.

I have just had twelve Prussian prisoners with a sergeant at their head remove twenty-five Russian and French corpses, which were in the house or around it, and take away more than four cartloads of waste from all around, which were making it revolting. It was necessary, at daybreak, to send two surgeons to the castle of Plirchten, where there are 300 wounded who have not yet received help; I gave them linen, lint, bread, candles and thread. In the morning, I sent two others to the castle of Mernitz, where there are as many of them in the same situation; they left with the same aid supplies. There are wounded men everywhere. Three hundred Russians are gathered in the town's church, next to our lodgings. This morning, twenty corpses were removed from this foul place, where these wretches are pressed in like herrings in a barrel, and where those who are not injured are making a terrible fire, from which the thick smoke suffocates any Frenchman who tries to enter this den. So far, it has been impossible for our surgeons to bring the slightest help to these people, so packed in and piled up are they, and so the smoke from their fires obscures the poor church. They are burning pews, partition walls, organs, the altar, everything in fact, and even the tombstones in the cemeteries, which in this country are made of wood and resemble a large box, or rather an encasement of earth, as if one were to plant flowers or make a planting box there. To remove a corpse from this church, it is necessary to have a living person roll to the ground, who is arranged and stretched out over the dead person to keep them warm. One cannot imagine how tough and without care these soldiers are, not that they are stupid and brutish as is claimed; I know few who are more shrewd, more cunning, more brazen, more forward; but, entirely occupied with saving themselves, they do everything to succeed and think nothing of other people. We have just distributed bread to them; I am employing some of them for the manual tasks in the houses where we have wounded. I have had the order of the sentry who guards them relaxed; they go to the water, seek their food in the abandoned bivouacs, strip their dead to cover themselves with their spoils, chop wood and make do with the most basic food. I do not know if they help their compatriots who cannot leave.

Twenty-seven officers of the ... regiment of the line are currently being buried in the same pit. The peasants have been ordered to open twenty pits during the coming night, each of which must be able to contain no fewer than sixty bodies; at least as many again will be needed to clear the battlefield and the town. As for the dead horses, of which there are almost as many as there are men, I do not know how they will be disposed of: the dogs, the wolves and the crows, which do not touch human corpses, will destroy them in part.

11th – The thaw is still increasing; it is creating a horrible mud in the town and, unfortunately, the shoes and boots of the army are in very poor condition. The wind was extremely fierce last night: I believe that the country is prone to it, because of its proximity to the sea, and that the towns and villages are planted with dense trees such as limes to temper its effect.

I slept badly. Last night we were busy and extremely tired; all of our surgeons were exhausted. The I Corps passed through the town; I had many visits and no assistance; the surgeons of this corps were obliged to follow it.

We were given 200 soldiers to serve as *infirmiers*. I allocated them to the various houses where the wounded are and placed them under the orders of the surgeons; but, although one finds a few among them who are good, there will be many more who will not want to do anything and who will perhaps devour the little sustenance that we can procure for our wounded. I am sending some of them to the villages and castles where I know there are wounded; they protect them, prevent the foreign soldiers from looting what remains in the houses, and go to search for something to feed them and to eat themselves. This morning, one of our surgeons, whom I had sent to help sixty wounded men half a league from here, brought me back an excellent ox tied to his sledge, which I had slaughtered immediately by His Majesty's guards, to whom I gave a quarter of it. With this meat, we will make broth for the wounded in the houses close to ours for two days; I found two large cauldrons, tripods and good, obedient and intelligent conscripts. I, as is only right, had the tongue. I was given some coffee found in the ruins of a beautiful house where everything has been upturned and looted; I was delighted to find a grinder, with which I ground it, and the two cups that I have drunk already have done me much good. All our men have diarrhoea; the water is foul in this country, and they eat only meat, potatoes and a bit of bad rye bread, which is still very rare. Happy is he who has schnapps, to drink a drop from time to time!

12th – *Longin: Three pages have been left blank.*

13th – The wind was dreadful during the night and the cold was biting. We had hung a goose weighing more than 20lb out of our window; this morning, it was no longer there; the wind or our brigands had taken it away and I will not be able to make up for this loss for a long time. I slept poorly. After eating a country soup, I went to make my rounds in the town. His Majesty ordered that all the wounded be evacuated from there to Heilsberg during the day, 7 leagues from here, where *M.* Boudet, principal pharmacist of the III Corps, present in the town, informed me by letter that 1,500 of them could be placed in the castle alone; there are already 400 beds in this castle. The Emperor had sixteen large wagons and more than sixty sledges procured for us, on which 494 wounded were loaded somewhat hastily, several of whom were amputees and unfortunates who had suffered fractures. This evacuation was to be completed by noon. I took twenty Russians, prisoners and able-bodied, to carry the wounded onto the means of transport. It was a harrowing spectacle: there was no straw; hardly could any litter be found to put under these poor people who, according to a statement falsely attributed to His Majesty, had to be loaded to the number of ten on each open wagon. Heaping them up like that was not even possible and I would never have consented to going along with it. My heart bled when I saw these unfortunates being lifted on a ladder over the sides of the wagon, to set them down almost naked on the boards: it was almost like torture on the wheel. I did not spare our leaving wounded the feather quilts and pillows: if they travel quickly, they will not be cold; they were given broth and eight of our surgeons accompanied the convoy formed by the wagons and sledges. His Majesty, seeing some empty sledges pass by his window at about three o'clock, shouted, saying that the evacuations had not been sufficiently hurried and gave orders for them to be resumed. Despite the state of weariness and exhaustion in which our surgeons find themselves, they returned to the sad duty that they had suspended; but this has not resolved the fact that there still remain nearly 450 wounded in the town, who will no doubt have their turn tomorrow. When they have all left, what will be done with those from the villages 1, 2 or 3 leagues from Eylau?

Everything suggests that we will soon be on the move; the *carabiniers* passed through this morning, we are expecting Oudinot's *grenadiers* and we have been assured that Marshal Lefebvre is marching great distances every day with 30,000 men, as many French as Polish.

I received eight Russian surgeons, a Prussian *chirurgien-major* and two Orthodox priests, all of whom looked well and all speaking Latin and German. I led them to the church, where the wounded of their nation are gathered; they stepped backwards with fear and repugnance on entering this smoky, foul place, cluttered with bodies as many dead as alive. Seeing that they were hesitating, I threatened them and consigned them to guarding the post, which humiliated them greatly; but, as it is necessary to have friends even among the Russians, I softened my stance and provided them with 30lb of bread and a pint of unpleasant brandy, which, by proving to them the interest I took in them, gave them a little more courage. But they did not fulfil my expectations: no sooner had they used the linen and oakum that I had provided for them, than they withdrew to a room from which the wounded had just been evacuated and busied themselves there settling down and eating. I gave them 25lb of the fine ox that I had slaughtered yesterday and which our *sous-aide* Poté had brought me from the area around Eylau.

To distract myself and while I waited for the soup, I sewed pieces of thick white cloth to a pair of grey woollen socks, the heel of which was worn. I sent our young men out to join the plundering; they brought back sugar, coffee, white bread, and I procured a cask of good white wine that I chanced upon an hour or two ago; I needed no less than this precious find to revive me and give heart to all my dejected colleagues. The sun has been warm and bright today; no more wind; it is freezing tonight.

Tomorrow I will have a few hundred corpses that were scattered around the town buried. Nearly 200 Russians have left on foot, which gave those in the church more space. We fed twenty-five of these unfortunates in a nearby barn, which none of them can leave to find food for themselves. That church where the Russians are is a dreadful thing: ten corpses were again removed from it this evening. The streets are being partly cleaned, which is to say that the bodies that most obstruct them are being removed. A few more days, and it will be a horrible cesspool, a hotbed of pestilence; I have had His Majesty warned of this. Everywhere excrement, manure, beasts' innards, crushed corpses of horses, rotten and foul debris; every house exudes a gangrenous odour and all the streets smell like a hospital. Our surgeons devote themselves with a zeal beyond all praise; we cry out at not being able to help the poor wounded more effectively.

The ambulance of the Dupont division, where Vanderbach is, was burned last night: carriages, horses, belongings, boxes of instruments, of lint, everything perished. Ten soldiers lost their lives and sixty horses were scorched by the fire which, from a house on fire, spread to the barn where all the men and animals had retired. On the following day, one of our carts, which was carrying a cask of wine, two packs of lint and many other effects, was stolen in front of a guardhouse.

13th – The thaw has made great progress; the snow has already partly disappeared, the wind is light and the sky is very overcast. The stench of the town is increasing in a frightening way. I slept badly because of the wind, which was very violent.

This morning some Russians were harnessed after the sledges to remove the rest of the dead: these unfortunates are exhausted and look like corpses themselves; it would have been simpler to take advantage of the horses that wander around the town and two of which would have done more work than all the prisoners made weak by destitution. In the doorway of the church there are twenty-five Russian corpses; the surgeons of this nation have not yet been able to help the four or five hundred wounded piled up in this church.

His Majesty has ordered the prompt and complete evacuation of the wounded behind the army's lines: we are all out of bed; the sledges are arriving; the surgeons are putting the wounded who could not leave yesterday on them. The

Emperor has stood at his window to make sure that his orders are executed; he is extremely keen that we should leave no one here, but such a thing is impossible for they return as we send them away. Everyone sees the efforts we are making to fulfil His Majesty's intention; he himself is forced to applaud it, all while insisting on the need to finish this difficult evacuation before nightfall. The town is constantly full of troops passing through and returning; our sledges loaded with wounded are mixed haphazardly with the cavalry. The wounded cry out; some of them scream, but it is necessary to leave, and the surgeons who are accompanying them are obliged to use violence against the peasants to make the horses go. We dress, we amputate, we set broken limbs and immediately we load either the carriages or the sledges. How many will not die on the way? And what horrible anguish and torture will those who arrive alive not have been exposed to by rugged paths, through woods and fields where, since there is little snow, the sledges can hardly go? There is no food on the way. I do not know whether they all had some broth before their departure: the evacuation surgeon has nothing to give them, not even a drop of very bad brandy. Most of the sledges, perhaps even some of the carriages, will overturn: what a harrowing thought! The pain of these sad victims of war is reflected on the faces of our surgeons: they are pale, defeated, depressed and extremely tired. From the notes that they provided during the day, it transpires that around 600 wounded were evacuated yesterday and today and that there are still 500 of them left in the town; that 300 amputations were made; that there were around 500 comminuted fractures and 200 serious injuries, to the head, to the lower abdomen or to the chest, caused either by firearms or by the sabre and blade.

*M.* Poté brought me back two live oxen from the surrounding area, one of which will be given to the Russians tomorrow. I gathered eight officers of this army together in the same room, among whom is a major: the Grand Squire[13] strongly recommended them to me and I had already rendered them all sorts of services.

His Majesty, talking with Marshal Soult, praised the conduct of the surgeons with a sort of enthusiasm, whom he described as beings ...

---

13. A member of the Royal Household in charge of the royal stables. Although originally a position under the French monarchy, it was revived by Napoleon.

Longin: These final words finish the second notebook of the *Campaign Journal* of 1807: the third notebook is unfortunately lost. The narration restarts with the fourth notebook, only after the day of 21 February. There would therefore be a complete gap from the 17th until the 21st if the chief physician Dionis du Séjour, librarian of the Technical Committee of Health, had not been very keen to make known to the physician inspector-general Dujardin-Beaumetz that the National Library possessed an extract from the *Journal des Campagnes* relating to the Battle of Eylau. Indeed, one finds there, in the 'French Manuscripts' under the number 12315, an original manuscript of eighteen pages *in-quarto*, without an author named, listed as belonging to *M.* Monteil and acquired on 3 May 1837 by the State. It is entitled *Notice chirurgicale sur la bataille de Preuss-Eylau* ['Surgical Notice on the Battle of Preuss-Eylau']. The author presents this text as 'an extract from the journal that Baron Percy held strictly and that his friendship for us has seen him entrust to us'.

One cannot doubt that this anonymous author is Laurent, nephew and colleague of Baron Percy, who published, in 1827, the history of his life and his works. It begins, in fact, with these words: 'We have shown in the last issue of our Annals, in the *Military Jubilee* article, how much the surgery of the Prussian armies has been honoured in the person of *M.* Goercke, at the time when this respectable old man had just completed his fiftieth year of service ... .' If one would like to refer to pages 184–190 of the fourth volume of the *Annales des faits et des sciences militaires* ['Annals of Military Events and Sciences'], Paris, 1819, you will see there that the article on the *Military Jubilee* of Surgeon General Goercke bears Laurent's signature. The title page of the volume mentions Percy among the contributors who wrote the Annals, which succeeds in giving an absolute authenticity to the text that Laurent intended to publish in the fifth volume of this collection. It simultaneously concerns extracts from the second, third and fourth notebooks: we believe we must compensate, as far as possible, for the loss of the third by reproducing here what Laurent has preserved of it for us in manuscript 12315 of the National Library, which has remained unpublished.

---

'Content with the zeal and efforts of the surgeons, the Emperor bore witness in writing to his satisfaction to Baron Percy, tasking him with telling his colleagues that he had found everything in them, courage, bravery, zeal, devotion, and above all patience and acceptance; that he was thinking more seriously than ever of having a well-organized surgery in his armies, and that he was inclined to welcome all the plans and projects that could be presented to him on this subject. Never, perhaps, had circumstances been more favourable for appreciating the necessity of having many good surgeons. It is they who had done almost everything for this army. Nothing was too hard for them, nothing stopped them from better fulfilling their duties. They carried the wounded, took care of the straw, the food, and often made them broth. Finally, it can be said that it was among them that boundless humanity, that pity, stifled by selfishness and personal hardship, seemed to have retreated. And while they were endeavouring to console, to help the unfortunates for whom, since their injury, they had taken the place of relatives, friends and comrades, their horses, their baggage and even their hats were stolen.

'The evacuation continued until the 17th. Only sixty wounded were left in the town of Eylau and fifty in the castle of Molwitz, because the gravity of their wounds did not allow them to be transported. They were reassigned to the Russian and Prussian surgeons. The army withdrew to Thorn.

'When they arrived at Landsberg, they found the town full of wounded, whom it was necessary to evacuate. The Emperor placed his vehicles at the disposal of *M.* Percy, as well as all those that passed on the road. The wounded were immediately loaded into the carriages of the general officers and into the sutlers' carts, and, in spite of this aggressive measure, only 250 of them were able to leave. Around twice as many remained.

'The army was almost completely afflicted by diarrhoea, which could be attributed to cold feet, the use of meltwater and the excess of meat, especially from pigs. However, nothing could be proposed or done to men who lacked everything, who sought their subsistence and gorged themselves on potatoes when they could find them, and who sometimes went for twenty-four hours without drinking anything but water from the gullies or ponds. Some of the wounded died on the carts and wagons; some of them were thrown into the mud and water, and there was nothing with which to dry them and feed them.

'When they arrived at Liebstadt, the most seriously wounded were dressed, and *M.* Percy himself took responsibility for distributing a small glass of brandy and plenty of bread to them, which they devoured, although it was of the most detestable quality; in each convoy of fifteen vehicles there was a surgeon who was personally tasked with going to look for bread for the sick, since they had no servants with them, and the cart drivers being unable to leave their horses. The passage of all these unfortunate people who had not been able to be treated for several days left a lingering of cadaverous stench in its wake. Everyone looked at them and no one offered them assistance or solace. They seemed only to pity them. Some friends or comrades cooked potatoes that they distributed to them. A huge number of men with fever or diarrhoea passed by. They were lean and so feeble that one could not imagine how they were able to walk. They were gaunt, wrinkled, yellow, covered with spots and a sorry sight. Three hundred and fifty wounded remained in Landsberg for lack of vehicles to transport them. Three surgeons were left with them.'

---

*Continued from* 21st – ... I consoled him, gave him some brandy and bread, and recommended that his comrades have the wagon enter the shed. A captain was in this shed or in this stable; he had just arrived on a sledge that he is yet to leave since his operation; he is lying there on the bed and covered in feather blankets, having had his leg blown off by a cannonball; a surgeon, who had not been able to obtain instruments for the amputation, had removed the shreds and splinters with a simple scalpel. Soon afterwards, the amputation case arrived and his thigh was amputated. This brave officer is well; he is safe and has courage; he will recover. I have given him half a boiled chicken, a bit of white bread and a bottle of white wine; he will be in Osterode tomorrow, where I will bandage him.

Just outside this village, on the way to Osterode, we crossed a magnificent forest of pine trees that look like endless colonnades; the road is beautiful, wide and, it would appear, well maintained; but the snow, the ice and the passing of many horses and vehicles have made it almost impassable. Our horses have fallen twenty times; their feet fail them at every step; they slip and skid, which tires them as much as it torments and afflicts those who are witness to it. The forest is 3½ leagues long: what torture! One very often encounters horses dying of starvation or having broken a leg as they fell; they are still breathing and we pass over their legs with the vehicles, which crushes them, without completely killing these poor animals. Finally, one leaves the wood and can then see Osterode. The wind is unbearable; it whips the snow and covers the paths. Our coachman did not recognize the road, tipping us into a ditch filled with snow, and our fall was very soft, but very cold; we fell to the left, I on my nephew, and without falling out of the carriage, which we evacuated as best we could. It was righted without difficulty and without damage; the bags were placed back onto it and we continued our way towards Osterode. One of our surgeons was at the town gate to lead us to our lodgings, which the Grand Squire, he told us, was fighting over with us. It has, however, remained ours; it was well cleaned of the manure and waste of which it was full; five good bundles of hay were already gathered there; the stove was hot. All this relaxed and delighted me. We melted two large tablets of broth, which my host in Warsaw had given to me, in a large pot of boiling water: I found this soup good and tasty. We spread out the straw, my sheets on top, my blanket, etc., and I went to bed thanking heaven for having saved and protected me until this day and reflecting sadly on our situation.

22nd – Although I was lying on a bit of straw that hardly preserved me from the excremental humidity of a floor soiled by the waste and filth of a hundred Russian prisoners, I slept reasonably well. The wind has been blowing all night; it is thawing; this sudden contrast does a lot of harm.

I went to the three buildings marked as hospitals: what hospitals, great God! Some brown bread will be given to the wounded there, with a little hastily made broth. I demanded that there always be a pot of it, kept very hot, to distribute to the wounded, for there are convoys of them passing ceaselessly in front of the house where the cooking is underway; this cup of broth warms them, comforts them and makes them see that we have thought of them. Most of the surgeons assigned to the convoys were industrious and provided their wounded with fire, shelter and broth that they made themselves; the young *sous-aide* Lecat particularly distinguished himself through his generous and humane care. The road is so slippery that the vehicles can only arrive separated from each other. There is no bread in the town, neither for the wounded who are passing through, nor for anyone else; we have been promised some for this evening, but in the meantime we are crying out in hunger and everyone is suffering. Twenty ovens are to be set up by order of His Majesty, who must remain for some time in this miserable town of Osterode, already so many times pillaged and plundered again. I consider myself fortunate to have lodgings there. We have put our horses in a room that is uninhabitable because of the smoke; we are well enough, except that there is no hay, no straw, no bread and no meat – in a word, nothing.

I saw several wounded and had them dressed, including Lieutenant-Colonel Legrand, who has not left his wagon since the battle on the 8th: he has fractured the middle part of his right thigh, without displacement, caused by a shell fragment that struck the upper and lateral part of this thigh without causing any damage other than three small wounds; this wounded man is very well. I had the captain with the thigh amputation, whom I met yesterday on his sled, dressed; his stump is fine; it was the *chirurgien-major* Lampet who operated on him. A certain *aide-major* had wanted to disarticulate his foot and had sawn the bones through the shredded remnants of a leg that the cannonball had blown away with a bad saw: it was necessary, in order to save this brave officer who had already suffered so much, to amputate his thigh the same or the following day. This *aide-major* is a foul surgeon and ought to be dismissed for his immorality.

It is raining; an icy sleet is falling; the thaw is coming fast. We tried to purchase rice, sugar, coffee, etc.; they are sold by a grocer, whose shop is crowded with admirers, half of whom do not pay.

Through importunity, we have 2lb of sugar candy, which cost nearly 5 *francs* per pound; the rice cost 4 *francs* and the coffee more than 8. We still consider ourselves lucky that we have been able to afford to obtain a little of these commodities.

Our young men arrive one after another, all wet, shivering, telling me that the convoys to which I have attached them were passing or about to pass, or that they had lost them. They are not well received: I threaten them with dismissal and force them to retrace their steps, until they have found their vehicles. They are having it very hard, these good young people, and it costs me very dearly when I am reduced to pushing them around. I am keeping many surgeons with me, and have sent word to those who are scattered in the staging towns from here to Thorn, that if the headquarters move to any other place than this town they are to fall back to me early.

M. d'Albavie left after dinner with very detailed instructions from me regarding the services of Thorn and of Warsaw, where he is going.

The VII Corps has been disbanded: I have already taken back the surgeons to use them in the other corps; the principal, *M.* Blanquet, will go to lead the service of the hospitals of Thorn and its surroundings, in place of *M.* Tissot, whom I am sending back to his VI Corps.

23rd – Quite a good night; only two bouts of coughing, but my friend Beauquet coughs frighteningly and does not let anyone sleep.

The convoys of wounded arrive one after the other; the surgeons who accompany them always return depressed; I revitalize them a little, give them time to warm themselves. While waiting, we give a little hot broth to a few of the wounded passing by. I say *a few*; the vast majority have not had any of it in the past few days and it was only this morning that I was able to have a second cooking pot established. Bread is entirely lacking here; we live here as best we can and nobody is dying of hunger. After a short stay, the convoys set off again, followed by the surgeons, to whom this service seems very hard. On the 25th or 26th, everything will have passed through: His Majesty is keen for it to be done, and seems to be staying in Osterode only to wait for the end of the evacuation and the news that the bridges over the Vistula river are finished. Not as many wounded died as we were entitled to fear, and yet their misery is extreme. Diarrhoea had emptied the first passages and the forced fasting has averted the outbreaks of the first period. No tetanus, except in the case of the young and unfortunate Darmagnac, whose left arm was amputated, who had always seemed very likely to recover, a child of 18, full of gaiety, wit and vivacity, whose father will soon mourn his loss: *M.* Larrey has had a patch of vesicatory plaster applied around his stump, on the skin; but the disease is still getting worse and his head is already drawn painfully backwards; the laudanum has done nothing; he is sweating abundantly, as always happens in this macabre illness.

I am making *M.* d'Albavie leave for Thorn and Warsaw; he will be able to have my equipages sent, if the Intendant-general leaves this city, which I strongly doubt. His Majesty could well go there in a straight line, without passing through Thorn, which, whatever is done, will be littered with wounded and sick for a long time. If that is the case, I will not delay in going to Warsaw myself; I will only remain a short time in Thorn and my first act in this place will be to send back *M.* Tissot, the principal surgeon, to the VI Corps, given that he has been improperly left far from his true post; this man has not yet seen a fuse burn.

24th – I had an excellent soup of rice and mashed potatoes for supper yesterday, which our good Mayot had made for us. Quite a good night: six hours of good sleep. Some nausea when I rose, but besides that I am quite well. I shaved: I find myself very yellow and much older. Yesterday I made a statement of proposal for the rewards to be given to the surgeons of Eylau. His Majesty is very willing to compensate them for their troubles: I asked for decoration for eight, promotion for ten and a pecuniary bonus for all the rest; my statement was finished a little late yesterday.

At this moment, I am receiving orders to go on duty to Thorn with *M.* Lombard, the *ordonnateur*. Before leaving, it is a question of presenting my statement or having it presented; *M.* Lombard, who saw the Emperor this morning, also has one to give to him; I have convinced him to return to His Majesty and we are going there together. We were introduced at once by General Bertrand: the Emperor, who had in his apartment the Major-General, the Grand Duke of Berg and Marshal Bessières, welcomed us perfectly; he asked me many questions about our wounded, our convoys and our surgeons, about whom he spoke to me with interest. I thanked him for the approval with which he had been kind enough to honour us, and gave him my statement, which he glanced at while saying: 'That is fair', which is a very good sign for my success. He asked me if we were losing many wounded. I responded to him that in bad hospitals we were losing more; that still fewer of them will die, in spite of all the difficulties and miseries of the long-distance evacuation that we have been forced to undertake, than if we had left them at Eylau, Landsberg and everywhere where the Russians were bound to replace us. I told him that the open air, that the cold, that the snow even, were less dangerous than the poisoned air they would have breathed everywhere else, and that, misfortune for misfortune, suffering for suffering, it was infinitely better to have removed them, as we had done, than to have abandoned them to the enemy. 'Is tetanus ravaging your wounded?' he asked me again. I replied that we had only a single case of it, that of young Darmagnac, in whom a heightened sensitivity and excessive irritability had done more to cause it than the cold and the distress he had experienced. I added that the contrast of great cold and great heat most often gave rise to this terrible attack and that our wounded were not exposed to a contrast of this nature: 'Fasting, forced abstinence, frailty and the state of exhaustion are also contributing to averting this terrible scourge. However, I will never give such a secret for protecting oneself from tetanus; but it is good that the art makes the most of such an observation.' His Majesty, pleased with us as much as we were with him, bade us farewell and thanked us.

Returning to my lodgings, I packed my small bags and, after half an hour, I was in a carriage with *M.* Lombard. Our men will set off tomorrow.

I am finishing with this reflection, which is that there are many sick people in the army, and yet there are no diseases: it would be difficult to find a single adynamic fever there, a single case of peri-pneumonia; diarrhoea has partially prevented the development of these diseases; fasting has done the rest. For that matter, no one has yet entered a hospital: it is there that fevers of a serious nature arise, reproduce and spread. Must we admit that a sick person exposed to the bad weather of the harshest season is safer than if he were thrown with 500 others into a large building that we call a hospital?

More than 2,000 men are in no fit state to walk because of chilblains on their toes and heels. There are many of them whose feet are torn by the icicles. One sees fluxions of the jaw, ophthalmia, but they are rare. Hardly does one meet anyone coughing, except in two or three regiments, where everyone is coughing from the colonel to the drummer. But the appearance of our troops is dreadful: their uniforms are in tatters, they are covered with mud and they are distressingly thin. Many soldiers have their feet wrapped in old linen and walk like that; there are some who take the horses of the peasants, and one sees only such people on the roads, perched on a small *cogni* that they have bridled with bits of string and that they strike as the locals do to make it go. The Poles call a horse *cogni*: their whip to make it walk is usually a large cane with which they hit it repeatedly.

The convoys of wounded march slowly. There is no food anywhere, either for the wounded or for the carters. In Löbau, it has not yet been possible to establish a cooking pot. A young man acting as bookkeeper is having meat rations given to the inhabitants on whom we or some of the wounded are descending; soup is made for them; those who can support themselves carry a little broth to their comrades who have remained in the covered wagons or on the carts, and it will be necessary tomorrow, for lack of bread, to distribute potatoes to all of them. The covered wagons stink of pus and excrement; our surgeons can hardly tolerate this stench, and yet it is nonetheless necessary that they dress these unfortunate people.

We are lodged with three of the surgeons whom I sent on the 22nd to Löbau; our host is a Jew of good appearance, with eight children. He is a very honest man. Boyer, the *chirurgien-major*, is ill; his fever is continuous; I hope it will be nothing. I will sleep on a bedstead and on a feather mattress, even if I am at risk of being assailed by some of the animals that are very common in Judea.

Today there was a biting cold wind; this evening sleet is falling; tonight it will freeze.

25th – I was not mistaken: more than one parasite visited my poor body last night and fed itself at my expense. However, I had four or five hours of good sleep, and my cough did not torment me much. This particular town is sad. The road to Strasburg, where we are going, is dreadful: it is 6 or 7 miles long. We arrived at Neumarkt, a small town halfway along the route, at half past nine; we continued on our way so as not to be overtaken by the convoys, trains and a long column of equipages, which are behind us; ahead of us we had several trains, beside which it was difficult for us to pass in order to reach the front. At around two o'clock, believing ourselves to be still 3 leagues from Strasburg, we stopped in a deserted village to give our horses a handful of hay, and some water to eat and drink. A train being just about to overtake us, we immediately set off again and saw Strasburg ahead of us. After an hour, we arrived in this town, which is quite large and which, in another season and another time, must be quite beautiful. We are well housed; it is snowing; a horrible mud is beginning to form.

A kind of hospital has been established in the poor convent of the very poor Capuchin monks. Here we are back in the domain of Jesus; for quite a long time, we have been in that of Calvin and Luther. In this hospital, which hardly has any straw, only sixty wounded people are received at once, and these are the coldest, those who are suffering the most, who are warmed and soothed a little until the next day; most of the others are left with the townspeople, who are distributed some food to feed them; the next day, they are reloaded onto the carriages and caissons. There are no resources in Strasburg, because they have been exhausted there: we have been lodged with the best inhabitants who have given us plenty of tea and sugar and who tomorrow will give us coffee with milk, but it would be impossible for them to provide us with bread. We will each have a bed. It is the local custom to prepare the beds outside the room and to bring them in there all covered, as one brings an armchair: I have arranged mine well. From my room, I hear the rain, which is falling in torrents: the roads will deteriorate and our wounded will be all the more unhappy for it, even though the mild weather suits them well enough.

Staging post after staging post, we find surgeons who are very useful to us for our lodgings and positions; they are there to aid the wounded who are passing through, to renew the most urgent tools, to see that food, etc. is distributed. But they are lacking linen and lint: it is impossible to find any in the devastated towns, and we must wait for our caissons carrying what remains of these items to pass by; those of the VII Corps will be able to provide some, as it makes its way past.

26th – It rained all night: I spent it well enough, despite the importunity of the hosts who, without my permission, took over my vest and my shirt; they upset me, but I certainly gave it back to them, for I disturbed them terribly in their errands and meals, and scratched myself according to expert judgement. This morning it rained heavily. The road up to a league short of Gotleube is beautiful, especially in a wood 3 leagues long, where it has not entirely thawed; but the approach to the town is terrible, because of the mud, and it will be much worse still tomorrow.

Gotleube is a fairly pretty little town, which is overlooked by a castle that is still inhabited and beautiful. On entering the town, we saw the shops for bread rolls, cakes and brandy set up by the Jews, which is a good sign; everything is to be found there if one is willing to pay, and the inhabitants, who have suffered without having been pillaged as elsewhere, can feed the troops; our wounded find all kinds of aid among them. The three surgeons whom I sent here in advance are running from house to house to dress them, and the local people are fairly willing to assist them. It has not ceased raining; the wind is south-westerly and the air is heavy with moisture. We are lodged with a good baker who has accommodated and fed us well; our beds have been reasonably good; we have done marvellously, and 26 February is the happiest day that we have had for a month. The *commissaire* Quillet, from Strasburg, had given us five excellent white loaves of bread; we had the same with our *bœcker*,[14] baked like brioche. We requested and obtained, not without difficulty, four post horses for six o'clock tomorrow morning: this will allow mine to rest, and we will arrive in Thorn a few hours early.

The lark has certainly sung today; the sparrows, the greenfinches and the chaffinches are stirring and are already making the air resound with their amorous cries. *Here comes the sweet spring*:[15] Will it be necessary to spend it again in Poland, far from our homes, from our gardens, from our pleasant solitude?

27th – We were well lodged, well fed and provided with good beds: God bless our good hosts! I have slept for as long as I needed and I feel marvellous this morning. It has frozen very hard, but the mud is still not firm enough to support us; it is only more exhausting because of it. Our four little horses are very brave; they have led us well. The paths are detestable; we cross five or six streams, where the wheels of the carriages disappear. The lark sang, made what is called the Holy Spirit;[16] the sun shone with all its radiance, but it only appeared for a short time and it rained a little. What a pity to squander one's life in such a miserable profession! The road continues to be covered with wounded coming, some limping, others on small horses and the majority on carts.

We saw Thorn from a great distance. It is a fairly beautiful town, but it is cluttered with people, waste, etc., and all the houses there are full of wounded or of soldiers of all ranks, passing through, staying there or assigned to the

---

14. Longin: *bœcker*, baker.
15. Percy's original line, '*Voici venir le doux printemps*', is the opening line of a song by the French poet and novelist Jean-Pierre Claris de Florian, published in 1788.
16. To '*faire le Saint-Esprit*', or 'make the Holy Spirit', refers to the stationary hovering flight of some bird species.

town. There are already eight hospitals there. It is a frightening thing to see the state of dissolution to which the army has fallen; everyone seems to be running away; it is a question of who will retreat the fastest. I was four hours without being able to find lodgings; I argued at the office of General Jordy, who is the officer in charge of the town, and I was given two pleasant rooms in a good house. I saw to the most urgent aspects of my service, dined beautifully at the house of the *ordonnateur* Géant and went to sleep in a good bed, which I made the most of, to the great advantage of my health. My faithful companions are to arrive tomorrow with the small equipages and our horses; but there is no fodder here and they do not even sign the coupons, so that the horses fast like the men, for they too lack bread and supplies.

28th – I have not seen myself so well for a month; I slept. This morning I had a wash, and that rejuvenated me a little. I hurried about the town, first to see our good Laurenchet, *chirurgien-major*, who is in his ninth day of an adynamic fever, with which he arrived almost dying on the evening of the 24th. Yesterday we believed him to be irretrievably lost: the vesicants did not take hold and his bladder was painfully affected. Hardly conscious; a fatal despondency; the most frightening symptoms: his tongue is burned, his teeth are encrusted and his skin is burning. He recognized my voice and, clasping my hand, exclaimed: 'Here is the best medicine for me.' His face changed; his pulse seemed good to me. I had the vesicants reapplied to him, which unfortunately have again carried to the bladder. An emulsified herbal tea calmed the dysuria; vinous water, lemonade and barley juice will be what he will take above all; he will pull through.

I saw General Leval, who was wounded by a shot from which the musket ball passed under the Achilles tendon, which is being gradually worn away. Nothing will remain of it, but the calf does not contract, or rather does not retract; the leg has been put in a state of half-flexion, in the manner of a Pott's fracture.[17] The scar will form and little by little the ends of the tendon will bond to the neighbouring parts and will contract solid adhesions; the movements of the foot will suffer from this; the general will limp.

General Varé, who suffers from catarrh, with a large face, a large belly, small thighs and bad legs, has a minor gunshot wound in the outer part of his left foot, despite which he was able to walk and to ride on horseback the day

---

17. A Pott's fracture is a type of ankle fracture, named after the mid-eighteenth-century English orthopaedic physician Percivall Pott.

of the Battle of Eylau. After a few days, he developed phlegmonous erysipelas that spread across the whole of the same leg; two enormous gangrenous sores have formed, one on the lower outer part of this leg and the other on the middle part. His knee is shiny and purple; I fear that a sore is forming there again, which would be terrible. I insisted on the use of quinine in a decoction, and I have prescribed a resolutive flour poultice for the knee in the same decoction, which will be sprinkled with camphor and with powdered quinine; two emetic pastilles will be given tomorrow and one on the following days.

General Heudelet is doing well. The musket ball is under the skin in the lumbar region; it will be extracted tomorrow. Having hit the spine obliquely, it changed direction and, instead of passing through the lower abdomen, it traced a curve without affecting any of the viscera.

Lieutenant-Colonel Villeneuve of the artillery, who has a stray musket ball in his thigh, will be fine; the pus is abundant; when the cellular tissue is worn away, the laxity of the skin and the limpness of the flesh will make it possible to feel the projectile.

I saw many other wounded and several sick; I also visited half of the hospitals and met most of the surgeons.

I was dining peacefully when I was brought a very pressing order on behalf of His Majesty, who has remained in Osterode, to return there with as many surgeons as I can; I am even expected to relieve those in the staging posts between Thorn and the headquarters. This order dismayed me. I have gathered my colleagues and ordered thirty of them to leave tomorrow without fail, and to do it under their personal responsibility. The poor people are for the most part without boots, linen and money; many have been robbed of their possessions and their misery is extreme: they will leave no less miserable tomorrow. I would be so close to staying here, for what we are being made to do is too much; we are being run into the ground and no one is rewarded; everything is couched in empty promises and useless compliments. This sacrifice again, and we will leave. My horses, which arrived this evening, are beleaguered; perhaps they should be left to rest tomorrow. I am deeply saddened: I had hoped to enjoy a few days' rest, and now we have to go back to the mud, the filth, the vermin, the hunger and the suffering. There is nothing in Osterode; they fight over potatoes and they no longer know of bread there. We will take supplies with us and make do as best we can. My colleagues are going from door to door asking to buy knee-high boots and cannot find any.

The weather has been superb.

1 *Mars* – Good night, good rest. The weather is quite mild, although it has been freezing. Today is Sunday: our horses are unshod; it is impossible to find a farrier. After making tempting offers to several, it was necessary to resort to military force and the job was done at bayonet point.

This morning I extracted the musket ball from General Heudelet: having entered through the left side, it had stopped under the aponeurosis and the lumbar region on the right. I roamed the town again, saw some wounded and visited our *chirurgien-major* Laurenchet, whose illness has settled; his tongue is now clean and moist; his consciousness has returned; indeed everything suggests an imminent convalescence. The wounded are still arriving in their droves, and there is no space to receive them and no means of transport to make them go any further. A bridge is being built over the Vistula, on the other side of Thorn, and another on the other side of Marienwerder. We will see what will be decided in Osterode, if we still meet the headquarters there after all; it is said that Russian and Prussian envoys have arrived there, but what will they do there? I see no hope of making peace; the army is uneasy and, for my part, I have made up my mind to leave on 1 May.

There are more than forty complicated fractures and more than thirty amputees in Thorn, which, despite the fatigues and the incredible misery of a very long journey, are in fairly good condition. There are no instrument cases in Thorn: *M.* Tissot is rightly complaining about this. This principal surgeon makes a great deal of noise; he dictates laws, has regulatory measures printed, attaches the duties of the surgeons to the doors of the hospitals, hurries about, grows restless, goes twenty times a day to the *commissaires* and is terribly afraid to return to the VI Corps, where he has not yet seen a single fuse burn. The principal Beauquet, whose VII Corps has been dissolved, is to replace him and it will not be easy to move the stubborn Tissot aside.

We have an order to return to the main general headquarters. I am leaving *M.* Beauquet in charge of the service, and I am installing in my lodgings; *M.* Tissot is not happy about that.

We arrived early in Gotleube.

3rd – Our journey begins under good auspices. This morning the weather is superb. We are having a wheel on the carriage mended, which gives us time to have a good breakfast; our lodgings have been excellent. It is a spring day:

it is warm, the sun is shining, the birds are singing and the roads are drying out well.

We passed through the forest for 4 leagues and met several small columns of Russian prisoners there, who had earlier been taken prisoner.

I learned that the Russians, on their arrival at Eylau and Landsberg, had behaved well towards the wounded left in these two towns, and particularly in the latter; they are not barbaric, as we attempt to promote by attributing to them acts of cruelty of which no nation in modern Europe is now capable.

We made our 8 leagues very pleasantly because of the fine weather and the variety of the scenery before and after the forest. We have taken lodgings in a good house, no. 207; the commandant Pépin gave me a good dinner; all of this is making me feel better. There is talk here of peace, the first rudiments of which are to be thrashed out on the 12th of this month, according to the report of an old Russian general who was taken prisoner on the 27th while in bed. He passed through Strasburg yesterday and spoke of this news as if it were guaranteed; but personally, I regard it as very doubtful. Our army has taken unassailable positions; all its forces are united: either there will be peace or a terrible battle.

4th – I had a good night; we are all cheerful, fit and well. We are all on horseback; I went on foot to the Recollects' convent,[18] where the hospital is, crossing the brick ruins of the fortified castle built by William, or Willelm, known as the Fearless, captain of the Guards of Othon. Hoffmann, a young writer, died at the age of 30 and was buried in Strasburg with this simple epitaph in German: 'He had genius by the grace of God'; Hoffmann wrote, in his book on ancient wars, the almost romantic and tragic story of this hero.

Moinard, our *aide-major*, gave me splints, cloth, sugar, a small amount of cinnamon; thus, we are back on our feet and we are leaving.

It is a true spring day, but the road is long and sometimes bad. We only meet soldiers going back behind the lines. From time to time we see in the sun, on the grass, at the edge of the forest, Jews who have laid out bread rolls and schnapps: the soldiers who have money buy and pay for them; those who have no money sell some item either stolen or belonging to them, and, strangely enough, these markets come to pass quite amicably and to the satisfaction of the Jews, since they start again the following day.

---

18. A reform branch of the Franciscan Order, originally established in France.

Having travelled 5 leagues, we rested at the entrance to an unfortunate village that had been completely devastated; we found in the barns of the first house some bad remains of fodder and had lunch there sheltered from the cold wind. I gave half a loaf of bread to the old man of the house; he thanked me well and devoured this basic food; in his room, on the rotten straw, there were some wounded people waiting for a wagon to pass by to take them further along.

In Neumarkt, we even found General Walther with two strong detachments of mounted *grenadiers* of the Guard: this town is extremely miserable. Between Neumarkt and Löbau, we met more than fifty wagons of wounded soldiers, to each of which were harnessed two horses from the artillery train of the Guard; this convoy was going to Neumarkt and the horses were not to go any further. It was General Lariboisière who took this good step to evacuate the wounded who were filling the houses of Löbau, where he is billeted with the artillery of the Guard; but how will these unfortunates be treated in Neumarkt? I have quickly sent two surgeons there. Tomorrow, the same general will have all the wounded and sick who remain there leave his headquarters in the same way. It will soon be filled with them again, if twenty-five or thirty wagons are not made to leave every day.

We are lodged with the fat Jew with whom our surgeons are staying. Poor Boyer, *chirurgien-major*, whom I left sick there six days ago, was in a bad way: I found him very unwell, with a high fever, spitting with a lot of effort and complaining of pains in his left side. His tongue was wet, but of a red colour mixed with a yellowish tint at its tip and along the sides. *M.* Thérin, *chirurgien-major* of the artillery of the Guard, a charming young man, full of kindness, tenderness and politeness, has been caring for him assiduously: he could not apply a vesicatory to him, because the heat and irritation were too great; he had made a lohoch with a little scillitic oxymel and *kermès*[19] for him, and ensured that he used a bechic tisane. *M.* Thérin helped the surgeon Beauquet a great deal with the many dressings with which he has been overburdened. He is the only surgeon that the *commissaire des guerres* has agreed to leave in Löbau, where at least four of them are needed; but His Majesty's order, literally interpreted, was that all the surgeons placed by me in the four evacuation staging posts should be made to fall back on the main headquarters, and that has been done to the great damage of the service, for, since this wrong step or misinterpretation,

---

19. *Kermès* is a cough medicine made from Kermesite (antimony oxysulfide).

everything has gone from bad to worse across the board. We saw the corpses of some wounded who had died on the way strewn along the side of the road.

Our Jew received us well; Miss Rebecca, his daughter, smiled and simpered at us. We were given a very grubby supper, on an even grimier tablecloth, so I had to go to cut a length of cloth to make the horrible tablecloth disappear; otherwise it would have been impossible for me to eat anything. No matter how hard I tried to prevent the stove in the foul room where we were to sleep from being lit, it was heated until red-hot. I was given a detestable pallet near this blazing fire; having some p..., I was not afraid to win some; I have as much to give back as to acquire. A bitch, a mother to four puppies, risked disturbing my rest: Miss Rebecca was kind enough to shoo this bothersome family and I thanked her for this kindness by taking her chin and making her some compliments that flattered her. I doubt that it is possible to be any less clean than this girl, who is otherwise sweet. She is Jewish: that says it all.

We were sweltering, roasting. I slept until two o'clock; then I woke up with a start, with a dry tongue, burning skin and my body covered with flea and p... bites; not being able to find any water, I drank a little of our white wine, but immediately I began to cough horribly and did not stop until daybreak, which bothered my companions greatly.

5th – The weather is gloomy; it will snow. Having had a vesicatory applied to poor Boyer, who had a very bad night, I left at seven in the morning.

The road from Löbau to Osterode is poor and quite long. We found a barn in which we discovered a lot of beaten oats under thousands of bales of straw; we filled three sacks with them and gave plenty to the horses. I mounted Coco and made the cart into a transport wagon. I arrived on horseback at three o'clock and had the good fortune to find my lodgings, which Ackermann, one of our *sous-aides*, had kept for me, having argued over it with several generals and other pretenders. We have settled in there; the pot was immediately put on the fire and, to top it all off, our surgeons brought me hay and food supplies for several days. This good hay gave me the idea of making my bed from it in a neighbouring room, all lined with pieces of raw meat hanging against the wall, and filled with effects, saddles and bags of clothing. I arranged it well and thought that I had made the most beautiful thing in the world; but during the night, which was icy, the north wind hit me from all sides, so that I found myself very uncomfortable in my wonderful bed. Moreover, I had a bad supper: the broth was bad, the potatoes too peppery and the meat tough.

His Majesty asked this morning when he rose what the weather was like, and was told that it had frozen solid. 'It is strange,' he responded, 'the day before yesterday it was a summer day, yesterday a spring day, and today it is a winter's day. But what can be done about that?' He added, 'I do not command the stars, unfortunately.'

6th – My head and shoulders were cold and I was coughing. I cannot get warm.

*M.* Dufresne, secretary to His Serene Highness the Prince of Neufchâtel, our Major-General, was kind enough to announce to us that His Majesty had granted all that I had asked of him with regard to the medals, ranks and bonuses for our surgeons at Preuss-Eylau. Never had a message so flattered me. The Emperor has included a charming grace in this act of benevolence: Beauquet, Le Vert, Mornac, Laurenchet, Tainturier, Thomas, Béclard and Affré, *chirurgiens-majors*, have been decorated; five *aides-majors* have been named *chirurgiens-majors*, and four *sous-aides* have been named surgeons-lieutenant; forty surgeons of all ranks have 300, 200 or 100 *francs* each as a reward; this is a great triumph for military surgery. Ribes and Yvan, surgeons in the retinue of His Majesty's household, but supposed to be serving with us, also received the cross, which makes ten. 'His Majesty,' reads the preamble to the decree, 'wishing to reward the services rendered by the surgery of the Grande Armée, particularly during this campaign, etc.'

I sent twenty surgeons back to Thorn. *M.* Coste claimed fifteen for Warsaw and he had the Intendant-general play a role in this unusual claim, to which I replied. I sent details of the service to *M.* Daru, who, giving me a lot of detail on certain aspects of my competence, seemed to reproach me for my silence.

Our boys have gone out to forage and have brought back or taken food for our horses for six days; it is thought that at the end of that time we shall leave here; we have supplies for two good weeks. My appetite has diminished; I have a cough and a sore nose and throat. My bed has been made for me in the room with the stove, where it is pleasant. I have been drinking sugared water and milk all evening.

7th – Bad night: I only slept until two o'clock. My dry cough has made me very tired; my eyes are sticky; my whole head is congested with catarrh. I have procured for myself twenty-four pastilles of jalap powder; I have taken half of them, which have purged me perfectly; the other half will be for tomorrow.

In the morning, after the departure of the *chirurgien-major* Louetier, who is lodged with us and who has a heavy heart for having been omitted, I added the ribbon to the buttonholes of seven of our new *chevaliers* and embraced them. Beauquet will receive my letter notifying him of the news tomorrow with his little length of ribbon. I have formed six surgical divisions and have sent two of them immediately to be stationed 3 leagues from here, where there is still some food and fodder.

My little purgative did me good. The evening was tumultuous: I coughed a lot and had fits of impatience of which I was ashamed; the fear of falling seriously ill, so far from home and in such a miserable country, caused me this short-lived gloominess.

His Majesty's beneficence and justice towards surgery are causing a great stir in the army. The proposal of the *ordonnateur*-in-chief Lombard in favour of two *commissaires des guerres* and two hospital workers was dismissed, which must have given rise to a great deal of jealousy against us; but, without insulting anyone's misfortune, we are forging ahead and preparing to do even better, if possible.

The wounded from Guttstadt and from the VI Corps, which fought there, have come to us. The enemy is all around us; they are manoeuvring at full speed and have designs on the V Corps, which is in the area of Wittenberg or Ostrolenska; but our Emperor has certainly foreseen that and we are manoeuvring on our side accordingly.

We are quite well off here: there is no longer any shortage of food; we have fodder; the barns are being demolished to reclaim the wood; our hostess is washing our laundry; we are sleeping on good hay. Once I am feeling better, we will all be quite happy.

8th – I had terrible fits and yet slept for six hours in two parts. This morning I took another twelve jalap pastilles in well-sugared water, which is not bad at all. I had to work hard in the morning.

The weather is superb; the sun is shining as it does in June. Our cavalry reserve is at Soldau; the Guard is beginning to move.

I am not coughing much anymore; my eyes are better too; I was lost without my jalap. This proves to me more and more that my cough was again dependent this time on the bad state of the important respiratory canals, and especially of the stomach.

9th – It was very cold last night; it is snowing heavily this morning. Yesterday we thought we were in June; today we have returned to December. The troops are marching no less for it. I coughed a little, but I slept very well and this morning I find myself feeling more or less recovered. I had to work, write and send to the eight newly created regiments, which we plan to garrison behind the lines and to then be incorporated, sixteen surgeons-lieutenant and sixteen *sous-aides*, who will return with me when these corps are disbanded.

Ten Cossacks and a Russian officer arrived, all mounted on good horses and of good appearance; they brought back to us one of our generals who had been sent as an envoy to the Russian general. I believe that Marshal Ney, who was due to receive this general officer and to send back his Cossack escort, was quite glad of the occasion to manoeuvre his army corps to show these people the main headquarters and the numerous well-dressed troops spread along the route, so that they could say that our army is still in very good shape. The Cossacks are well-dressed, well-armed; their pikes are 10ft long, with a red two-pointed banner and a quadrilateral iron head; one of them has the horse and clothing bags of a dragoon from the 12th.

Warsaw is under threat; there is talk of evacuating all the wounded who are difficult to transport from there to Breslau; 1,500 would be left who, at the first signal, would leave. The Intendant-general is in Thorn, as is *M.* Mouron; the wagon with my personal effects should arrive there any day now; I am very worried about it, despite d'Albavie having taken charge of it. We must wait.

Our surgeons from the billets have brought us three hens and a goose, so we have dined well. Everything is going well now; our boys have brought back six enormous bundles of fodder.

The Emperor asked yesterday if I had returned. He was told that I had. 'That is good,' he added, 'I am counting on him.'

*M.* Samson wrote to me that all was well on my estate. I have received two letters from my wife, who is still feeling well.

10th – The night was not very cold; the snow stopped and there has been a fine frost.

General Varé died, covered with gangrenous sores.

11th and 12th – It froze slightly these past two days; the weather has been quite fine; it has been sunny; but the town is so dirty and there is so much mud there, as much outside as inside, that it is difficult to walk around. We gathered to discuss surgery: I gave two long lessons on the subject of instruments; tomorrow we will begin a course in bandaging. Our young men have not been taught and I do not think that they are very willing to teach themselves; they are busy for half of the day foraging 3 or 4 leagues away to feed their horses and concerned with finding ways to survive themselves.

Yesterday, I learned with sorrow of the death of our good Laurenchet. This *chirurgien-major*, whom His Majesty had decorated on the 5th, perished on the 6th, at four o'clock, a victim of the excessive amount of work that he undertook at Preuss-Eylau. His colleague Boyer will pull through. One had an adynamic fever, and the other was on the brink of death with a catarrhal fever with stitch pains, anxiety and extreme chest pains.

The orders for the payment of the bonuses granted by the Emperor have already arrived; most of the surgeons have received them today.

13th and 14th – Excellent night: beautiful frost; the most beautiful weather in the world. Food continues to be distributed; one can find some to buy, but at an exorbitant price. We have to go 4 leagues away to find some fodder.

The dragoons of the 9th were beaten and lost their élite company; those of the 16th lost a captain and a dragoon, killed and left pierced by lance blows on the small battlefield, as well as thirty prisoners. Eight squadrons of Cossacks played a dirty trick on them. Such skirmishes happen every day; the enemy is all around us.

15th – The night was cold and foggy; it snowed a little this morning. I have here the adjutant inspector Denié, who has an eruptive fever, which looks very much like smallpox. I had him vomit a lot and the eruption is quite a sight.

I saw His Highness the Prince Major-General and expressed to him all our gratitude for the enthusiasm with which he passed to us the generous decision of His Majesty regarding the decorations, promotions and bonuses that I had requested of him for my colleagues. The supplies are arriving in large quantities; the sutlers bring wine, brandy, etc. It seems that we will spend another fortnight here; we are covering the siege of Graudenz and Dantzig; this latter has yet to begin.

It is snowing heavily; everything is covered with snow and it is very cold.

16th – The night was very cold: I was well. There are 6 inches of snow everywhere and it is still falling; the sun is trying to emerge. I will go for a walk.

17th – It is extremely cold: the thermometer must show at least 6 or 7 degrees; it has frozen solid; the snow has stopped. I slept wonderfully. My patients are going well. *M.* Denié's smallpox is doing marvellously. I feel quite well.

Today 5,000 bottles of wine are being distributed to the Guard, to the general headquarters and to some army corps; the Guard will also have a ration of rum this morning. We are building new ovens. Abundance reigns here for the men, but more than ever there is a shortage of food for the horses.

18th – The frost mixed with a little snow continues, but the weather is fine. The sun is strong; it is pleasant to enjoy its brightness and its rays in places where one can take shelter from the north wind; I enjoyed this from two to four o'clock. The weather turned gloomy in the evening; there will be a change in the air and that is a pity, because everyone is fine with the cold weather, most of all me. His Majesty has been riding, and always at a gallop, according to his custom; he is dealing seriously with the military organization of his administrations; he sent for *M.* Thevenin, head of the transport administration, yesterday and today, and kept him for two long hours each day. I expect that it will be my turn one of these mornings, and I am going to prepare myself for it.

19th – The wind is south-westerly; it is thawing, it is raining, it is hot. We are slow, lazy; the roads have become dreadful again. I slept well. When I rose, I received a pleasant letter from my wife. His Majesty does not want the soldiers who are not seriously ill to go further than Strasburg, where he has ordered a large hospital to be established to hold them until they recover: I will send surgeons there. He has also ordered that a hospital of 600 beds be formed in Elbing and two staging posts established, with one in Dirschau and the other in Mewe, in case it becomes necessary to evacuate Elbing. His Majesty involves himself in everything, does or orders everything, and is worth as much as all the administrations on his own.

20th – Bad weather: it is snowing hard and the cold has returned. We slept well on our hay; overall, I am well and happy. Here comes the sweet spring! No doubt, there will be some political changes in our affairs. Austria is arming: is it against or for us? I believe that this power will line up on our side. Then peace will soon be made. Amen and a thousand amens!

21st, 22nd, 23rd, and 24th – These four days have offered nothing of note; we had a complete thaw on the first day, fine sunshine the second and a very heavy frost during the last two days. This frost is continuing; the thermometer must be at 7 or 8 degrees during the night because, during the day, the sun emerges and it is strong. We are all doing well and are writing a lot, for, when there is no fighting and there is no more blood to be shed, it is necessary to spill the ink. I have not yet been able to provide the Intendant-general with an exact inspection: all my papers have remained in Warsaw, from where I await them day after day. Moreover, every day I call for new subjects; the hospitals behind the lines are all going to be taken down; I will try to have those of Wurzburg remain for one more month. The orders of the 15th and 17th will make the indolent surgeons march and join the *chirurgiens-majors* who have remained with their colonel or simply with wounded officers, whether they be in Leipzig or in Warsaw, Thorn, etc. His Majesty has ordered that hospitals be established on both banks of the Vistula and within range of the army corps; I am having our surgeons advance.

There is talk of departure. It is said that the Emperor will establish himself in a beautiful castle that William II often visited; the general headquarters will be in the village of thirty houses that depends on this castle.

The 25th, 26th, 27th, 28th, 29th, 30th and 31st March, as well as 1 April, did not present anything in particular. His Majesty's wagons have been seen leaving, and yet we are staying. It has fluctuated between hot and cold; the frost has even been very strong from one day to the next. I sent six divisions of mounted surgeons to Elbing, Marienbourg, Marienwerder, Christbourg, Dirschau and Mewe, not counting the surgeons whom I directed to Saalfeld. *M.* Coste has requested his leave of absence and obtained it; but only, it would appear, on condition that he would stay until the arrival of his successor. Now, it was said that this successor would be *M.* Gilbert who, being already present, would not have delayed him: it is more likely that it will be Desgenettes, who is in Paris, which is going to cause our poor homesick man to die of impatience, since he is so anxious to see his home, his family and his garden. He thought for a moment that I had tried to keep him back and that I was the cause of the delay that he was enduring; he had even written me letters of complaint; but he is convinced today that I have not interfered in any way with his business. He will leave when he is able to.

At this very moment, the Emperor is climbing into his carriage. Our turn will soon come.

2 *Avril* – Superb weather; beautiful sun. I have an order to leave for Rosenberg, 14 leagues from Osterode. My companions will leave tomorrow. I will stay until the 7th to continue my care of *M.* Denié, who, following a terrible bout of smallpox, is in a sorry and very worrying state: an intense, nervous, burning fever is consuming him; his body is covered with phlegmons; purulent coughing fatigues him day and night; terrible spasms threaten him at every moment with suffocation. I cannot guess what will become of this consequent illness.

I have written a lot, laboriously made several inspections and answered 200 overdue letters.

3rd – It froze as in January; this morning there were 4 inches of snow; the day has been dark, foggy and sad. At nine o'clock, *M. Le Vert* left to set up our lodgings in Rosenberg; he took our wagon with the biggest of our bags. I was bored and had a headache without otherwise suffering.

4th – The night was cold; it froze and it is cold this morning. I slept wonderfully. Our patient, for whom I am staying a few more days in Osterode, is getting worse and worse. Yesterday he offered a lot of hope; an energetic, broad, fairly regular and slow pulse seemed to herald a happy conclusion; the vesicatory had done well; he had not slept at all, but his strength remained and his mind was very sharp. Yesterday, at nine o'clock in the evening, he took twenty drops of laudanum: he spent the night without sleeping and in an alarmingly listless, passive, silent and frail state. Today, his face is crumpled, his urine is suppressed; he will require a catheter, if the poultice of raw onions does nothing. He was given a catheter without difficulty; three or four other abscesses were opened; he has started to take quinquina wine[20] in the evening.

5th – A beautiful and good night; it has brought a beautiful frost.

Our patient is really quite unwell: I have opened a large collection of pus near the edge of his anus; several phlegmons that have arisen in the past few days have also been opened; he has begun to use a partially wine-like tincture of quinine; I have put him back on the barley juice, which he takes alternately with his broths. He is extremely weak.

I walked around the surroundings of Osterode. Not a field has been sown, not a single man preparing to plant a potato. Yet, they are hardly ever eaten anymore, because they are mostly sprouting and hence very much in a state to be planted. The ground consists of pure and fine sand; the manure has turned it brown in some places, but the sand has remained no less dry and arid; the potatoes are excellent and grow well in this sand. There are two large lakes around the town; fish must be common there. In general, the landscape is beautiful, but the orchards have been devastated and more than sixty good barns perished in the flames with the horses and livestock that were there.

6th – It froze last night. This morning it is windy and the weather is stormy.

---

20. Quinquina is a fortified wine that contains quinine, which was used to treat various diseases in Europe from as early as the seventeenth century. It is still used, though increasingly rarely, to treat malaria.

My patient did not sleep, but his pulse is good and his breathing is almost natural. New abscesses under his chin and on his forearms had to be opened; the one on his anus provided more than a glass of pus with a pad of wadding, or discharge, as thick and long as a finger. Besides that, he is calm, trusting and resigned; his emaciation and weakness are extreme.

I have been reading all day, first some unpublished letters from Frederick II to *Madame* de Lamarck, and then his memoirs, which served as a history of the state of Brandenburg. Time is dragging for me, because there is no post here.

7th – The westerly wind blew throughout the night. Yesterday, at eight o'clock in the evening, unable to resist the need to sleep, I lay down on my hay and I fell asleep so quickly and so deeply that my young companion, *M.* Mayot, having brought me tea, thinking that he would find me still reading, left it on my chair and did not wake me. It is raining, but it is the kind of rain that is perfect for vegetation; it is not cold and, in a few days, everything will grow. Alas! What will grow in these sad regions? Nothing has been sown there; the poor inhabitants will die of hunger. In 1710, with the armies of Russia, Sweden and Brandenburg having exhausted the food as they passed through and remained here, the scarcity of food added to epidemic diseases and a third of the population died. Frederick I, King of Prussia, lost 200,000 souls, having failed to provide any support to this unfortunate land, and while his States were becoming depopulated, he indulged in all the most lavish extravagances at his court.

We are at present in the theatre of the bloody wars that took place in the last century and in those that preceded it. Frederick William forged a great legacy here. On the first day of 1679, he set out from Berlin, and on 15 January he crossed the Vistula and on the 19th found himself with 9,000 men 3 miles from Tilse, where the Swedes had their headquarters; he made his army travel on sledges, across the Gulf of Frische-Haff,[21] and made his infantry travel 15 and 18 leagues a day. He defeated the Swedes, who had already burned the suburbs of Memel and were threatening Kœnigsberg. We are going to Braunsberg, Marienbourg, Elbing and to all these cities made famous by the treaties that were concluded there or the sieges that they endured. Soon, without doubt, we will enter Dantzig and Graudenz: it is to cover the very slow and very

---

21. Also known as the Vistula Lagoon, it is separated by the Vistula Spit from the Gulf of Gdańsk.

cold siege of these places that we remain here. The abbey of Oliva, famous in Prussia for a treaty, is close to Dantzig.[22]

*One page has remained blank.*

10th and 11th – Left this morning, at half-past eleven, in very cold weather; the road is rather bad at times. We crossed a forest 2 leagues long in which we were sheltered from the chill wind, which was icy cold; there are 7 leagues between Osterode and Deutsch-Eylau. We arrived at five o'clock. We found good accommodation; General Ruffin gave me dinner. We made the road to Rosenberg rather swiftly, despite the very bad going and rather poor weather. The country is picturesque: one encounters a lake with every half a league that passes, and there are always forests, in which there are many oak and beech trees. I am well lodged in Rosenberg and have a good little table there.

12th and 13th – I have a camp bed with feather bedclothes and many pillows, which simply keep me awake when in Osterode, on my hay, I slept so well. Yesterday I had a very small room. Today I have been given a very large one next door, where I feel infinitely better.

It has rained a lot; the weather is extremely mild and fine at present; the greenery, which has not yet appeared at all, is about to show and prove to us at last that spring, in these climes, is not impossible.

Rosenberg is a pretty little town on a hill, near a lake rich in fish; the inhabitants are good people; the surroundings are pleasant. In walking along what remains of the surrounding wall, one can enjoy several charming vantage points. The houses are clean and of good taste; in front of most of them a few lime trees shaped into spheres have been planted, creating a good effect. They like flowers a lot in this country: everyone has his windows lined with pots of geraniums, rosebushes, etc. Yesterday I saw a superb carnation, dame's rocket and double violets in flower.

14th – Superb weather. I will go for another walk; I find myself well here, may I stay a good month!

---

22. The 1660 Treaty of Oliva contributed to the end of the Second Northern War, between Sweden and their opponents in the Baltic region, including Russia, Poland-Lithuania and Denmark-Norway.

15th – The weather is warm: the earth is going to enter into love,[23] as the gardeners say. We are all astonished, in Poland, to see such beautiful weather: usually, on 15 April, the ground is still covered with snow; the lakes and rivers with ice. Admittedly, it has only been a few days since this has all melted, but still, one does not see such beautiful days in this season. There are many fruit trees around the beautiful little town of Rosenberg; the inhabitants are honest and good-natured people; there are charming women, very well and very elegantly dressed. Good fish is eaten there, which one can go to see being caught in the two nearby lakes. Under the square is a huge vaulted cistern, where good spring water arrives via canals from the surrounding area: it is a beautiful structure.

Here is what I am going to present to the Emperor one of these days:

'Sire,

'I have the honour of proposing to Your Majesty the project of an institution of which he had the first thought, which under his august eyes has already proven itself and which, in a short time, at little cost and without much effort, can occur, because the elements for it are all in the army and it is only a question of gathering and modifying them.

'There is no service as complex and as poorly organized as that of the hospitals. In the state in which it is and in the circumstances in which we find ourselves, nothing would be more time-consuming or more difficult than to set it on a better footing. Your Majesty would sooner have a specific service created for the active army and leave the other such as it is for what he has called the *territory of the army*; this will be the *subsequent service*.

'In this I present to Your Majesty his own ideas, his own expressions: he himself has divided the medical service in this way; it is he who, speaking of the surgeons, said: "They are no less necessary in the *territory* than the physicians and pharmacists, who must never go beyond it; but they belong

---

23. The French phrase '*entrer en amour*', meaning 'to enter into love', alludes to the beginning of spring, when animals are in heat and beginning to reproduce.

more particularly with the army, which goes onto the *field* to fight, and they must follow it there, as well as in its camps and bivouacs."

'It is therefore necessary to have an entirely military surgery on the front line. By calling it *battlefield surgery*, Your Majesty will fix its use and will avert any jealousy, any claims on the part of the other medical officers who, sharing neither its perils, nor its work, will not be able to complain of not being associated with its prerogatives.

'But this battlefield surgery must be so composed that it is self-sufficient in everything and everywhere, that it can take charge of everything that concerns the health matters of the active (or campaigning) army, that it has its own independent administration and that it is provided with soldier-*infirmiers* of sufficient quality and in sufficient number to escort its convoys and evacuations, to guard its wagon parks, to raise the wounded from the battlefields and to have the dead buried, to treat the sick in the ambulances; to carry out orders relating to the sanitation, cleanliness and hygiene of the camps, hospitals and headquarters.

'By establishing battlefield surgery in this way, Your Majesty will be sure to keep all the soldiers in the ranks and will remove any pretext for diverting any of them for the service of the wounded in the hospitals and the convoys; it will remove this confusion, this disorder that the competition between several administrations and the plurality and conflict of different authorities adds to a service that, in order to perform well, must have its own leaders, be subject to a single will and be formed of similar parts acting under the same guide and by a direct and immediate impetus.

'At the heart of the surgery of the Grande Armée, of this surgery ennobled by your generosity, distinguished by your honourable rewards, you will find, Sire, men who to the great talents of their profession marry the character and the qualities necessary to lead successfully and administer the new battlefield surgery with order and to spare Your Majesty these cares, these afflictions of a

## 1807 – The Campaign of Eylau

sensitive soul, which the bad state, or rather the inexistence of the hospital service, has so often caused to interfere with your most arduous war-related tasks.

'But, Sire, in professing to you the devotion and unbounded zeal of the surgeons slated to become part of the battlefield surgery, I dare to propose to Your Majesty that it is both just and indispensable to grant them military ranks, as he has already deigned to confer on several the distinction of the Legion of Honour.

PROPOSAL

'1. There will be a permanent corps of military surgery formed under the distinctive title of *battlefield surgery*.

'2. The battlefield surgery will have a general staff composed of a *chirurgien-major* general who is the commander in chief, of two inspecting *chirurgiens-majors-généraux*, of a paymaster and senior manager-bookkeeper.

'3. The battlefield surgery will be divided into several centuries each with its own number. There will be at the head of each century a *chirurgien-major* centurion or century leader. A managing-bookkeeper will be attached to each.

'The century of battlefield surgery will be divided into ten decuries. Each decury will be composed of a *chirurgien-major* decurion, or decury leader, two *aides-majors*, seven *sous-aides*, an adjutant-manager, a sergeant-purser, a police sergeant, a corporal in charge of spending, a police corporal and twenty-five servants (soldiers, hospital workers, *infirmiers*). The decury will be able to be divided into two maniples.

'Each decury of battlefield surgery will have with it two light wagons loaded with aid supplies of all kinds, two horses with packsaddles to carry the urgent aid supplies rapidly to the field of battle, and fifteen rustic carts to take the wounded back from the field of battle to the first military hospital and to transport them successively further.

'The surgeons of the regiments, legions and battalions will be affiliated by right to the battlefield surgery. The number of *aides-major* and *sous-aides* will be reduced by at least half by their admission to the battlefield surgery or their return to the medical service that is following the army.

'In order to be eligible for the battlefield surgery, it will be necessary to have served one campaign in the active army or to have been employed for one year in the territorial hospitals.'

17th – I left this morning for Finckenstein Palace, where the Emperor is staying. My project weighed on me, worried me; I had to rid my heart of it. Having written it up neatly yesterday, I got dressed, arranged my affairs and climbed into the carriage at half past nine. The road is 2½ leagues long and is at times detestable, at times very good; we are crossing a good area, well cultivated, well sown; we also cross some beautiful forests. We saw several ploughs harnessed to oxen and driven by farmers who feel totally safe; some of these ploughs have no wheels; it is difficult to steer them; the oxen that pull them are harnessed more than 8 or 10ft apart and the farmer draws his furrow very straight. Herds of cows, heifers and sheep were quietly scouring the land for the first patch of greenery.

The palace of Finckenstein is beautiful for the country: it only emerges once one has left a beautiful wood that is only fifteen minutes from it. The village is superb, but everywhere there is full of lodgers; generals, officers and soldiers, everyone is crammed in. The Royal Prince of Bavaria is staying in the school. The palace is also very full; the Major-General has fine lodgings there; Boyer, Yvan and other officers of the household have theirs there too. The former had just climbed into a carriage in order to visit General Savary, who is very ill, this side of Dantzig; *M.* Renoux, his *chirurgien-major* and friend, is as ill as he is.

It was a question of seeing the Prince Major-General. I saw him without difficulty and communicated my project to him, which he read from beginning to end: he would have liked me to create some tables and to fill them with the names of those to be involved before proposing anything to His Majesty; but I made him feel that it was necessary above all to know if the Emperor would adopt the fundamentals that I wished to present to him. He told me to go to see him, and that if I could not obtain an audience, I should come back to him. Having gone up to see His Majesty, General Bertrand, whom I did not know until I was obliged of it with a lot of grace, kindly told him that I was there and that it was the Major-General who had sent me there. The Emperor was not yet in his study. As I was warming myself with the general, a door was partially opened and I saw His Majesty, who said to me with an affable air: 'Ah! It is you. How have you been?' And there we were, chatting and walking side by side for twenty minutes. I had left my papers on my hat, far from the corner of the large room in which we were walking diagonally: I went to take them and presented them to the Emperor, having briefly explained their subject to him. He took one look at them and said: 'We will see to this', before putting them in his pocket. He continued to ask me questions and speak about one thing or another, but always concerning my service and my responsibilities, or relating to the great battles and their consequences for surgery. He reiterated to me the testimonies of satisfaction that he has so often given to us and told me that the surgeons of the Grande Armée were performing their duties well and serving excellently. He spoke to me of this good man *M.* Coste, of his homesickness, of the weakness of his soul, of his fear of death, etc. When I asked him if this colleague would be replaced, he replied that he would, 'Because after all,' he added, 'it is customary to have a physician-in-chief in an army.' I endeavoured to paint our young surgeons as well-born adolescents, sons or brothers of officers, who could also have gone to Fontainebleau, but who had a vocation for army surgery, and I made sure to emphasize to him the hope that they all have of obtaining a rank in the military hierarchy; I often returned to this wish, to this need, to the necessity of this act of policy and justice, and, if I do not win my case, it will not be for lack of having pleaded it well. His Majesty welcomed me and treated me with a kindness and familiarity that emboldened me and rendered me almost eloquent. As he was speaking to me of Preuss-Eylau, I confessed to him that *M.* Goercke, my colleague in the Prussian army, had written to me and had *M.* Loiseau, one of our *aides-majors*, who had been made prisoner and taken to Kœnigsberg, tell me that in the twenty-four hours that had followed the battle 13,000 wounded Russians had been brought to this place; we had at least 7,000 of them, both in the church of the town and in the surrounding area. 'Sire,' I said to him, 'that therefore already accounts for 20,000 wounded whom the enemy cannot refute, and Your Majesty's army has not had more than 6,000, three-quarters of whom will recover or have already recovered, while almost all the Russian wounded have perished.' 'How many wounded do you think we have had,' the Emperor asked me, 'since we returned to campaigning?' I hesitated, and he answered himself: 'Ten thousand, or hardly more.' I had to be of this opinion, and yet it would be possible to count three or four thousand more. Suddenly His Majesty escaped and left me alone in the room with General Bertrand, whom I thanked very much, who spoke to me at length of my nephew whom he knew in Egypt, and whose name I did not know until I returned to the lodgings of *M.* Yvan, to whom I had communicated my project and to whom I came to tell of the greeting that His Majesty had deigned to extend to him.

At four o'clock, I climbed back into the carriage, and as the coachman was about to set off, a messenger came to give me 8 *ducats*[24] for the *berlingot*,[25] which I immediately promised to deliver to him the next day. I can no longer feed so many horses; I only want three strong ones for my caisson and one saddle horse to ride; it is fortunate if they are not yet dying of starvation, because we are not being given hay, nor oats, nor straw. I was horribly cold on my way back: the weather is snowy and freezing.

I found the *ordonnateur*-in-chief Lombard very ill. For three days, he has stayed in bed: I had made him take 2 ounces of cream of tartar and the next day a pastille of antimony potassium tartrate, which had produced several stools. Today I find his tongue rough, his mood distracted, his ideas disparate; he is going to endure a pernicious fever.

18th – The weather is very cold: it has frozen; it is raining; it is snowing a little.

*M.* Lombard is not well; his pulse is faint; he is completely delirious and his eyelids are swollen; I had a vesicatory applied to him and a potion of quinine made.

19th – The weather was terrible last night; the wind is still blowing fiercely; it is north-westerly. It has snowed; everything is white in the town and in the country and we have a real need to keep warm. The troops who arrive are

---

24. A gold coin used for trade throughout Europe.
25. A '*berlingot*' was a two-seat variation on the four-seat Berline carriage, which had an exposed seat for the driver and covered seats for the passengers.

frozen. Here we are at 4 degrees of cold and the day before yesterday we had 4 degrees of heat.

*M.* Lombard's condition has deteriorated further; he no longer feels the need to drink; he fills his mouth and does not always think of swallowing; he is only faintly delirious; his face is very different; this evening he was sweating heavily; his pulse is irregular. We applied a second vesicatory; vinous and aqueous infusion of polygala and quinine, with a little ether. His son arrived this morning: the father did not recognize him. I announced that he is likely to die and wrote to the intendant; he has neither a black tongue, teeth nor lips; it really is an ataxic fever.

20th – Wintry weather; there is a heavy frost and snow 4 inches high. It is fortunate for this country that nothing had yet grown. I slept wonderfully and for a long time; on the whole I am well; may Providence preserve this health for me until the end, for it would be a very great misfortune for me and for the surgery of the army, if an illness were to take me away or force me to follow *M.* Coste. I would rather die of a shrapnel shot than leave as this respectable colleague is leaving. His condition inspires only humiliating pity.

Poor *M.* Lombard died at four o'clock in the morning, without agony and without having recovered a single moment of consciousness.

21st – Extremely cold weather; frost with snow and ice, as in January. A glacial wind from the north-east; this will set us back a few weeks again. I passed the night well.

It is good that I remember the names of the surgeons of the Prussian Army. Here they are:

General Stabs-Chirurgus und Ober-Medicinalrath.[26] Doctor Goercke (who is now in Kœnigsberg).

Ober-Stabs-Chirurgus.[27] Better.

Stabs-Chirurgi. 1. Bruckert; 2. Stein; 3. Rebentisch; 4. Krantz.

Ober-Chirurgi. 1. Horlacher; 2. Lohmeyer; 3. Winckler; 4. Tiesse; 5. Escheggen; 6. Bennoit; 7. Lœsch; 8. Schilling; 9. Muller.

There are seventeen senior army surgeons, who have a pension of 2,000 *thalers*. The *chirurgiens-majors* receive 500 Prussian crowns; in addition, they receive one *groschen* per month for each soldier and an invitation to the table of the colonel who is in charge of the regiment for as long as they are boys;

---

26. 'General Staff Surgeon and Chief Medical Officer'.
27. 'Chief Staff Surgeon'.

it seems that they are well respected and that in general they are worthy of respect.

The successful academy for army surgeons in Berlin is the source from which they will now be drawn; they are taught very good things. I do not know if they are prepared well for surgical practice. There are some very well-educated surgeons in Prussia.

22nd until the 30th – It remained cold until the 24th; but, from that day forward, the weather turned fine and we had the pleasure of seeing the first signs of spring. Nothing has yet come into flower; the plum and apple trees are barely budding; there are a few violets. In this country, they only grow hardy trees, almost-wild pear trees, common apple trees; no espaliers, no peach trees or apricot trees; few vegetables. It would be impossible to offer a *mai*[28] here, as we do in our country, other than a beautiful bunch of twigs. However, the customs of the inhabitants differ little from our own: same clothing, same way of cultivating, etc.

Dantzig is being bombarded fiercely. We will only be able to take it in a fortnight's time, and we will still lose a lot of men.

Beyderet and Steiner, *sous-aides*, returning from the VIII Corps, were murdered at the entrance to a wood; their colleague Desfriches only escaped by running away.

Our surgeons are falling ill in large numbers and some are dying. Hospital fever is wreaking devastation; up to 600 patients are lost every month in the army. It is said that the *chirurgien-major* Renoux, of the élite *grenadiers*, has succumbed.

I have never been in better health; may God grant that it lasts! I am content: His Majesty has just awarded another twenty-five honours to us; surgery is winning fame as a result, even if those imbeciles who oppose it should die of bitterness.

---

28. A '*mai*' signifies a tree or branch planted and decorated in ribbons in front of a person's house as a means of honouring or wooing them. It was customary to plant such trees during the night of 30 April – before the arrival of May, after which the tradition is named.

# 1807 (continued) – Dantzig

1 *Mai* – Superb weather; southern constitution; we seek shade and coolness. We have many patients: most of the surgeons are affected to some extent by nosocomial fever; several of them have died. In the past month, nearly 200 patients have been lost at the Crown Hospital in Warsaw. The months of March and April cost the army 4,000 sick; the packs of death certificates are enormous. I was not afraid to admit to His Majesty that the proportion of sick people was one in seven, and that for deaths it was one in sixteen. It is a pity to see the evacuation wagons arrive; one sees hardly anyone but young people there; the old soldiers are still resisting. My young manservant has just fallen ill: he was stupid enough to purge himself in secret with a powder that our pharmacist gave him.

2nd, 3rd and 4th – The 2nd was hot and dark; it was thought that there would be a storm; the wounded were suffering more; the men with scars said that they felt the pains that presage a change in the weather. On the 3rd, it was very cold. It was yesterday, Sunday; I went to Finckenstein to see Marshal Duroc, the Secretary of State Maret and some friends; I was very cold in the carriage, especially on the way there. The Persian ambassador is there with his entourage; everyone is lodged on top of each other. I did not see His Majesty there, but he is in the best of health. The Major-General received me well.

My Pètre[1] had an alarming haemorrhage the day before yesterday, which so deformed his face that one might have feared a gruesome end for him. He is doing better today, the 4th.

The weather is almost icy; a wind from the north-east is blowing; it has been necessary to re-light the stoves and put on our winter clothes again. These contrasts of great heat and glacial cold do a lot of harm.

---

1. Longin: Percy's domestic servant.

I sent the *chirurgien-major* Le-Clerc to Löbau with the *aide-major* Baltz with the intention of verifying the extent to which the rumour that is circulating in the country that there is a very deadly epidemic in this town is well founded. The administrative chamber of Marienwerder having informed the Intendant Gondot of the existence of this plague, and he having reported it to the Intendant-general, I had to send knowledgeable men to the place, so that I could receive a truly accurate report of what is happening. Thirty-six sick people of all ages and sexes were found at Löbau, some with merely a catarrhal fever, others with catarrhal-bilious peripneumonia. Since 1 January, this disease, which has not changed in nature, has caused the death of thirty-two people out of a very miserable population of 1,200; the Lutheran ministers and Jewish rabbis have declared that the disease is subsiding and the number of patients is decreasing. The German surgeons have overused bloodletting horribly. In general, the disease was misjudged and poorly treated: our *chirurgien-major* Boyer even had it in Löbau itself; emetic first, incisive and slightly diaphoretic drinks, lohochs with oxymel and red antimony oxide, and in particular large vesicatories on any pains in the side has almost always led to a positive outcome from the disease in the hands of the French. The bailiwick of Gotleube is struck by the same epidemic, for there is a real epidemic, but without any contagion. The physician from Marienwerder visited the scene and gave the inhabitants basic advice on cleanliness.

5th, 6th, 7th and 8th – All these days were beautiful. The sun has hastened the growth of the vegetation a little; however, there are still no leaves on the trees; they have hardly any buds and are without a single flower. Yet the countryside is quickly turning green and the meadows are beginning to carpet themselves with beautiful grass, which we await impatiently, as fodder is becoming increasingly scarce; we are still receiving a small amount of oats; as for the hay, it has almost run out.

I left today, the 8th, for Marienwerder, having packed up all my belongings and received the visit of *M.* Boyer; I had also sent to Marshal Duroc and to the Councillor of State Maret a copy of my letter to His Majesty and my project. We climbed into a sort of covered *vögele* at two o'clock, *M.* Le Vert and I: the road is superb; we are crossing beautiful forests, half oak and beech and half pine. We made 6 leagues, but it only took us three short hours to reach Marienwerder. This town is elegantly built and very lively. Today is Ascension Day; everyone is dressed well and out walking; Prussians and

French, everyone is mingling and getting along together in order to enjoy themselves. The women are milling around the town and appear pretty and immaculately dressed. Never, in such a small town, have I met so many of them; they are kind and well clothed. The town was once fortified: you can see the remains there of a huge fortified castle, situated on the side of the Vistula and built in brick; its extremely tall square tower is still there, and one can access it through a building supported by four arches or arcades running as far as the eye can see. This work is worthy of the Romans; it is more than five centuries old and looks as though it was built only a year ago. The convicts are held in this gallery-like structure. The hospital is established in a magnificent building said to be from the Regency, on the left as you enter the town; it contains 250 patients, who are all lying on bedsteads, on straw mattresses, with new sheets and blankets. This service is good. *M.* Desgenettes visited it before me and upon his arrival. I did not see this colleague, who has taken a very long route to go to Thorn, where *M.* Coste is awaiting his arrival so impatiently.

We had a pleasant evening, had a good supper and found a fairly good bed.

9th – I slept well and had a good night. The weather is cold. We left for Mewe, 6 short leagues away, because of the bridge over the Vistula, which it is necessary to go quite far to find and which forces us to take detours. This river is superb: the bridge is magnificent; it is very long and in two parts. I have never seen one so clean; it is swept constantly. The commander of the pontoon engineers is our captain from Rastadt. On leaving the second bridge, which is the longest, one takes a left; we saw, on the banks of the Vistula, barrels of biscuits in large quantities; there are enough in the nearby castles to feed the army for two months. I saw willows or poplars that were 24 or 30ft in circumference. On the Marienwerder side, we are making entrenchments and a bridgehead that will be extremely strong: if something were to happen, the army could pass over the Vistula without disruption.

We arrived in Mewe at a quarter to twelve. The town appears rather beautiful from afar: it is on a hill or slope that makes it visible from more than 3 leagues. Once one is close to it, it is a very ordinary small town: there is an old fortified castle belonging to the Templars; its fortifications are partly destroyed; the castle itself is standing and perfectly preserved; it is built of brick and has four floors. It is a warehouse for the trade in Polish wheat along the Vistula, which brings this rich and abundant harvest to Dantzig. Within the walls of this ancient stronghold, a munitions store with twelve ovens has been built.

The hospital is situated in the same enclosure; it was also a large magazine; the rooms are vast and very long, but low and dark; there are bedsteads and provisions. This service is one of the least bad among those of the line: I saw a nice little pharmacist's there; the bread is good and, overall, it can work fine in this way.

We left at two o'clock, for Stargard, a good 6 leagues away. The surface is still sandy but the road is quite good. Having travelled 3 leagues, we found the village of Pelplin, famous in the area for its beautiful Bernadine abbey. I dismounted there and found the courtyard filled with the Saxons' ambulance carriages: the army of this confederate state has its hospital in this abbey. I met its Ober-Chirurgus, who told me that he had only ninety-nine sick; it seemed to me that we could, if necessary, assemble more than 200 wounded in the cloister and dormitory, if the siege of Dantzig were to leave us overloaded. The church of this abbey is vast, although it is built in brick.

We arrived at seven o'clock, at Stargard, a small town consisting of a vast square with rather pretty houses all around, which one enters by seven or eight steps or stages made of granite or sandstone blocks; they have been raised because of the floods, I believe. The hospital has been established in a very beautiful barracks building parallel to another building that is just as beautiful, where the Badeners have theirs. These hospitals are composed of small wards, because the dividing walls have not been knocked down, which would perhaps be difficult because of the building's fragility, since it is made of wood and tiles. In these unhappy hospitals, especially in ours, there are no provisions, sheets or blankets; we have obtained a few bedsteads that were built with wooden boards sawn the same day from a tree cut down in the morning in the forest and assembled the same evening in the form of a bed. We had 500 fairly good straw mattresses, on which the sick lie on the ground or in their pallet beds; they are fully clothed or naked; the wounded live in these conditions and the cold torments them greatly. The bread they are given is very bad: they used to be given white bread rolls, which the *commissaire* David, it is said, had taken away. There are no utensils for drinking or urinating; it is terribly dirty; the service is bad. The bookkeeper is ill: before him, there were always *infirmiers* drawn from the Prussian and Polish classes; he drove them out and has not been able to find any others. A simple clerk remains in charge of this hospital. Doctor Delavallée is very ill; Doctor Meyer, from Baden, is also ill; two of our young surgeons are sick too, and all of them have a hospital-acquired fever, which is causing the service to stall even more. I saw forty patients with venereal diseases occupying the best places; I have ordered that they be sent back.

We are leaving for the surroundings of Praust, where we have a hospital in a nearby castle.

10th – I visited our sick and climbed into my carriage: the commanding officer had ordered that two horses be placed there to relieve ours, and it was a recruit of the Legion of the North who was to drive them. Thus, we set off, having given alms to some of the poor people who were surrounding the equipage. This was the way to travel without problems. Yet, as we were leaving the square, our postilion turned short; the coachman, still asleep, let him do it; a rather deep stream was there, and hence we were tipped upside down, through the broken bottles and a considerable amount of baggage. I was covered with vinegar, an excellent bottle of which I had received in Marienwerder: it is worse than a gherkin; my whole uniform is wet. I feared for my companion, who was on the left, as it is on this side that the carriage fell. Wine, vinegar, brandy, everything hit him. I climbed out of it as best I could and pulled my young friend from it; we looked at each other and began to laugh, instead of shouting and ranting, as one tends to do in such cases. I was bleeding from a finger that had been caught on a shard of bottle. It was nothing. The baggage was repositioned, the unbroken bottles were put back in place; we went to dry ourselves, and all was said and done. Indeed, we made our journey in safety and with happiness, thanks to the prayers of the poor people whom we assisted and the merit of our alms.

It is 8 leagues from Stargard to the castle of Rusoschin, at which we arrived quite swiftly. It is a charming dwelling: the house is elegant, laid out well, decorated with care and tastefully adorned. General Tiedmann, formerly in the service of Poland, an old man of 75, made the foolish mistake of abandoning it to retire to Dantzig: it has been turned upside down from the attic to the cellar; the library, which must have been quite beautiful, has been entirely squandered. We have space there for 300 wounded, who are on straw, in charming rooms; 125 wounded Russians, captured on a small island near Dantzig, with seventeen pieces of cannon, were brought there yesterday.

We arrived before this city at eleven o'clock. It is only a league and a half in a straight line: we travelled four because of the detours. We passed through the small town of Praust, where we saw the canal that turns the mills of the town and that our people have cut off, and we came to Langfuhr, a charming place, in which the rich inhabitants of Dantzig all have very pleasant country houses. I saw the siege hospitals[2] on the left, which support Langfuhr; those on the right support Ohra. Those on the left are established in very pretty country houses; the wounded are on straw, but they have enough of it; they are fed and treated as well as possible.

*M.* Canin, who is in charge of the hospital of the artillery and the engineer corps, had just amputated the leg of a sapper when I entered. He consulted me on the injury of another, which was produced by a musket shot, the musket ball from which, having hit the femur at its widest diameter and in the middle part of the thigh, shattered it and exited 5 inches from where it entered. He had just made a large incision that had allowed him to see the internal disorder; he was hesitating to perform the amputation. I dissuaded him from it and, having made him make the incision even larger, I invited him to remove all the fragments, which he did; there were some the size and length of a thumb. The exit of the musket ball was widened; the limb, which was in a state of half-flexion, was kept there; the man can recover, but with a shortening of the limb, which is still better than having a wooden leg.

In these cases, Desault's counter-extensive splints are fatal to the injured: the muscles swell, stiffen, fill with blood and can only be stretched painfully and violently. The wounded usually remove this bothersome apparatus, which then becomes more than useless. If they are forced to leave it in place, the cruelly extended leg and thigh soon give rise to a burning fever, often to convulsions and tetanus, and always to dreadful insomnia: this is where the best is the enemy of the good.[3]

I am returning again to the beauty of the surroundings of Dantzig. Everything there is enchanting; the plain of Oliva is delightful; from the top of the hillocks that overlook this charming area, one finds magnificent views. Our army is making its huts on the slope of these hills; the houses of Langfuhr, these beautiful lands, are abandoned and without furnishings; everything has been taken into Dantzig.

11th – It rained yesterday; it is raining today; the vegetation is growing well. There was not much fighting last night.

I went to the trench with *M.* Ramonet, *chirurgien-major* of the 19th Line Infantry. It is incredible how the surroundings have been ploughed up by the

---

2. A hospital established in anticipation of a siege.
3. This aphorism has been attributed to Voltaire.

cannonballs. One sees unfortunate women with their children looking for these dangerous projectiles, as well as biscayans, to earn a few coins that they are given for each; it is 5 *sous* per cannonball and 1 *sou* per biscayan. Our soldiers risk their lives much more still to earn these miserable 5 *sous*; they are constantly busy rummaging with a spade or a mattock around the places where a cannonball has fallen, and all those that are falling next to them do not prevent them from continuing. We saw eight or ten soldiers butchering a dead horse to eat its meat; it had surely been killed. We went to the second parallel line: it was eleven o'clock, and at that time the enemy fires little; they save their fire for the night and for the moments when they know that we relieve the men from the trench. I saw our batteries and was able to examine the enemy's forts, batteries and earthworks, though not comfortably, for fear that they would shoot at me. It would have been imprudent for me to go as far as the third parallel line, which is almost at the foot of the fort of ...; it is there that one sees large rollers ready to be launched at our men, if they were to mount an assault. On the side facing our earthworks, this fort presents a very steep embankment, strewn with innumerable cannonballs launched by us; it is all earth, without a single brick or stone.

Yesterday, at two o'clock, the assault was to take place; the *grenadiers* had already arrived, but there was a counter-order. The assault can only be attempted by day, because beyond the sap everything is bristling with caltrops and stakes that hardly protrude from the ground, with a sharp iron point, which, during the night would cripple any attacker. We would have lost many people if the assault had been attempted; the fort would have been taken, but we could not have kept hold of it. What a spectacle is that of a besieged place and a besieging army! The trenches are stained with blood; a sombre silence reigns there; everyone seems to be awaiting death. They position themselves against the ledges, without daring to show their heads, because the enemy, who is observing everything, immediately turns a wall gun towards them and kills them. This is what happened the day before yesterday to an officer of the sappers, whose skull bones were broken by the musket ball which entered between the frontal sinuses and exited through the occipital. The soldiers hold still, rarely standing; they lie down in niches carved into the earth that serves as the walls of the narrow passage; they try to take cover from the rain and from the enemy's cannonballs and musket balls, but the shells and the shrapnel manage to find them everywhere. There is not a day that passes without some of them dying or being wounded: a company thinks itself very lucky when, in the twenty-four hours that it spends in its turn in the trench, it loses only two or three men; thus, the regiments are growing alarmingly weaker; it is an unimaginable life. The fort that shows its embankment to our people and at the top of which we see so many rollers is called the Hagelsberg; the enemy has four or six constructions similar to a square pavilion; they are built of thick, well-bonded planks, have crenulations and can hold fifty men, who arrive there from below ground, for the construction has no door; these are called *blockhausen*. From the inside of these forts, they can pelt our men mounting an assault from the sides, to the right and left, which is extremely dangerous. The middle fort is called the Stolberg and the other is called the Bischofsberg. These have as yet been attacked only very lightly, for they are covered with beautiful green turf, while the Hagelsberg is entirely ruined. The enemy is hurling pots of fire at our skirmishers, throwing shells, rolling bombs and launching stones that do a lot of harm: these are what our men call 'partridges'. There are several very dangerous places in our parallels, because they can be threaded by musket balls and cannonballs: we passed through them quickly. Our sappers have set fire to the enemy's fences and they are working in the middle of a fire that is terrible at times; the poor people, while eating soup, are always on the lookout to avoid the bombs and other projectiles that are constantly thrown at them; they are relieved every twenty-four hours, as well as the officers of the artillery and the engineers, adjutants-general and generals. The trench surgeons, three in number, also relieved every twenty-four hours, stay in a rather bad house, which contains the major from Baden who permanently commands the trench. One had been built expressly for them; but just as it was finished, the engineers took it over to secure the sappers' tools and said they had neither the time nor the workers to build another, so that of the three trench surgeons only one remains with the major; the other two are in a house a cannon's range behind the line; it is to here that the wounded are carried.

After dinner, I mounted my horse to go to see Marshal Lefebvre half a league from Langfurh:[4] he had gone on reconnaissance to the area where some thousands of Russians sent to the rescue of Dantzig are to disembark; I could only greet General Drouet. On our way back, we saw the Baltic Sea, near Fort Wasser, covered with more or less considerable ships, each able to carry between 100 and 150 men, which made us estimate that the reinforcement must be around 10,000 men. The Emperor of Russia did not know at the time,

---

4. Percy transposes the 'r' and 'h' here. 'Langfuhr' is the correct Germanic spelling.

when he had these men embark at Memel, that communication was intercepted between Dantzig and Fort Wasser, which is three-quarters of an hour away from it. On the 9th, at two o'clock in the morning, the French seized the redoubts and the 700 men who were creating and protecting this communication, beyond the Vistula, which they passed on boats without anyone noticing; they killed a few hundred Russians and wounded 125, whom I saw at the castle of Tiedmann. Today, therefore, the garrison of Dantzig can no longer give a hand to the landing troops, and the coup has failed: what will become of these 10,000 men?

At five o'clock, part of the XIX Corps was made to march. We were curious to go as far as the bank of the Vistula to see the place where it had been crossed on the 9th and to observe the troops that were beginning to pass; but the enemy began to fire with all their might at a battalion and the 23rd Mounted *Chasseurs*, with whom we were waiting, and since the cannonballs were falling close to us, we had to take refuge first behind a pile of planks and then behind a house, before beating a retreat and returning to our lines. No one was hurt, because the cannonballs do not ricochet in this soft, marshy ground.

A battle is expected and everyone has been ordered to hold themselves ready. All our surgeons will sleep dressed and with their horses saddled. We will see tonight or early tomorrow.

12th – There is nothing new to report. The enemy is disembarking at Fort Wasser, on the banks of the Vistula, from where it is easy for them to push us back; we do not even try to worry them. This fort is now isolated; it contains 1,200 soldiers of poor quality and they can do us no harm. The commanding officer, *M.* de Croko,[5] a sad character, an intemperate man, was taken on the night of the 9th; he was drunk; our people disdained to kill him, but they beat him with blows from a lance shaft. This Prussian officer has long plagued the neighbouring area of Kustrin with partisans. Up to sixty sails were counted this morning; it is thought that more than 7,000 men have landed and a great battle is expected tomorrow, in the morning or at night. The troops are bivouacking on the plain of Oliva, along the woods that are dotted across it. I dined with General Savary at his lodgings in this abbey, which is more famous than it is beautiful; it is of the Cistercian Order; I returned from it on foot. On my way there, I visited the colonel of the 44th Infantry, who was wounded the day before yesterday: the musket ball entered through the scapular region

---

5. Longin: The officer that Percy calls Croko is the famous partisan baron of Kakow.

and fractured, according to the surgeon, the vertebral extremity of the fourth rib and was lost under the clavicle, without damaging either this bone or the joint. I saw the former system rise: the upper arm or, rather, the space between the joint and the neck, was very swollen and very badly bruised; I found œdema there, from which I infer that this is where the musket ball is, with a few bone fragments or shreds of clothing, etc. I advised *M.* Florence, *chirurgien-major*, to plunge a scalpel into it in two days' time to empty this collection of blood and foreign bodies. I would have done well to advise this operation for today itself.

We are firing fiercely and the sound of the cannon will not let me sleep.

I witnessed the amputation of a sapper's thigh by the *chirurgien-major* who, not having a retractor, did it badly, which is to say performed it like everyone else, in a sickening and awkward manner.

These poor sappers are suffering a great deal: one of them had his coronoid apophysis fractured by a shell fragment; another has had his thigh fractured; five were killed today. We are losing many people. The artillery complains about the engineers and the latter complain about the artillery, which nonetheless has, by all accounts, succeeded in silencing the enemy's fire on the 7th, 8th and 9th, and which suggested that we mount an assault, against the advice of the engineers, whose work is said to be slow. We will have news tomorrow. The night is beautiful, but a little cool.

13th – The loud noise of the artillery disturbed me during the night; our 24-pound guns made a dreadful noise and those of the enemy made no less of a roar in response. We feared an attack and the Marshal bivouacked. He told me this morning that he had been in cruel torment all night, not for the fate of his troops, which he had spread over the plain, in case of a sortie by the Russians and the Prussians who landed yesterday, but for that of the siege works, which the enemy, leaving Dantzig, could have destroyed for lack of enough people to guard them. Fortunately, Marshal Lannes and General Oudinot have arrived having undertaken forced marches with seven or eight thousand *grenadiers* and élite skirmishers: there is nothing to fear now with regard to the forts Wasser and Weichselmünde. We fired a lot today. The day was superb. We lost fifteen or twenty men: one of General Bertrand's aides-de-camp, whom I had seen arrive yesterday at the lodgings of the general of the engineers Kirgener, was killed at four o'clock by a musket ball that entered his skull through the lambdoid suture on the left side; he died after quarter of an hour.

I saw at the engineers' ambulance, which is managed by the *chirurgien-major* Canin, a sapper who was shot in his left knee, with the musket ball lost; five days have passed; his leg is swollen; the thigh is even more so and, on its inner part, on the side of the entry of the musket ball, one can see this purplish redness that always indicates imminent gangrene. This shot is the most awkward for us. How do you persuade a wounded man to allow his thigh to be cut open for such a seemingly minor wound? None of them will consent, seeing the knee in its integrity and the leg healthy; the surgeon himself hesitates. Yet, as I have often said, out of a hundred with wounds of this kind, ninety-five die without the aid of amputation, unless the musket ball has passed through both condyles, spongy parts that it can penetrate without splintering and without affecting the joint. When one cannot or does not believe that one can take the decision to amputate the wounded man, it is necessary to make a deep incision, cutting the ligaments in all directions, the capsule and the whole joint system: in this way one can improve one's chances of being fortunate, save the ankylosis, which is inevitable in such cases. Several times, I have seen the leg separated from the thigh as a result of gangrene, which had destroyed all its linking tissue.

The *chirurgien-majors* Fizelbrand and Dupont have seen, in recent days, a Russian who had been struck by a bayonet through the lower abdomen; a considerable length of omentum was coming out of both wounds, which they reduced. However, here is what was so unique about this wound: it is that in this unfortunate man's breeches was a mass as big as a fist of a tapeworm, which, laid out (it was separated into two pieces), was more than 10 ells long. This wounded man was evacuated to Dirschau, from where it will be difficult for news of him to reach me; he will no doubt have died there.

The *chirurgien-major* Dupont told us that he had seen a gunner who had just been killed by a large cannonball that had passed through his chest from left to right and in the path of which the left forearm was found embedded, in such a way that the fingers were partly protruding through the huge opening on the right side. How had this forearm been pulled into this terrible wound? We do not understand this at all.

The enemy threw broken bottles and old scrap metal at our men, and murdered a wounded man 4 feet from the trench as he was escaping. The Marshal complained about it to *M.* Kalkreuth. The famous French engineer Boussemard, an *émigré* who has remained in the service of Prussia, where he was a major, and who directed the superb works of Dantzig, was killed a few days ago by a musket shot to the head: this is a great loss for the Prussians. The garrison and the inhabitants of Dantzig are dismayed, according to the report of tonight's deserters, to see that the Russians and Prussians, who landed yesterday, cannot save them, the communication having been intercepted between the city and the sea.

14th – Nothing new. We did not fire much today. The deserters agree that there are a great number of sick and wounded in the city and that most of the forts are mined. That of Stackelberg is certainly so, since the other day one of our sappers took seven Prussian miners from a well itself, whom *M.* Kalkreuth wanted to have returned to him in exchange for whomever the Marshal would have liked. Our wounded are well treated by this honest governor: he is, it seems, very generous and very humane. When he learns that we have taken prisoners, he immediately sends money for them; he recently sent 200 *louis d'or* to the eleven Prussian officers who had been taken and kept alive in the night expedition that put the island in our power.

The weather is cold; our troops are suffering; however, there are few sick among them.

15th – I am fortunate to feel well: the air is so pure, the landscape so beautiful and the distractions so powerful that I am holding up wonderfully. This morning the enemy, 8,000 men strong, left the forts of Weichselmünde and Wasser and attacked our men facing these forts, in the forest that borders the sea; the bombardment and the gunfire were lively on both sides. We sent carriages, stretchers and surgeons to the banks of the Vistula in order to reduce by half the distance that the soldiers had to make to bring the wounded back to the ambulance; they were all dressed on the battlefield by the surgeons of the 2nd Battalion of the 2nd Light Infantry Regiment and the first battalions of the Legion of the North, but there were major operations to be performed at the ambulance stationed in a house on the left bank of the river, where there was a decury of battlefield surgeons. It seems that the enemy's intention was to retake the island that they had lost a few days ago, and to enter Dantzig; they were beaten completely; we took only twelve prisoners; the rest were killed. General Oudinot told me that more than 1,500 had been killed. This brave general had his horse (he had bought it yesterday for 30 *louis d'or*) killed under him when a cannonball struck it; he is limping a little, because the animal fell with all its weight on his left leg.

I visited all the hospitals and ambulances; I saw twelve complicated leg or thigh fractures, very well dressed. A soldier of the Garde de Paris was struck by a musket ball that entered next to his right nipple and was extracted under the inferior angle of the scapula on the same side. Dyspnoea, not being able to lie down, a need to remain seated, difficulty spitting, most painful anguish and much altered features: it is a fatal wound.

An aide-de-camp was bayoneted in the region of the liver. The *chirurgien-major* who dressed him says that the viscus was damaged; however, he has a good face, clear conjunctival mucosa, strong pulse, no hiccups, no sharp pains and no anxiety attacks.

Lost musket ball in a foot, below the malleolus: a serious case. I advised to make an incision in all directions, to heed neither the capsule nor the ligament and to treat not the foot that is lost, which is to say that it will remain at least ankylosed, but the life of the injured person; for why take so much care of the joint system? Why spare the tendons, ligaments, etc., since none of them will serve any further purpose? If one does not believe one should amputate, it is therefore necessary to cut from the bottom, slice in all directions, and to open a wide path for the investigating finger to retrieve the musket ball.

A musket shot that caused a fracture of the spinal column, paralysis of the abdominal limbs: certain and imminent death.

In all, we had around 200 wounded: they are all lying on good straw, in good houses, where a fire has been lit, because it is raining and the weather is cold. Most of these brave men are wet through, either from the rain or from having passed through the gullies and fallen into the *trous-de-loup*[6] that are strewn around the surroundings of the forts.

I have ordered that there should be six stretchers at each of the outposts; they will be numbered so that we know which ones have been left there. We have everything we need to provide first aid; but nowhere is there an *infirmier* and we are reduced to a single casual worker, who does what he can. Tomorrow, M. Kalkreuth is to be summoned, and if he refuses, the day after tomorrow we will mount an assault to take the Hagelsberg.

16th – There was not much noise last night. I left this morning for Ohra, a superb suburb of Dantzig, on the road to Warsaw: we made a large detour to

---

6. A style of fortification in which a stake is placed vertically in a sloped hole, so that a soldier falling in might be impaled. They were designed to control attackers' movements, forcing them to navigate around the pits.

get there, hoping to avoid the fire of the batteries; the one that overlooks this suburb is called the Bischofsberg; it often pounds it and disturbs it greatly. Three days ago, four large cannonballs pierced the walls of the house where M. Lacretelle, *chirurgien-major* of the 2nd Light Infantry Regiment, is living; by an incredible stroke of luck, they hit no one. The houses on the right are more covered, so it is on this side that the market is held and everyone chooses to walk. Moreover, the people of the country are, like us, used to the racket and danger and go about their daily lives no less despite the fiercest bombardment; I even find that they fear it less than we do, and I am always astonished when I see the women and children hurrying through the streets almost in the midst of the cannonballs.

I dined sumptuously at our surgeons' and walked in the ruined but still pleasant gardens that surround this beautiful suburb. The ambulance at Ohra is very good: the *chirurgien-major* Dupont showed me eight amputations that he had performed there, which are recovering perfectly well. I will send 100 wounded to this ambulance to be treated there indefinitely.

We came to sleep in the castle of Rusoschin, among the sick and wounded, which is not salubrious; but this establishment affords the charm of a beautiful garden, whose many cherry trees are all in flower, of a fishing pond that is always full of gudgeons and other excellent fish, and of hunting, which the day before yesterday produced a good hare and a splendid quail.

My young companion has left for Riesembourg, from where he will bring me my letters and papers.

17th – This morning the engineers tried to blow up one of the *blockhausen* at the Hagelsberg fort, but they mined it insufficiently and we laughed at the sputtering explosions. The work is very slow and we are losing many people: de Toloze, an officer of the engineers, was killed this morning. We received 180 wounded at our castle in three waves; they were bandaged and fed as best we could; we have only *kommißbrot* to give them; the broth made from an old cow is very mediocre and we lack the utensils to distribute it. I visited the wards and saw the most seriously wounded men: there are a few fractures of the arm, three of the leg, an amputation of the arm, a fracture of the coronoid apophysis of the jawbone, several men shot in the chest and in the lower abdomen. I saw a Polish man, a fairly large area of whose coronal suture had been driven in by a musket ball, so that the part held by its base resembled a valve or a lid: we will put the upper edge back in place; the detached edge has sunk more than three lines deep.[7] The wounded man is not in the least bothered; it seems that the musket ball did not enter beneath the skull.

The weather is superb; the vegetation is going strong. I caught about forty gudgeons, which we ate with a hundred others; we have here only what we can procure through industry or with money; a Jew comes to sell us eggs, butter, wine and white bread. The Polish soldiers, a coarse and starving race, have taken the market of Ohra and scattered the small village merchants who are such a great resource to us.

18th – It is raining: I can feel it in my lethargy and the painful heaviness of my arms. I slept excellently and took a delightful walk along the beautiful paths of flowering cherry trees that lead to my small office. It is said that our cavalry have taken three Russian battalions, who were unable to return to the fort at Weichselmünde, as prisoners. It is raining at the moment. The carriages for the evacuation are not coming; we are in danger of becoming overcrowded. Yesterday I directed 120 wounded to Dirschau, who will remain there; tomorrow a place will be found to put 200 of them, who will not be evacuated; I am sending for surgeons.

19th – Last night, from nine o'clock until eleven, there was a terrible exchange of gunfire; during the day, the enemy had fired incessantly, yet there were very few wounded. The Prussians had broken through some fences and had entered our covered walkway: we must have killed and wounded many of them. A dynamic fever is becoming commonplace in our hospitals. In this one we have the captains Salomon and Tugnot who have been struck down by it to an alarming degree; unfortunately we do not have a grain of quinine, nor a drop of wine, and these are the two remedies par excellence, for camphor and all the drugs that we dispense for this disease are, to say the least, useless. Nothing is more harmful than to purge too strongly at the onset of these fevers. In general, they should only be treated with acidic, vinous and slightly bitter drinks; resort to epispastics early; keep the patient as clean as possible; open doors and windows often; admit light and sunshine and wait for the stomach to bloat and for diarrhoea to occur: then the illness can be assessed.

I have just learned with sorrow of the death of my poor friend Beauquet, whom I had entrusted with the service in Thorn. He died of catarrhal peripneumonia. He was always coughing and spitting. For some time he had

---

7. A line ('*ligne*' in French) was a measure of length, equivalent to a twelfth of an inch.

had epidemic diarrhoea and I saw him coughing until he gave up his food. I was told that he had been coughing up rust-coloured, even blood-streaked sputum, and that he had all the symptoms of those mucous engorgements of the lungs that kill people subject to coughing and abundant sputation. He was treated in a way that is not generally considered correct; he was constantly given lemonade and other similar drinks; no ipecacuanha at the onset of the disease; no light purgatives to bring back the diarrhoea and to bring a point of irritation to the intestinal system, which has so many sympathetic connections to the lungs; no simple oxymel, nor oxymel of squill; no red antimony oxide; no vesicatories, and in this case it is necessary to flood the thorax with them. At any rate, my poor friend is no more; it was the 7th when he ended his career.

I have just learned that on the 12th of this month His Majesty did me the honour of appointing me one of the commanders of the Legion of Honour.

I have also learned from *M.* Husson and *M.* Dupuytren that on the 5th of this month the Institute appointed me to the place left vacant by the death of *M.* Lassus. *M.* Heurteloup, *M.* Larrey, *M.* Deschamps, *M.* Boyer, *M.* Dubois, *M.* Dufouart, *M.* Thouret, *M.* Corvisart and *M.* Leclerc were on the list, and they were torn between *M.* Corvisart and me: I got thirty-six votes and my competitor, nineteen.

This is therefore an overwhelming mixture of bad and good news. I was informed at the same time that poor Lepecq, *chirurgien-major*, has perished in Warsaw, as well as several *sous-aides*.

20th – Nothing is advancing before Dantzig; it will be necessary to attempt the assault; it is expected. *M.* Philippe warned me enigmatically that it would be this evening or tomorrow. I will leave early. It will be hard work; fortunately, six surgeons arrived this evening, whom I will send tomorrow to Langfuhr. It is very windy; the weather is otherwise clear and quite fine.

Yesterday, a corvette carrying twenty-four carronades, 18,000 measures of powder, wine, oats and a crew of 150 Englishmen had the temerity to enter the Vistula with a good wind and with the intention of destroying the bridge and going to Dantzig. Having travelled around half a league from the fort of Weichselmünde, it was necessary to manoeuvre to follow the curves of the river; our people came running, we pelted the cabin boys and sailors; they could not manage the manoeuvre and the vessel was cast into a small cove, where the captain lowered the sails. The musket fire from the city and the two forts was terrible for the whole time. The crew was taken, with not a man killed and only twelve wounded. Our men flung themselves onto the corvette, drank a lot of rum, took whatever they wanted and they were left to it. The enemy fired heated shots to blow the powder and burn the ship, but they were not able to succeed.

21st – Very windy and the air is very cold. We have been fighting fiercely. I arrived in Ohra at ten o'clock, and in Langfuhr at eleven. The troops from Wurzbourg were arriving there: superb troops, dressed entirely like those of Austria. I saw the wagon train file past, among which was the *Medicin-wagen*; all of our neighbours and allies have caissons for pharmacy and ambulance equipment.

At six o'clock, the 2nd Light Infantry and the 19th, 44th, 72nd and 12th of the line must go to the trench; everyone else is also to go there; the assault on the Hagelsberg fort has been decided. I have brought with me three surgeons who will run the service today and during the expedition. The divisions on duty in the Langfuhr ambulances will remain at their posts and will wait there for the wounded; thirty stretchers have been carried and distributed to the trenches; four surgeons will be in the first parallel; the other four will take their positions in the surgery shed; they have little linen, few aid supplies; a case and splints have been procured for them. At the moment, the gunfire is terrible.

At half past six, I left with the principal Capiomont. All our colleagues are in position; we found them, some in the shed and others in the trench; the gunfire is continuing, the cannonballs fall in great number and the musket balls and biscayans whistle and wail on all sides. We are sitting next to His Serene Highness the Prince of Baden against a fascine ledge, where there is no risk except for the bombs and shells that will come. The wounded are to be carried from the trench to a lone house that remains standing, quarter of an hour behind the line; there are two or four surgeons permanently on duty there. There should be six or eight carriages in front of this house to transport the wounded to the Langfuhr ambulances as they arrive and are dressed or operated on, but such is the state of our miserable service that we have not even obtained this support. The wounded will therefore be left to gather in the house and in some of the barns that are not entirely destroyed. After the battle, the regimental surgeons will go to identify their men; the Badeners will take the wounded from Baden to their ambulance; the Saxons, likewise; we will do the same, and in this way the line will not be weakened, for the six or eight *grenadiers* or soldiers who will carry a wounded man on a stretcher will not go further than the house and will soon be able to return to their post with the stretcher, which, like them, would be lost to the battle without this precaution and if they had to go as far as Langfuhr.

However, the gunfire grew quieter towards half past eight and suddenly ceased on both sides. General Drouet, according to what was said in the trench, entered the city on diplomatic grounds; General Kalkreuth admitted him for negotiations: it is hoped that the assault will not take place and that the governor, desperate to be rescued, is prepared to surrender. This is good news. I returned at ten o'clock, having made this long journey and duty on foot. Everything is quiet: I think the troops will return.

22nd – The most beautiful weather in the world, although it is windy. The garden adjacent to my lodgings is delightful. This property belongs to *M.* Fromm, an agent of the King of Denmark: we have been good stewards of it for him. I walk with delight in the garden and cannot satisfy my appetite for the beauties of this country. I have never seen anything fresher, more picturesque, more attractive: the Baltic Sea cuts the horizon on one side; the plain of Oliva surrounded by green hills, charming forests, small shadowy woods, magnificent country houses, copses, gardens and orchards, most of them terraced and divided into tiers of greenery; well-cultivated and sowed fields; a beautiful meadow; the road to Dantzig, planted regularly with very symmetrical trees; the impressive view of this beautiful city; the forts Wasser and Weichselmünde; the Vistula carrying its waters to the sea; all of this is pleasing to the eye, astonishing, leads to contemplation and makes one wish that the people who own this land will soon be able to return to it.

I have just written the following letter to His Highness the Minister Major-General:

'Your Highness,

'The notice which you were good enough to give me of my appointment to the rank of commander of the Legion of Honour only reached me this morning before Dantzig, where the service will keep me until the city surrenders, unless you order otherwise.

'I would try in vain, Your Highness, to express to you with what sensibility, what gratitude the new proof that I receive of the honourable trust of His Majesty and of the particular kindness of Your Highness fills me. I regret more than ever that age and nature have brought my work to an end by limiting the duration of my strength; but my zeal, my loyalty, my gratitude and my admiration are beyond their reach, and, as long as I breathe, I will feel with equal intensity the feelings that our august sovereign and his worthy minister know so well how to inspire.'

I went to see the siege works and travelled through them from one end to the other: the enemy has not been firing since yesterday evening; we are at the proposal stage. Marshal Lannes went in all haste to His Majesty to inform him that *M.* Kalkreuth wants to be treated as he treated the French in Mainz: it is hoped that this condition will be accepted; tomorrow, at ten o'clock, the Marshal will return. What a beautiful thing these works are! We walked down as far as the fences, sixteen of which were torn down during the previous night by a young skirmisher, who was paid sixteen six-pound crowns, just as he had been promised; there is therefore a large breach and we could easily mount an assault. We are surprised, when we see all this, that there are still so few injured. With what skill everyone manages to kill and not be killed! How the gabions, fascines and sandbags are arranged! The trenches are strewn with shell fragments, bombs, stone cannonballs, rocks, pots of fire, grenades; everything has been pounded; the fences are riddled with musket balls and biscayans. In the space between the third parallel and the enemy's fences, one walks on stones, musket balls, fragments, etc.; the ground is covered with them. I saw the sentries and was two steps away from them. The *blockhausen* are fortifications with huge palisades, on which rests a reinforced roof bearing a mass of earth 3 or 4ft thick; the soldiers fire through the opening left by the points of two palisades; this type of bunker is only 2ft above ground. Many Prussians and Russians mixed with curious townsmen and women were on the parapets and works of the enemy.

23rd – The weather is the best in the world. Everyone is running to see the works, while *M.* Kalkreuth and Marshal Lefebvre are discussing or disputing the terms of the surrender. It seems that an agreement will be reached: the Prussian general is highly respected and regarded and much will be done for him personally; already His Majesty, it is said, has agreed to let him take his colours. The good man wants more: he demands that his garrison not be disarmed, and perhaps he will obtain it.

24th – It is expected that we will learn this evening that the surrender has been signed. The French are going in advance to drink at the gates of the city, where wine merchants are selling them good wine at 32 *sous* a bottle; our officers are friendly with those of the garrison; they mingle and get drunk together.

This morning I saw *M.* Barthélemy, captain of the engineers, with General Kirgener. The former was wounded twelve days ago in the trench by a musket ball that entered through the posterior, upper and internal part of the left arm, pierced it at this point, and when it emerged, tore the skin that covers the breast on the same side. The direction of the wound made the *chirurgien-major* Dupont assume that the brachial artery might have been affected and that there was reason to fear that the loss of the bedsore might cause a sudden haemorrhage and kill the wounded man; nonetheless, his pulse was as strong as usual and no complication has developed. On the 21st, which is to say ten days after the injury, the patient felt a sharp pain in the wound and tension with beating in all of the surrounding area, and suddenly the blood came spurting and gushing out from it, so much so that a fainting fit occurred, during which the brave man was thought to be lost. This event, on the contrary, saved his life; the blood spontaneously ceased to flow and everything returned to normal. The surgeon applied a ball of wool under the armpit, which had been lined previously with lint, and made an appropriate compression bandage. Since then his pulse has become imperceptible, and still this morning it was impossible for me to find the slightest trace of it, for the tingling sensation that one feels at the tips of the fingers, when one pushes quite firmly on the skin, is only the result of the muffled and simultaneous beating of all the arterioles in these parts. Moreover, the arm and the hand are well-served and warm; there is no swelling or œdema; the colour of the skin is a little more pale than on the other arm, which always happens to parts that have suffered severe blood loss; the wounded man is not suffering at all, hunger bothers him and in all he is very well; but it is necessary to remain vigilant around him: a surgeon will always remain in the room or in the building.

This evening, General Kirgener, of the engineers, gave me the good news that the surrender has been signed.

25th and 26th – The most superb weather in the world. I am doing wonderfully well. It is very hot and the vegetation is growing quickly. Nothing is as beautiful, as pleasant and as fresh as the garden of my small lodgings, which in front and behind seems to blend its greenery with that of the forests between which it is situated.

We are entering Dantzig, but without permission and by pure complacency on the part of the Prussian officers; everyone is soon weary of this town, which, it is said, is ugly, gothic, not very open, badly paved and built in the manner of the ancient Iberians. It belonged for a long time to the Teutonic Order, which did not cede it until 1443. Everything there is unaffordable, except for the wine. One of the articles of the surrender states that the sick members of the garrison will remain in the city until they are no longer unwell and that they will be treated there by Prussian surgeons: this gives me great pleasure; it is one fewer terrible worry and difficulty for me. The city being still dirty and crowded, our wounded and sick from the suburbs of Ohra, Langfuhr, etc. will remain where they are, and they are well there, until a good hospital can be prepared for them in Dantzig.

The forts of Weichselmünde and Wasser are evacuating their men and their weapons and munitions. There are only a few ships left in the harbour. The Prussians and the Russians had a great brawl between themselves in these forts; the latter struck the blows and the others almost all deserted; there is a continual procession of deserters, all fine men and well dressed, from the aforementioned forts to the headquarters. We can be sure that before leaving they nailed shut the cannon so that they would not be fired upon.

I already have my lodgings in Dantzig.

There is a Polish *grenadier* in the ambulance of the Legion of the North who has been shot in the forehead; the musket ball has made what is called a 'concameration' or 'vaulting' because of the vitreous table of the skull, which has become separated from the diploë and been pushed inside the skull; the wounded man is not complaining at all; he is drinking and eating well. What is to be done in this case? A reasonable man would allow a crown trephine to be applied; our *grenadier* may die of convulsions on the first day, as happens all too often on the fortieth.

27th – The weather is extremely warm. All our men have taken up arms: a battalion and a squadron from each of the regiments of the X Corps have been made to enter Dantzig. At dawn, we took possession of the forts Weichselmünde and Wasser, where there are only sick and wounded, still very few in number. The Russians have left by boat and the Prussians have all deserted: this is a great fortune for us.

At nine o'clock, we entered the town. What a spectacle of desolation! The houses that form the first streets have been ruined by the cannonballs and are uninhabitable; the walls of several, already remarkable because of the cannonballs of all calibres that became embedded there after the siege of 1733, have been riddled with those of the siege of 1807 and some have even inserted themselves and remain there, set like the jewels of a ring; one sees this most at the arsenal. In these districts, there is not a single pane of glass left; everything is shattered. Everywhere they have a disgusting appearance; they are foul areas, badly built, terribly paved; today they are dreadful. Thirty or forty townspeople have been killed in their houses or in the streets. Beyond the arsenal begins the beautiful half of Dantzig: it contains some attractive houses, for the area outside it is neither elegant nor in good taste; they belong to rich merchants, who have covered them with mahogany, chandeliers and all the furniture that England provides. There is no other type in this country: fabrics, engravings, mantelpiece ornaments, etc., everything is English; the inhabitants' customs are also English. We went to see the canal, which is stinking, loaded with rafts and littered with beautiful merchant ships. At half past twelve, the weather being very hot and the sun having been suddenly hidden by thick clouds, we saw the air obscured by very large flying creatures, which we at first took to be locusts and which we then recognized to be damselflies. I have kept one of them; they all look alike: they are the damselflies from the lakes, marshes and pools, and the most common; only they have a hairy body and especially the midsection. Swarms of them have passed by, all travelling in the same direction, coming from the sea and going from north-east to south-west. This unusual migration lasted a quarter of an hour: we concluded from it that there would be some change in the atmosphere and perhaps a big storm. The local people told us that in England, in the month of August, this astonishing passage of insects has sometimes been seen. At about two o'clock, we could hear the thunder, the heat intensified and the rain started: a real thundershower.

I visited some houses where Prussian-style lazarettos have been established: the sick and wounded, numbering 1,800, others say 3,000, are lying on boards and trestles, with a thin straw mattress under them; they are in a bad way. There are still quite a large number of Prussian medical officers to treat them. Tomorrow we will see to our own service.

Everyone is hurrying to Dantzig; the *ordonnateurs*, *commissaires*, workers, and tradespeople are arriving there from all directions; we call out with taunts and jibes when we see them coming. Our people drank and ate well today; some got drunk and decided to cause a commotion, but nothing came of it. I rebuked two officers of the 2nd Light Infantry, who, having already drunk too much, were demanding more wine and threatening their host with sabres. General Rapp is the governor of the town and General Ménard is the commanding officer. Everything is very expensive there.

28th – It rained last night and it is still raining: there is no time to lose. From the morning, the squares and streets are full of merchants selling butter, eggs and other foodstuffs, which is a good omen. I am lodged in one of the best houses in Dantzig, no. 433, with *M.* Weichbrot, a sugar refiner; he is an honest young man, whose wife, sisters and female friends are good and charming people. I had a visit from *M.* Lichtenberger, *chirurgien-major* of a Prussian regiment, in charge of the service for the hospitals of this nation: he is an old man of very good appearance, well-kempt, and who introduced himself nobly; he has several battalion and company surgeons to assist him; with him was an infantry captain in charge of the administrative service. I hurried to obtain premises; I think we will take the house at no. 395. The conference hall is superb and can hold 300 patients. The Stock Exchange offers some resources from which we can profit. I have seen the arsenal and found little there, except for some enormous copper boilers that can be put to good use; I have set aside a helmet, an armlet, a shield and some other items, which will be brought to me tomorrow.[8] The building is vast and beautiful, given the time and the country: one could make a magnificent hospital there; in the cellars, there are half a million wines belonging to a gentleman who is in Berlin. The main church is immense and very imposing, but has nothing more to offer. They drink porter and Oporto wine here: these are two very strong liqueurs and I can hardly stand them; the English find the Portuguese wine still too weak and mix it with arrack. Dinner tables in this country glisten with silverware, beautiful linen and *pâtisserie* as a starter, but they make bad food.

29th – Cool, rainy, stormy weather. I did not go out. All the shops, the doors of all the large cellars, etc., have been sealed; nobody can buy anything; to get an ell of cloth, you have to win over a merchant and hide it well. How this poor town will be squeezed! We are not yet seeing to the hospitals there. I had the building known as the Stock Exchange arranged for 200 patients; already forty or fifty scabies sufferers had been placed there and were lying on good beds; I had them moved; it is for our amputees and those with fractures from

---

8. Percy had a real interest in armour, and collected items of interest while on campaign. The collection was valued, after his death, at 60,000 *francs*.

the siege, whom we are still keeping in Langfuhr. It would certainly be a good thing to have a hospital of 500 patients with venereal diseases here, but this establishment would be detrimental to the views of certain people who have a commission to exploit the city. Marshal Lefebvre has promised a reward to the surgeons; we will see if he keeps his word. Each soldier will receive 10 *francs*. The sub-inspector Lacroix did not agree that they should be given to the men absent because of injury, saying that the funds should be distributed according to the number of troops remaining on the day after the end of the siege: the marshal became furiously angry, called him all the most insulting names and wanted that, notwithstanding the special instruction of the Intendant-general, our poor wounded men should receive their 10 *francs*, which, indeed, is of the greatest justice. Each soldier will also receive a bottle of wine.

30th – It is very cold and we are forced to cover up as if it were winter; the wind is from the north-west. Our hospital at the Stock Exchange is coming along well; there we have a patient with a strangulated hernia, which has withstood two bloodlettings until the man faints, and bathing; it will have to be operated on tomorrow if during the night, by the means of taxis, it does not re-enter. The X Corps has been disbanded; the marshal is leaving for Paris.

Since Grand-Marshal Duroc replied to me that my project of battlefield surgery had the potential to be good, but that he regretted that it was only partial and did not encompass the whole service, I wrote the following letter to him:

> 'Dear Grand-Marshal,
>
> 'The disadvantages that my project of battlefield surgery seems to present would disappear in your eyes if I could give you all the developments of this institution, of which I only had the honour of giving the simple text and the general rudiments to His Majesty and Your Excellency. I am increasingly anxious that battlefield surgery, or élite surgery, should cease to be a project and that it should be established on a footing worthy of it and of the services that it is to render. His Majesty has just honoured a large number of surgeons with rewards and distinctions; but surgery remains in no less of a precarious state, in which, having endured great fatigues and frequent dangers, worthy and valuable men will find in peacetime, instead of a viable existence, a dismissal that is

disheartening to them and fatal to the interests of the armies, from which disdain and disappointment will ultimately drive them away forever. My colleagues fear this fate so much that several of them, even those with ranks, have taken service as officers, and have been received by His Majesty, who has shown surprise and displeasure at it. Sixty-four are asking at this moment to retire because in their absence, although they have served in five or six campaigns, they have been drawn for conscription, which has happened to more than two-thirds of them. Eighteen or twenty were condemned in absentia, as refusing conscription or deserters, and the parents paid a fine of 1,500 *francs* for these young men, at the very time that they were sacrificing themselves in the armies and that some lost their lives there, either in the hospitals or on the battlefield. We have some who, having become unfit to continue serving as a result of their injuries or the contagious diseases that they had contracted, were handed over by the minister director under the authority of conscription in order to be incorporated into a regiment or converted into soldiers.

'You are well aware, Grand-Marshal, that things cannot continue in this way. As long as His Majesty personally commands the armies, there will be no lack of surgeons, because this class cherishes, reveres and admires him with enthusiasm; as long as I am in charge of the service, confidence, custom and curiosity will attract them around me: but what will they do there? What will I do myself if we are left there as we are? For my part, I am extremely reluctant to remain there under the administrative regime and it would be impossible for me to return to campaign if I had to be there in the state of shortage, suffering, and shameful and cruel destitution in which we found ourselves. The surgeons do everything: His Majesty knows it well; he is well informed that we have neither administrators nor *infirmiers* to help us. During the siege of Dantzig, where we had 1,600 wounded and 2,000 sick, we did not have a single sack of straw, not a single straw bed, no bowls, no *infirmiers*, nobody in fact. Being in the trench, I pointed out to the generals that, in order to take a wounded man out of the range of the cannon, it was necessary to have at least six soldiers or *grenadiers*, which would soon have left the lines bare. Why not give us some servants of battlefield surgery? We would have needed twenty-five of them every day on duty in the trench with our surgeons. On the day that the assault was to take place, there should have been a hundred or more in the lines to gather the wounded and take away the dead. We have in the army more than 500 soldiers who have lost or cut off a finger; recently there were 162 disabled in this way in the hospitals of Posen; these men should be put at our disposal to make surgical servants of them.

'Our service is terrible; it is barbaric. His Majesty was quite right to say that we were below the Cossacks where it concerns the hospitals. I offer the most efficient and simplest means of ensuring the aid due to the wounded and sick of the active army: see to it, therefore, Grand-Marshal, that it is adopted. That is all that can be done at present, because to want to improve everything together, to reinvent everything at once, is to confirm the loss of everything and to risk having no more service of any kind.

'I have the honour …'

Our man with the strangulated hernia is fine; it has partly re-entered.

31st – The day was very beautiful; it is Sunday; everyone is taking a walk. There was a great parade. I saw General Rapp at his lodgings, and he spoke to me with the greatest indignation about Tissot. I introduced him to the major-director and the surgeon-in-chief of the Prussian hospitals, inviting him to be favourable to them; I also introduced them to the *ordonnateur*-in-chief Mathieu-Faviers. The besieged army, according to what they said, lost 8,000 men to injuries, illnesses or being killed, a number that included eighty-eight officers: the most distinguished of which were the general of the engineers Delaurentz, who was crushed by a poorly fixed blindage,[9] and Major Boussemard, who was killed by a shot to the head. There are still 1,400 sick Prussians and 168 Russians; two-thirds are wounded. His Majesty arrived at Oliva at four o'clock; he wants there to be space for 2,000 sick men in Dantzig; that will not suit General Ménard, the commanding officer of the

---

9. A blindage is an overhead cover for an advanced trench, often made from earthwork and a supporting wooden frame.

city, who said yesterday to our surgeons, who presented him with an invitation from me to find lodgings for them, that they were doing well in Dantzig and that they did not need any medical officers there. He is a fool, whom everyone laughs at: it is said aloud that, on the day when the assault was to be made, he made his will and asked several officers if mounting an assault was a very dangerous thing.

An artillery officer died this morning, on the eighth day since his injury; he had been hit in the forehead by a musket ball that had sunk and splintered the bone. A large crown trepan should have been applied to remove the depressed portion in its entirety, under which, according to custom, there were sharp points from the vitreous table. Desault, who does not like the trepan, which never worked for him at the Hôtel-Dieu,[10] very unwisely forbade this aid and thought that he could render it useless by using antimoniated drinks. This is a fatal error, which has taken root dangerously among our young surgeons.

Our hernia has re-entered and the unfortunate soldier died a few hours later. A cadaveric post-mortem was to be undertaken, but, because there is not even a corner free in a hospital that had just been established, it could not be done.

At the site of the arsenal, one can see a 27lb cannon, through the mouth of which one of our cannonballs entered when it was in battery. As it was loaded, the intruding cannonball compressed the other to such an extent that the flanks of the piece were bent wider by it.

His Majesty arrived at four o'clock; he is staying at the Abbey of Oliva.

1 *Juin* – The Emperor did not go to bed until four o'clock, in the morning. On seeing Marshal Lefebvre yesterday, he said to him: 'Come and embrace me, Lefebvre; I am pleased with your operations in Dantzig and I make you Duke of that name.' In the morning, he saw the siege works and made his grand entrance to the city at two o'clock, to cheering all around. I was returning from forts Wasser and Weichselmünde, where I was expecting to find premises for hospitals. In the first of these forts there are indeed some very large warehouses made from wood for wheat and salt; they have boarded floors and it would be easy to create casements there and to put them in a condition to receive the sick; this is the wish of the town and of the magistrate. But the country is insalubrious, covered with stagnant water, and the warehouses are on the very banks of the Vistula, which would make their stay damp, cold and stinking. Besides, how would one supply it? It is a league and a half from the city;

---

10. A Parisian hospital, close to Notre-Dame de Paris cathedral.

the river would be convenient for evacuating and bringing in foodstuffs, but one would risk being neglected at such a great distance. We will be able to treat a thousand patients with venereal diseases and scabies sufferers in Fort Wasser; as for the wounded and those with fevers, we must have them more within reach of the city and in a more salubrious place. I am requesting the arsenal; we will see if it is granted to us. The weather is fine, but the shores of the Baltic have made me cold. We overturned on our way and while passing a deep ravine; no one was hurt; it is true that we were able to set foot on the ground. The coachman ran risks: the front train separated, the horses became frightened, but our driver, who had been thrown to the ground, clung on to the reins and allowed himself to be dragged, his stomach on the ground, rather than let them go, which stopped the horses. The Weichselmünde is curious; the works are beautiful, fairly regular and old; the tower is from 1490, built under Casimir, King of Poland.[11] There are dungeons for prisoners of the State; there are some all around in a circular building, which leaves only a narrow courtyard between it and the tower, still filled with small wooden cells; in those above there are iron rings to tie up the prisoners who have been condemned to this extra discomfort or who expose themselves to it through their mutiny. If the enemies had lived together more peaceably and kept these forts, two months of siege would perhaps not have made them give them up to us.

On our return, we saw His Majesty's entrance into Dantzig. I believe that we have been granted the arsenal.

2nd – Lovely weather, good health, full of energy: they drink excellent wine here. I have just confirmed the arsenal: we will not have the ground floor; the artillery is keeping it. Tomorrow we will have beds on the first floor. I have removed some armour of little consequence; it has all been placed at my disposal, but it is so far from here to France that I cannot take advantage of such a good offer. I have only accepted a few articles, which I will try to send to Berlin, from where it will be easier to have them sent home.

3rd. – The weather has certainly cooled: I was restless last night. This morning we went to see the Abbey of Oliva, where the only curious thing is the Abbot's garden; even so, it is not particularly significant. The abbey building is quite beautiful, but it is modestly furnished. It was here that His Majesty spent one night. At the bottom of the main staircase of the cloister is an inscription on black marble relating to the signing of the peace treaty between Austria,

---

11. Casimir IV Jagiellon (1427–1492).

France, Sweden, etc. in 1660; we were led into a dirty, narrow refectory where this important ceremony had taken place, and we saw the rather crude table, with its inset in puddingstone marble, on which the ambassadors had signed. The library of the Bernardines is very poor, as is the mense of their prior, for they are poor. The church is curious; there are seventy-four chapels, one of which has four marble pilasters that, through their fluting, represent very beautiful heads of young women, old men and animals. I spoke a lot of Latin with the good clergymen; it was as if I were seeing my poor brother, who was also of this order.

The arsenal was a little contested, but tomorrow we will have the part that is due to us without fail.

This evening I went to the show and saw *The Caliph of Baghdad*: the opera house is quite beautiful and I found the music charming.

4th – The weather is still fine, but it is cold: I have a discomfort in my head; if it continues I will be forced to resort to my twenty grains of jalap. Our hospitals are not doing well; the arsenal is being evacuated only very slowly; I thought I could still take some armour there, and some has been put aside for our marshals. Everything is unaffordable in this city: a pound of meat is sold there for 1 *thaler* (3 *francs*, 12 *sous*); passable wine costs just as much; blue cloth is not sold for less than 56 or 60 *francs* per French ell; permission is still needed to buy some. Dantzig has been ordered to pay 20 million *francs*. The bells, according to an old ruling, belong to the artillery, which had them bought back by the town for 80,000 *francs*, a quarter of which, according to the same ruling, was to be given to *M.* Lariboisière, who was the chief commander of this division; but this gallant man gifted his share to his gunners.

One knows only to think of peace or of war: everyone speaks of it according to his wishes and hopes; but there is not a face on which one does not read the ardent desire to return to France. We are almost all becoming homesick. I believe that His Majesty will not spend the winter in this country; but the army will remain there for a long time still.

5th – The weather is fine; there is almost no night. Everyone is coming to see Dantzig; they drink good wine there for a day or two, and leave scarcely content with their trip.

Today I saw several wounded in the city. The colonel of the 44th Regiment, who was wounded a fortnight ago and for whom I had advised making a large incision above the clavicle to release the blood that was causing a tumour in that area, is doing very well; the clavicle was not fractured, as was said, nor the rib, but the spine of the scapula, and it is from there that the small splinters came. He was kept for a long time in a state of diarrhoea, which has been very helpful.

The lieutenant-colonel of the 12th Light Infantry had his olecranon fractured and the capsule torn; he is in great pain, but he will be fine. The suppuration seemed to me to be disgusting: it smelled of the mouldiest cheese; I forbade the use of fatty broths and food taken from animals, and only allowed the use of thin soups, fish, spinach, preserves, etc.

A sapper who had his thigh amputated has a large, extremely sensitive medullary fungus around the bone: this is a sign that the bone has been severely disturbed by the biscayan, and that the surrounding bony structure, or reticular substance that supports the marrow, has been badly damaged. Usually this mass contains little marrow; it is the tumefaction of the medullary membrane that gives rise to the volume of fungus; but almost always it is the sign of a more or less extensive exfoliation, which takes place in the form of a ring.

General Ménard, the commander of the place, came to my lodgings with the brave major from Baden who had been on trench duty during the whole siege. I proposed to him that he demand from the affluent inhabitants of the city 400 bunks equipped with their bedding to furnish our first two wards in the arsenal in forty-eight hours; they adopted this efficient method and tomorrow the requisition will be underway.

The pharmacists have rushed here to request medicines: they will, they say with an air of contentment, collect 100,000 *francs*' worth; but I intend that their statement be seen and signed by me, and this will upset them a little. I am also intending that one of our *chirurgiens-majors* will be present at the distribution of the items and will sign the expertise and visit reports; we will also call one of our physicians there.

6th – A letter has just been dispatched to General Rapp from the Major-General announcing that the Russians have attacked everywhere and that they have been more or less beaten back; it invites the general to make all the officers attached to the general headquarters leave at once; the headquarters will probably move. I will set out at five o'clock, for Rusoschin, where I will sleep; after tomorrow, I shall be at Riesenbourg;[12] I will take my ambulance or battlefield surgery divisions. The Major-General has agreed to include me in

---

12. Percy or Longin spells the name of this town with a middle 'm' or 'n' interchangeably.

a distribution of rum and Bordeaux wine that will be made to the army of the siege; I am to receive twenty-five pints of rum and 400 of wine; this souvenir flatters me a great deal, and the items granted will do me a lot of good. They had been informed at His Highness's lodgings that that I had been at the siege and that I had directed its surgical service.

His Majesty ordered that all the Russians and Prussians who remain sick in the city should leave it within twenty-four hours to be transferred to the surrounding area; but where should they be placed? I proposed Praust, in the church and barns. I did not dare speak of Oliva; General Rapp decided that it would be in this abbey that they would be placed, unless the abbot and monks can work to put them elsewhere. Thus, the evacuation will begin this evening or tomorrow: this news satisfies *M.* Lichtenberger, the Prussian *chirurgien-major*, who was afraid of going too far. General Ménard proposed sending all these patients to Pillau; but, besides the fact that we lack ships, how would we pass under the noses of the English fleets and what would we say about such a terrible violation of the surrender?

I am leaving all the surgeons of the first Legion of the North, those of the garrison and a reserve surgical division here: this is more than enough for the service of the city. We are arranging for the transport of our wine and rum; there is a shortage of carts, but we will have one. I am leaving at five o'clock, leaving honest souvenirs and sincere regrets in *M.* Weichbrot's house. I will see my castle of Rusoschin again, 3 short leagues from here; we will spend the night there; our host's horses will take us there in a rather pretty and new little carriage.

7th – We slept at the castle of Rusoschin, which has been completely evacuated. I was delighted to see the beautiful garden again; for supper we were given fresh gudgeons to eat, which were caught in a small river at the bottom of the garden; I slept well and this morning I again saw my dear garden. Again, we had excellent gudgeons for our breakfast. We left at half past eight in the burning sun and terrible dust. I am not so bad on my little Prussian carriage: the nice seat I have put there is comfortable and good; I am not sheltered from the sun or the dust, but I am going to war and, in these circumstances, I should not be so delicate.

We arrived in Dirschau at half past eleven. This little town, in which there is nothing remarkable, was ruined and pillaged in March by the Poles and the first Legion of the North, all of whom are Polish, while Marshal Lefebvre was on his way to Dantzig. There were only 500 Prussians in the place who, on the approach of our troops, had withdrawn, but who, having known that these troops were Poles, had returned to beat them. Dombrowski could have driven them out without harming the inhabitants; but he calculated that there would be no merit for him in such a victory, and he preferred to cause a commotion and attack the town with cannon fire. He destroyed it and, having pounded it with cannon it for a long time, with General Ménard assisting him, so it is said, he gradually and cautiously sent in his Polish troops, who fired on the inhabitants and killed thirty of them, broke doors and shattered windows with their gunfire and gorged themselves on the spoils. Dombrowski, since this awful and cowardly success, has fallen into disfavour; his son has been wounded in the arm. One cannot take a step in this sad town without encountering debris, broken glass, walls pulled down, burned houses, etc.

A hospital has finally been established in a church and an adjacent house. I was very pleased with it: each patient has a good little bedstead with straw bedding and linen; the food is not marvellous, but I am always astonished when I see that they are given passable bread, rice, prunes and eggs, even a little wine and enough beer. This establishment, already filled with 200 sick and wounded, can be cited for the regularity and generosity of its service; it has been organized under the direction of *chirurgien-major* Ristel-Huber, whom I am taking with his division. I dined well at the house of the host of this *chirurgien-major*, where I saw some beautiful women, one of whom was a brunette with concupiscent eyes and a lustful, bold look. We left at four o'clock, our wine cart following us very well.

The countryside between Dirschau and Marienbourg is superb, rich and well sown; the rye is in ears; the oats are large and the wheat beautiful. Nothing is as attractive as the plains I crossed; there are few woods; the edges of the road are planted with willow trees, but the villages are large and well built.

The town of Marienbourg is quite pretty. At the entrance to the town, on the Dirschau side, there is a considerable building, built in brick and surrounded by ditches: this is where the hospital has been established. This building once belonged to the Templars, who ceded it to the Teutonic knights; it was a very important fort in its time; you can still see the remains of fortifications that were fairly regular for the period. The King of Prussia had this place converted into warehouses for wheat and military effects; we have 500 sick and wounded there, all lying on a bedstead and with some straw bedding, but it smells terrible everywhere. The hospital is badly kept; we have not been able to open up air currents because of the thickness of the walls, or rather the *commissaires* and other people, who in my absence have presided over the establishment, have neither known nor wanted to do better; thus, in any room that one walks through, one is plagued by an unbearable smell of excrement.

It is a question of opening another hospital in Marienbourg: the battle that is due to take place in a few days' time will make it necessary; but this is a project about which they appear to have done very little.

Yesterday eighty wounded arrived from the I Corps, who were wounded in the combat on the 4th, when a large number of Russians launched themselves on this corps and on the IV Corps, which suffered greatly. Marshal Bernadotte was hit in the neck by a musket ball that only tore the teguments; he is due to arrive in Marienbourg today, but it is impossible for me to wait for him there, so much am I anxious to join the general headquarters to prepare myself for the great battle. The wounded are only mildly so; some of the Russian amputees whom I saw in Dirschau replied, when I asked them how they were: '*Vanbé, vanbé*, very well, very well.'

8th – I awoke very early in the morning, having slept quite well in a bad feather bed that made me very hot: the sun is extremely strong and the day superb. I directed the 2nd, 8th and 9th Divisions of battlefield surgeons to Christbourg; the others are going to Riesenbourg. Having written some orders and provided for the service of Marienbourg, from where the 2nd Division is leaving, I hastily drank a little coffee and set off. It was half past six. Marienbourg has the appearance of a strong city; it is being made into a defence point or a bridgehead; a crowd of peasants are working constantly. They have built a fence, dug ditches and made ramparts, so that in any event the French army will be at ease and will be able to protect itself from any surprise, if it crosses the Vistula again. There are 10 leagues from this place to Riesenbourg; the first three are beautiful and pleasant, because of the countryside, which is well cultivated; then one arrives at Stuhm, a small town that was once very heavily fortified, belonging to the Templars and Teutons and situated near a lake that teems with fish. The remains of walls and towers built of brick can be seen; the ditches are partly cultivated as gardens. We saw a fisherman whose pirogue[13] was full of fish; this skiff was a hollowed-out fir tree; we bought fish (perch)

---

13. A dugout canoe.

for 10 *kroches*,¹⁴ which we were able to enjoy in a large house, a quarter of a league further on. This is where our men stopped on their way; they were so satisfied that they encouraged me to stop there too; it is a beautiful house on high ground and surrounded by well-cultivated fields. There are many lakes in this country. The misery of the inhabitants is going to be brought to a head by the epizootic disease that is plaguing the stables and pastures; most of the cattle are perishing; I do not yet know the nature of this disease.

It appears, by what I learned on my way and after arriving in Riesenbourg, that the Russians did us a great deal of harm on the 4th. The VI Corps was crushed and driven out of Guttstadt; its cannon pieces were either taken away or nailed shut; most of the officers of the general staff lost their wagons; the treasure was plundered and, moreover, there are seven or eight hundred wounded. The IV and I Corps also suffered greatly.

His Majesty left before them at noon for Saalfeld; it is said that he is in Mohrungen. Our ambulance caissons left yesterday. There is no one left here: I am leaving on duty this evening for Saalfeld; tomorrow my wagons will come to join me. I am leaving two large trunks in Riesenbourg, one black and one with three keys; plus a small case full of porcelain; plus a *vitchoura*, a large woollen blanket, a bracelet, a large whip and a Spanish dagger: this will come to me when God wills it. We are taking wine, rum, ham, bread, flour, biscuits and oats with us.

9th – I had risen by 4 o'clock: I had a few cups of coffee, wrote a few orders, had the carriages loaded and set off in superb weather. The sun has been raging and we have been travelling through clouds of dust; the dust is horrible in this country and in this weather: nothing can save me from it, as I am sitting on a simple seat suspended at the end of a small wagon, which looks respectable enough. I am fairly well, except for the inconveniences of the heat and the dust; but I am bearing them wonderfully; neither hurts my eyes as much as I thought they would. I have kept my Rusoschin peasant, who has hitched three horses to my wagon and the fourth to my large caisson; this is fine, although the road, all sand, is very hard going.

At five hours from Riesenbourg, one comes across a sort of village called Preuss-Mark: one sees there the remains of an old citadel built by the Templars; the belfry or bell tower is still standing, as well as a part of the brick wall. This

---

14. Longin: *Groschen*, German money made from billon [typically an alloy of copper, zinc and silver or gold].

fort is surrounded on three sides by a beautiful watercourse that made it almost inaccessible; it is even probable that the water once went all the way around it, since there are supporting walls for a bridge that used to connect it to the mainland.

Two short leagues further on is the town of Saalfeld, which has suffered a little less than the others. I saw seven houses there that serve as hospitals. There are at the moment nearly 300 wounded, and we have little aid to give them; however, they are not lacking the bare necessities; the bread is quite good; the broth is, as everywhere else, very light and insipid, because of the young cow's meat that is usually distributed. I found five surgeons, including a young Prussian, whom I requisitioned on the invitation of Adjutant-General Levasseur, whom he had bandaged during and after his captivity among the Prussians and Russians. This officer had received a large sabre blow to his right arm at the Battle of Eylau, which had cut the olecranon and divided the condyles of the humerus by penetrating the joint; there is ankylosis, as can well be believed, but the arm was wisely held in a state of semi-flexion.

We had a good meal, to our great surprise and contentment, and climbed back onto the carriage at three o'clock to travel our 6 leagues and arrive at Mohrungen. Even more dust than there was in the morning, because of the wagon trains of all kinds, and the sun is truly burning; but we are passing through beautiful forests and travelling alongside a very long lake, which resembles the Vistula. I saw a mill that the waters of the source of this lake cause to turn; opposite is a delightful island, which can be reached by a bridge as flimsy as it is elegant: what a pity not to be able to go and take a breath of cool air in this beautiful place! However, the horrors of war are calling us; the convoys of wounded follow one after the other; we must make haste. These poor wounded are covered in blood and dust, and gasp from the thirst and heat. A league and a half short of Mohrungen, on the road itself, there is a fine castle where 200 wounded have been put, and they are doing well there; *M.* Torreilhe is in charge of the service there.

We entered Mohrungen at eight o'clock. During the whole journey, but especially as we approached this unfortunate town, we were poisoned by the smell of rotting corpses, not or badly buried. The town is overloaded with rotten and foul manure; all the barns are uncovered. Upon arriving I saw a man and two women who were loading three French corpses onto a sledge to take them to the cemetery; one of them had a horribly red, or rather purple, face, which happens to those who have been killed without having lost blood, and especially to those who have been struck in the chest; even the bones of the skull are bloodshot. The corpses of men killed with large wounds and with a large amount of blood loss are white. I visited the hospital, which is very foul and always full; the wounded are arriving there night and day; since the 4th, 800 of them have passed through Mohrungen. I saw *M. Marillon*, deputy chief of staff of the VI Corps: he was hit by a cannonball in the upper part of his right arm. The fracture is terrible and extends as far as the clavicle, which has also been affected. It was not possible to amputate at the joint; already his chest is engorged, as so often happens in this case; his fever is high; his face is burning because he is struggling to breathe, which is beginning to become wheezy; he is a lost man. The town is full of carriages. The general headquarters left yesterday. Tomorrow, at two o'clock, we will gather in the courtyard of the hospital to leave all together; there will be more than fifty of us.

My gums are hurting, I have hardly any teeth now and I cannot chew. It is quarter past eleven: I am sleeping in a room with four beds, one of which is occupied by one of our surgeons who snores horribly; I will hardly sleep. I have shaved and washed, which refreshed and soothed me greatly.

I am leaving Cols, Pierron and seven *sous-aides* in Mohrungen.

10th – At half past two I rose, having not slept a good hour because of my snorer. It was broad daylight and marvellously cool; already all the birds were singing and the sun was about to appear. At half past three, my company set off: the wind was fresh then and almost cold; this is what makes it necessary to take the precaution of covering oneself well in the bivouac. Mounted on my good seat, I made the journey like yesterday in the middle of a dust cloud through which it was impossible to see oneself. We had to travel in the wake of some wagon trains and convoys, the road being too narrow to move beyond them; however, we got through them, but not without an accident, for as we passed a small wooden bridge pitched over a cesspool, a wagon from the artillery train that we had cut off tried to join the line again and turned the wagon on which my young friend Le Vert was sitting upside down. No one was hurt by this fall, which was maliciously provoked by a corporal whom I wanted to punish; the officer of the train was mistreated by our surgeons; however, everything was arranged and in our presence the corporal was condemned to arrest (that is to say, to nothing, and even on campaign, arrests are less than nothing). What a poor country! Already it is dry and arid as if it were the end of the most scorching summer; it is hardly cultivated at all, and the few green meadows or fields that are to be found here and there have already been devoured by our army. Lakes are very common. There are also many forests; but on all sides one meets enormous blocks of granite, sandstone, flint, quartz, which resemble the remains of rocks that no longer exist or that were brought by the sea with which this country was covered, and it is with these blocks that the inhabitants surround their fields and make the foundations of their houses. The unfortunates have been dispersed in the past few days; they are returning little by little, bringing back some parcels of belongings that several of our men and especially the allies still are keen to see.

Having travelled a good 6 leagues, we found the small town of Deppen, which the Russians, on withdrawing, had reduced to ashes: it was not pleasant to pass in front of these houses, which were still smoking, so extreme were the smell and the heat. The Passarge flows there. It is a small river over which there is a bridge that the Russians were to destroy in order to cut off any retreat by the VI Corps, which they had forced to withdraw; fortunately they were unable to perform this operation and some companies of *voltigeurs* prevented them from doing so, without which it would have been the end of the VI Corps; the Russian general who had the mission of destroying this bridge has been dismissed. It is said that the Russians had nearly 60,000 men on the single point of Guttstadt. In this instance, they manoeuvred very badly, for the VI Corps retreated only 4 leagues during the first two days and held out against such a great number of enemies; it lost some men, but it saved its artillery, which was said to have been taken; it seems that it lost only two pieces. The surgeons-major were as exposed as the officers and the soldiers; they were in the middle of the infantry square that they continually formed. We fought again yesterday and the enemy suffered fairly heavy losses: they have murdered most of our sick left in Guttstadt and the wounded left on the battlefield; however, they have treated our captured officers well. They are withdrawing in great numbers: it is believed that they will cross the Pregel again and that it will be at Bartenstein that they will await us. It is to be desired that they should accept the battle; it would be terrible, but a great setback would knock their pride and perhaps bring peace, which is still very doubtful. In any case, if we were to remain more than a fortnight in this country, the army would risk being attacked by an epidemic, so unclean is the air, the land marshy and the water detestable here; so many corpses of men and horses are found rotting in the open air; so great is the misery and so constant is the boredom there. General Guyot, ex-colonel of the 9th Hussars, has been killed. General Dutaillis, chief of staff of the VI Corps, had his arm blown off very close to the joint; no resection was made and I do not know if the amputation at the joint was proposed; the *chirurgien-major* Jeantet has left with the wounded man.

The distress that pursues the poor inhabitants is a cruel and desolate thing. Three or 4 leagues from Guttstadt, we stopped this morning to graze our horses and refresh them. We were having something to eat; a young and beautiful girl approached me, opening her starving eyes on my bad bread. One of our surgeons unwisely threw her some change, which she picked up rather out of gratitude and decency than out of need. It was bread that she needed; I presented her with a good piece of bread; she blushed as she accepted it and immediately took it to her mouth; but as she ate it, she hid and cried. Alas! Perhaps it was the memory of her past fortune which allowed her to give relief to unfortunates, too. I gave her a good glass of brandy to drink: she swallowed it only with difficulty and out of deference. This poor village is absolutely devastated. So are all those through which we have passed; some of them have even been burned by the Russians.

We are leaving at once for Heilsberg, 7 leagues from here. It is seven o'clock in the evening: we will travel for part of the night, but by daybreak we must be close to the Emperor, who may give battle tomorrow. Farewell, rest and sleep for another night!

# 1807 (continued) – Friedland and Tilsit

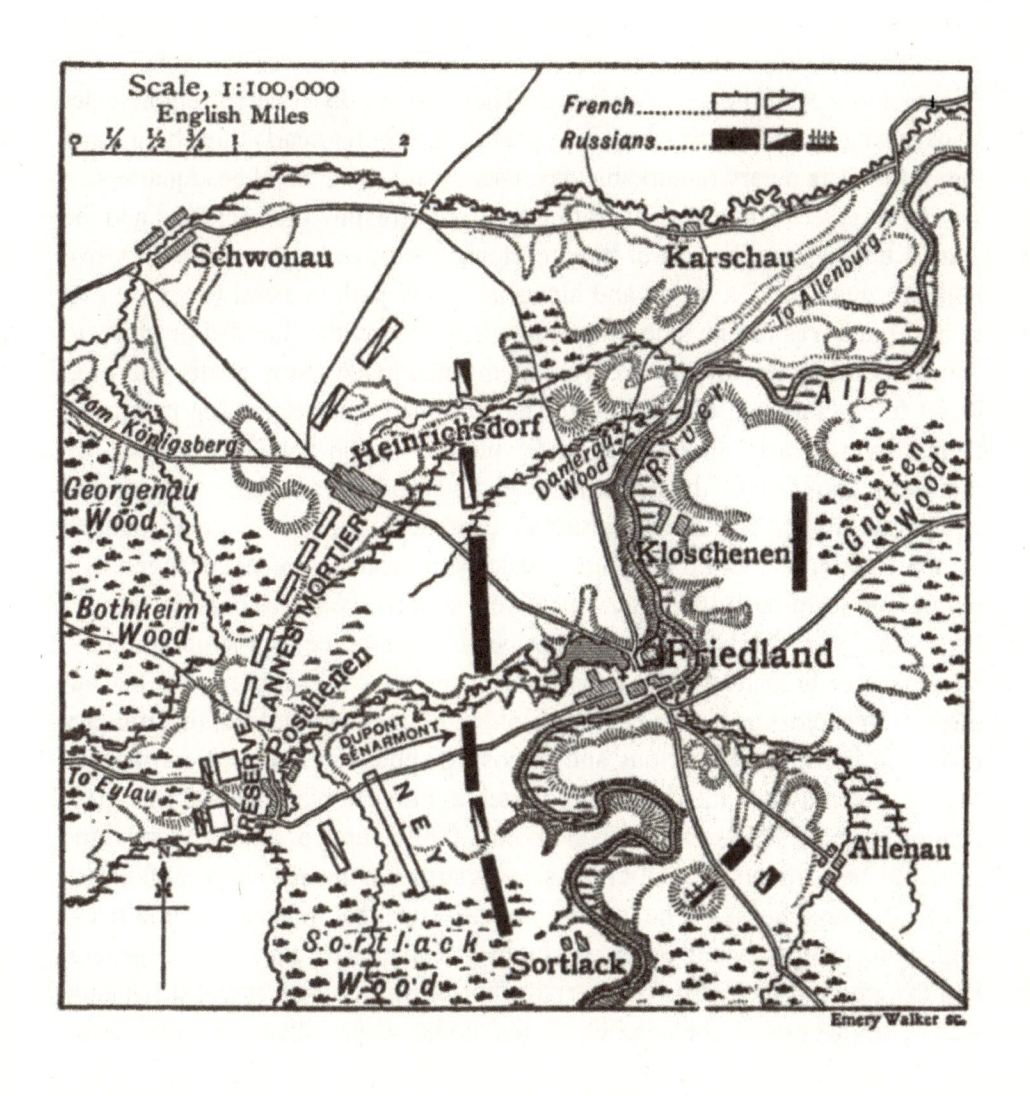

11th – We had left at ten o'clock for the main headquarters, which was to be, it was said, in Peterswalde, 4 leagues from Guttstadt; the dark night, the approach of a storm, nothing had been able to prevent us from leaving; forty surgeons were with me, but we had forgotten to take a guide. Having travelled a league, hardly able to see, we could not find our way; my caisson had followed an artillery train and was going in the right direction. Having headed left, I recognized that I was about to lose my way and, not knowing whom to blame, nor whom to address, I grew angry, which bothered me greatly. After shouting, hurling insults and cursing, because no-one could guide me or show me the way, I made the decision to return to Guttstadt, where the sentry at the gate was unwilling to let me enter. I ordered my men to be ready at three o'clock in the morning; I threw myself on the straw, fully dressed; it was midnight, it was raining and the darkness was profound. They had put my covered wagon under an overhanging roof and the horses in a stable. I slept for nearly three hours, and today, the 11th, a very remarkable day, I set off for the general headquarters.

The weather is dreadful; the rain is pouring down by the bucketful and the cold is unpleasant. We left at three o'clock; we travelled for more than two hours through a thick wood and along a narrow path; several times we had to hurl ourselves to one side to let wagons loaded with wounded or going to the munition stores to pass us. The enemy has made many abatis and tried to set fire to one end of the forest. The wounded were streaming past us in their droves, nearly all on foot, and wounded in the hand or forearm; we met more than 500 of them. On leaving the wood we saw the carriages and equipages of His Majesty assembled in a meadow, opposite a site abandoned by the Russians, a camp elegantly made with branches of fir arranged in a pyramid to form beautiful huts, which were covered with tree bark; in front of these houses, which have a protruding peristyle entrance, is a large umbrella, also made of branches of fir, under which the stack of weapons was placed; there is an enclosure for the horses, drinking houses, etc. Indeed, this military residence has a rather curious and imposing appearance. It is there that we fought yesterday and the day before yesterday: the Russians caused us a great deal of harm; it seems that we had about 2,000 wounded, among them some distinguished officers. General Roussel was struck in the head by a cannonball, which shattered his skull; he is in a comatose state that indicates a certain and impending death. General Ferey was hit by a dead musket ball. Another general had the external malleolus of his right foot blown away. General d'Espagne was lightly wounded; the colonel of the 55th has been killed; a host of senior officers have died or been put out of action. The Russians hold impregnable positions: at least that is what we will see tomorrow.

I left my caisson and cart with His Majesty's carriages and came on horseback onto the field, entering some unfortunate houses, most of them uncovered, abandoned, without straw or anything in the world, and all filled with wounded. In one, *M. C...*, a *chirurgien-major*, was finishing an amputation; he spoke to me about his salary, which is still owed to him, and about other personal subjects, without thinking to give me a report on his service. I reminded him of this duty, exhorting him, nevertheless, to always do his best. In the next building, there were fifty wounded, with whom I left three surgeons. A quarter of a league further on, I found four *chirurgiens-majors* of the *cuirassiers* dressing and operating on a large number of wounded: this is where poor General Roussel is; his secretary came to weep in my arms, holding the sabre and belt of this brave officer. Principal Chappe has established the ambulance of the IV Corps in a hut further on; he has many surgeons with him. Yesterday the divisions of Baudry and Béclard arrived, who performed the evening service on the far left of the army, not far from the houses where the principal Poussielgue has placed the ambulance of the general cavalry reserve.

A great number of troops are arriving and positioning themselves in a line; the cavalry is arranged in a line filling the high ground. Our line is formidable; that of the enemy is no less so. We have stopped firing and it seems that the day will be spent examining and gauging each other. The battle will take place tomorrow. Tomorrow a hundred thousand men placed opposite a hundred thousand men must attack each other with fury, kill or be killed, and decide, according to His Majesty's proclamation, the destinies of Europe. Alas! What happiness is that which can be established only on mounds of corpses and in torrents of blood! I tremble at the thought that we will have 8,000 or 10,000 wounded, to whom we will only be able to administer the sad and painful aid of surgery. We have no lack of linen and lint; there is broth on the fire in two vast cauldrons, but that is only for the ambulance where I am presently. The Intendant-general is here with us: I introduced him to the eight divisions of battlefield surgeons and took pleasure in briefing him about everything. We each ate soup in a bowl from the ambulance; he bivouacked last night; he has no other lodging than a caisson, on the shafts of which he sits and sleeps. I am no better lodged and am writing at present on the front chest of another caisson or cart; but the cart that I left behind is to be brought to me, with a basket of wine, two of rum, my woollen blanket, etc.; I shall sleep in it. I have had 15 or 20lb of good meat brought to my men in the bivouac of His Majesty's carriages, with which they can make an excellent soup.

His Majesty has a cabin on a very high hillock: I went for a walk there and saw *M.* Boyer and the Intendant-general, with whom I returned. Since the latter is here, I doubt that the Emperor will call me to give a report to him.

In the course of my visits, I saw a soldier of good appearance, who had been shot in the lower abdomen, through the opening of which had escaped red and bloodshot intestines as big as two fists, a true strangulated hernia, the opening of which I had enlarged and the neck cut. It is possible that death will spare this brave young man, but I have just learned that the intestine has been pierced; thus, there is infinitely less hope.

Everyone is working to find somewhere to spend the night, to feed themselves and their horses. I am free from these cares: I have already eaten plenty of soup, then a pound of good bread with butter. I have also drunk two glasses of good red wine, and (will posterity believe it?) I have had an excellent cup of coffee with water made in my rural *cafetière*; and I have even had a little drop of brandy. Now it is a question only of my bed. But my carriage is there. I removed the packages and the bad straw that were cluttering it, filled it with good dry straw, lifted the seat and tilted it back, and I lay down on it at ten o'clock in the evening; the cushion was put under my head, my saddlecloth over my feet, my blanket over my body, the leather apron over the blanket, and there I was, asleep after quarter of an hour until half past three, when the voices of Grand-Marshal Duroc and *M.* Daru woke me. The horses were very good. The whole army has been quiet. The bivouacs of our surgeons were beside me.

12th – I rose early to speak to *M.* Duroc and *M.* Daru about the service. I reminded the former of my project of battlefield surgery and made him feel how significant it would be for us if it were adopted; I complained about not having a single servant and recommended this article in particular to him, by speaking to him of our disabled men from Posen and the way in which we confirm that they voluntarily deprived themselves of a finger. When we dress them, we propose a small operation that has the wonderful advantage of making the lost finger grow back: they refuse, hide, run away, from which we conclude that these scoundrels have put themselves out of action. I drank some broth, went for a walk with *M.* Boyer, saw my men, gave orders and went back to bed, where I slept for two hours, which means that I am faring very well. The enemy has made great movements. Not a cannon shot has yet been fired.

## 1807 (continued) – Friedland and Tilsit

His Majesty has been on horseback for three hours. He is at Heilsberg. I think that we are going to leave.

We spoke at nine o'clock with the Intendant-general, followed by thirty fairly well-mounted surgeons, which seemed to please him. The weather was extremely hot and stormy. We crossed the various fields of the battlefield and saw many French horses and some corpses of our soldiers there; we cannot conceal the fact that we lost many people. The enemy's position was impregnable: it is a great fortune that they abandoned it. They made their retreat with order and in silence: one would have wished that our army worried them more and even that we tackled them yesterday evening and during the night, but our Emperor judged otherwise and one must believe that he had strong reasons for that.

Everything is going to Heilsberg. We arrived there at eleven o'clock, and from the first house in the suburb, we saw how much it had cost the Russians during the preceding days: 400 of their soldiers, wounded and left by them in the town, were found; undoubtedly they took four times as many, for none of these wretches could be transported, owing to the severity of their wounds. According to their habit, they were piled up in the houses; I had them all visited and thirty surgeons have been charged with dressing and operating on them. They will be brought together at a single site, which will be their hospital, and it will be the town that will feed them and have them treated under the inspection of one of our French surgeons. Among these wounded were eighty-two of our soldiers, almost all of them very badly wounded, whom the Russians had taken prisoner and treated fairly well. These brave men were in agreement in telling us that the surgeons of the Russian army had dressed them in preference to their own people, and indeed, we found three to whom they had applied a tourniquet, in the fear (rather vain) of a haemorrhage. Our wounded say that the Russians treat them better than the Prussians; that the latter put black and coarse linen on their wounds, while the others use fine and very white linen, which is generally true. Moreover, it is easy to understand the reason for this preference: it is that, in order to dispose the victor more favourably to spare the sick and wounded whom they are forced to leave to them, it is advisable to begin by taking good care of his own, whom one mixes expressly with the others. I also have this policy.

We lodged as best we could in Heilsberg, a small town that is quite good and from which we would have benefitted had we not started by pillaging it: the drunk and starving soldiers threw themselves upon it, took bread, flour, lard, wine, utensils, etc., and we saw them leave with their hands full and return to the camp loaded with provisions. The enemy left a great deal of flour and war munitions there. I entered and took over the home of a rich apothecary, where we found three officers of the Guard taking from the house and the dispensary with reasonable moderation; they found wine, beer and other foodstuffs that the pharmacist and his people took great pains to declare to them to be medicines, which did not bother them. I went about my business. I did not forget to take some paper, pins and Spanish wax, which were on the writing desk, and I even succumbed to the temptation of putting a small amount of muslin of very little value in my pocket, enough only to make two miserable ties; but I was certainly punished for this moment of weakness, for in my absence, my silver-rimmed spectacles were taken from me, which I believe I had left on the aforementioned desk, unless I lost them as I was going around the town. I was greatly affected by this loss, which, fortunately, was immediately repaired by *M.* Baltz, who provided me with another pair of spectacles that are at least as good. I accompanied the Intendant-general to the castle, which we visited together and where we are convinced that we could place 1,500 patients: it was a Russian storehouse and, after the Battle of Eylau, we had already made a large hospital from it.

I dined with *M.* Daru, who had, for an Intendant-general, a very poor dinner, which is the only fault of the circumstances. His Majesty left at half past two for Eylau, so they say. My colleagues procured for me a barrel of good white wine, some oil and two large bottles of good vinegar from our host, a very bad man who had gone to complain that everything was being taken from him for the hospitals. We all set off on horseback at half past five, my two carriages following slowly. At seven o'clock, lightning and a few thunderclaps heralded the storm, which came down on us like a shower and soaked the whole army. Having travelled without resting the horses until half past eleven in terrible weather and on terrible paths, without even a grain of oats or an ounce of bread, since our carriages were 3 leagues behind us, I took the decision to halt with my forty-six surgeons in an enormous stable, where we placed our horses and where I lay down with my wet clothes on a bit of old straw, with a root of dry wood for a pillow and my saddlecloth to cover my feet. I slept until half past four; as did all my men and none of us had anything to eat. We had found bulrushes, a bit of grass and straw torn from the roof to feed our horses. We were now only two leagues from Eylau. It was not cold in this miserable lodging and I tasted the sweetness of sleep, although when I rose this morning, my neck was stiff and sore.

13th – We left at half past five in the morning, without taking the trouble to wash and having saddled and bridled our horses in the absence of our servants, who had lost their way or stayed behind. The weather was quite fine. We crossed large forests and found a dreadful road, on which the carriages had trouble moving freely: a lot of mud, gullies almost as bad as in winter, and narrow and hilly paths delayed us on our journey, not to mention the fact that our horses had eaten almost nothing. Finally, we arrived at Eylau, a town of sorrowful and lamentable memory: His Majesty slept there. We saw neither corpses nor anything too revolting to remind us of the famous battle; the houses have been partly repaired, but the misery is deep there and several inhabitants fled as the army approached, which only arrived in its entirety this morning. We went straight to our pastor's house, where we had stayed last year: the poor minister had deserted it again this time, and we found dragoons and soldiers doing their cooking and going about their ordinary business there; I ordered them to evacuate. At ten o'clock, the bell was rung for the *chasseurs* of the Guard, who were also filling the lodgings, to mount, so that we were able to take up residence in a room on the ground floor, the only one where there was some furniture left over from the previous and present ravages, and we were fine there. The *chasseurs* had already partly cooked their soup, and they were obliged to knock over the pots as they left; having neither meat, nor fire, nor utensils, we took advantage of their leftovers to make our dinner, which was good, with a piece of ham, which was slightly rancid and which we added to the half-cooked cow that we found in the room, and some herrings bought from a *cantinière*. There was no shortage of good white wine from Heilsberg. We had *M.* Larrey and *M.* Marchand, the *ordonnateur*-in-chief of the VI Corps, for dinner. *M.* Yvan came too late; we could only give him butter and good bread with a bottle of good Bordeaux wine. Coffee and rum followed later.

It was said that the Emperor would leave at six o'clock; our surgeons had orders to leave in his wake.

In the evening, there was a terrible storm, mixed with rain and hail. Hail! The poor inhabitants of these regions have nothing to fear from this torment since their land has remained uncultivated and the few fields that they have been able to sow have been harvested to feed our horses. Our soldiers, sabre or bayonet in hand, are seen rummaging through the ground where potatoes have been planted and consider themselves happy to find some, which they revel in, in spite of their present poor quality; they lack food and the consignments are becoming more and more difficult because of the bad roads. As they churn up the earth, they often find hiding places, where the unfortunate peasants have buried chests full of belongings; I saw some this morning. In general, little escapes our skilful foragers, and if one gives spirit to women by locking them up, one is sure to give malice to men by sending them to the armies.

The Emperor, who was due to leave, is still here; he will spend the night at Eylau, and so will we, which will give us all a good rest.

14th – His Majesty spent the night at Eylau; everyone is ready to leave and we are waiting. The I Corps is filing out at six o'clock this morning. The whole army is going to Kœnigsberg, which will host it unhappily for more than a day. The wheat is being cut and harvested in great quantities; that spells the end for this poor area, but it will be even less to be pitied than some others because of its proximity to a large city and the sea. No food is being distributed: woe betide those who have not brought any! There is rain in the air; I can feel in my head, in my low mood, that there will be a storm.

We are leaving now. I do not know whom I will leave here.

We left after the rain, leaving *M. Geib, chirurgien-major* with two *sous-aides* in Eylau. The path is dreadful: there is no road; there are almost always woods and low-lying land filled with ravines and impassable pools. The equipages are suffering greatly.

At every moment, one meets nasty little bridges cast across muddy streams. We had to pass through the cannon, the carriages, the infantry, the cavalry, all mixed together and almost disorderly; it was turmoil not to know where we each were and to risk dying from the dangers into which we could be thrown with every step.

Having travelled a few leagues, we were joined by the *aide-major* Spouville, who was hurrying as fast as he could to obtain a box of instruments, saying that they had been fighting since dawn and that there were already many wounded who could not be helped, the ambulance caissons having been held up on the way. I gave him the box that he asked for, which fortunately I had on the carriage that was following us at a distance. We then saw wounded men arriving, on their way to the small town of Domnau, where two of our divisions of battlefield surgeons have established themselves, those of *M.* Baudry and *M.* Ristel-Huber; they were very useful there. We finally heard the cannon, but the shots were not very near. As the wounded were arriving in columns, I placed some surgeons at the corner of a wood to stop them, gather them there and have them bivouac, until they could be dressed and undergo their operations. Having seen the equipages of the VIII Corps stopped on this side of a small bridge and the surgeons Damiens and Berthod remaining with the ambulance caissons, which an aide-de-camp of His Majesty did not want to let cross in preference to the other vehicles – because the Emperor had prohibited it – with the exception of the artillery, I ordered these gentlemen to set to work treating the wounded that I was to send them, and it is indeed at this point that the majority of the dressings and operations were performed for three hours. On the other side, the principal Ulliac had put himself in a wood, closer to the battlefield, and it was there that the wounded of the VIII Corps were mostly directed. A few small divisional or regimental ambulances had been arranged in the surrounding area and the wounded were very good at telling us that they wanted to go to one place over another.

We arrived on the field where the Emperor was in the midst of his generals, following the movements of the troops that he had forward with his eye, giving orders and assembling a vast line of cavalry, ready to have it march; sometimes he walked alone, sometimes with one of his marshals. When a regiment arrived, he went to see it file past; his Foot Guard received his visit from one end to the other; he was wearing his grey redingote and seemed very busy. There was little gunfire then, but all the preparations were underway for a terrible battle. M. Maret was kind enough to come to me and tell me that he had presented my certificate of nomination to the Institute to His Majesty for his approval, which he had done with pleasure and enthusiasm. I could have gone to greet the Emperor, who always sees me with so much benevolence, but he was too busy with his preparations; for that matter, I had nothing very interesting to tell him of my arrangements, since our twelve ambulance caissons were halted as a result of his complete prohibition more than 3 leagues from the battlefield.

I visited a large red house, a cannon's range from the ground where the Emperor was stood and beyond the small river of ... I knew that the assembled *grenadiers* had their ambulance there under the direction of *M.* Bancel, who had dispatched young Spouville to me to obtain a case. Already the surgeons had received many wounded there on whom, because they were missing this case, they had been unable to operate; *M.* Bancel, having received it, had used it only once. I do not know why, since there were many cases that required its use around him. The divisions of battlefield surgeons under *M.* Dupont and *M.* Fizelbrand did not leave it idle: instead of one, they would have needed six, so much damage had been done to us by the cannonballs and grapeshot. The front of the house was strewn with the corpses of our wounded who had arrived at the ambulance dying; in the room on the ground floor, near and behind the door, was a heap of severed limbs; blood was streaming from all sides. The cries, the groans, the screams of the unfortunates brought in on ladders, muskets, poles, etc.; of those who asked to be operated on immediately; of those whom we were operating on. These signs of pain and distress, this heart-rending picture of misery, misfortune and suffering, which this haven of unhappy courage presented, all this was destined to upset me, and although for sixteen years I have seen nothing else, I cannot get used to these horrifying scenes. There were only surgeons everywhere, and no workers or *infirmiers*. The comrades of the poor wounded gave some of them something to drink, but most of them cried out because of thirst, and we could not assuage them. Almost all were on the ground or in the road, and yet roofs were already being disturbed for straw. A barn next to the bridge was beginning to fill up. I saw *M.* Dupont amputate the two legs of a young soldier, who is surviving.

After this visit, I returned to the field where I had left my horses. I saw the *fusiliers* of the Guard returning from the battlefield and feared that the centre would fold; *M.* Larrey, whom I met, told me that it was a feint to better manage the enemy's wings. He had imagined this measure, I believe; moreover, he was going forward to join the Guard and he was complaining greatly that he had not seen his caissons arrive. From the field where I had left my horses and my companions, we could see very clearly the movement of the troops, their manoeuvres and most of the details of the battle. The enemy lined the heights and had a line that stretched as far as the eye could see on the steep slope; our men faced them with a similar line, not including the forces arranged laterally and in all directions that were employed against them. At six o'clock, the gunfire, which at intervals had subsided, resumed with a renewed vigour; every weapon along the line was ablaze. Never has the bombardment been fiercer, nor the musketry more sustained. The enemy even threw fire pots to set fire to and blow up our caissons; they spared neither shells nor grapeshot. What artillery! And how well served it is! Our men have not ceded anything to it with respect to bravery; the Russians have only a courage of obedience, of servitude, of temperament; the French are fundamentally valiant.

The two sides attacked and defended themselves with incredible relentlessness; we held the battlefield, but it cost us quite dearly. General de Latour-Maubourg had his hand pierced by a high-calibre iron musket ball, which he then found in his glove. General Drouet received the same blow to his left foot. General Cohorn was struck in the thigh by a musket ball that was removed from under the skin. The aide-de-camp Huttin (of General Oudinot) was caught in the left shoulder by a cannonball that shattered everything, turned everything to pulp, and this brave young man will die in the night, for his lungs must have been crushed too. The colonel of the 76th was shot in the chest; the colonel of the 15th Regiment of the Line was shot in the leg. It would be impossible to count the number of wounded with which this battle has presented us: 100 surgeons worked all evening and all night; more than 160 amputations were performed, consuming a lot of linen and lint, taking an endless amount of work, and little by little we came to the end of this service, despite the weather and the difficulty posed by our location. Fortunately, at nine o'clock in the evening, one of our caissons came to us, which sustained us for more than an hour; the others followed during the night; those of the ambulances of the I Corps had lent us 30lb of lint and a good case of linen while we awaited the arrival of ours. The *chirurgien-major* Gama even had us drink beer in the middle of the fields, which was more fresh than pleasant; he gave us bread, cheese and ham, which made us feel better. Our principals are covered in blood and spent from fatigue: they have no food; I gave them a little brandy. All the houses, barns and stables in the surrounding area are full of wounded, all of whom have been dressed; we would need 500 wagons to transport them.

At eleven o'clock, I went with the *ordonnateur*-in-chief Mathieu-Faviers to ask His Highness the Major-General for fifty men on fatigue duty to serve as *infirmiers* and twenty-five *Gendarmes d'élite* for our armed force. His Majesty was walking on the wooden boards in front of a large fire, around which his officers and guards were standing, while sappers were hastily building him a small cabin of planks and straw, open at the front and facing the fire. I saw him put his handkerchief around his head, have his boots removed by his mamluk and lie down on his straw; he called me, greeted me very graciously, asked me how many wounded we had had, enquired about the generals who had been wounded and recommended all these brave men to me. I received the soldiers and *gendarmes*. His Majesty was exhausted; he chose only to have some broth that was warmed for him, accompanied by a glass of wine.

Amidst the hassle and chaos, we were lucky enough to find a room in the main ambulance, where we went to sleep at half past midnight. At three o'clock in the morning, all my men had risen and the dressings, which the night had caused us to suspend, were resumed everywhere.

15th – I have just encroached on today. I rose last, because, not being well covered and with a bundle of straw torn from the roofs for a pillow, I did not sleep well. The rest of the service is done: there are six large cauldrons on the fire; the wounded will have broth everywhere. I have seen many surgical cases. The cannonball wounds are almost all the same. A Russian major had his trachea torn open at the front by a musket ball; he is naked, speaks French well and is a very handsome man. He spent the night mixed in with our soldiers and theirs; I had them taken up to a room and laid down on good straw; he was dressed in front of me; already there is emphysema in his face and in his upper chest, but it will come to nothing and the wound is very curable. A few stitches could have been put in, but I preferred, given the state of contusion at the edges of the wound and how easy it was to close it by tilting the wounded man's head towards his chest, to keep to this position.

Yesterday we entered Friedland, a small town that has suffered horribly and near which was fought the memorable battle that will undoubtedly bear this name so contrary to the horrors of war.[1] It is full of dead and wounded Russians; the battlefield, which we are partly crossing in order to reach the town, is strewn with them; there must be no Guards left for the Russian emperor, for we found only the corpses of those killed. At this very moment, I am sending a division of surgeons to ensure that there are no more wounded Frenchmen on the field and to arrange a kind of service for the unfortunate Russians who remain in Friedland. *M.* Le Vert, who went with two surgeons-lieutenant to visit the battlefield, did not find a single wounded Frenchman there; he saw thirty or forty Russians among the thousands of corpses. The enemy has lost spectacularly; more than a hundred pieces of cannon have been taken from them. *M.* Le Vert gave a summary of his mission to Grand-Marshal Duroc, who was satisfied with it. We are moving three or four of our French wounded from the lodgings intended for His Majesty, after they settled there. This was a great event, and one that must, or never will, lead us towards peace. We are assured that we will be in Kœnigsberg tomorrow.

We left, after our rustic dinner made in the orchard of the ambulance, at around two o'clock. It is only a short league from the hospital to Friedland, and we have to cross, or rather travel alongside, the battlefield, which has hardly extended further than the road. So many dead, so many dying, so many corpses! One pities even the unfortunate horses, which die beside their masters, whose sad fate they share, having been part of their fatigues and dangers. I came across one of Emperor Alexander's Guards, whose two legs were broken and folded back on themselves; this unfortunate man was lying in a pool of blood and his head was resting on his cartridge box. He

---

1. Longin: *Friede*, peace, *land*, country.

wanted only to live and showed how thirsty he was; it is known that the wounded who have lost a lot of blood need something to drink above all else. A young postal clerk went to fetch him some water, which he drank with a kind of fury. I ordered that he should be lifted from the ground and have both his legs amputated, which may save him: *M.* Dupont performed this operation twice on the day of the battle. I cannot guess how many other unfortunates were in the same position as this one, nor the extent of the losses sustained by the Russian Guards, and the soldiers and cavalrymen of this army; the number of fatalities must approach that of Austerlitz. We found the headquarters gone and I was unable to enjoy my lodgings, which had been reserved for me in the morning at the home of *Madame* Fontheim, the wife of a Prussian surgeon who had remained in Dantzig. This lady has four pretty daughters of 16, 15, 14 and 13 years of age; our men have broken and looted everything in her house. This devastated family began to cry again when they saw me, for they have not stopped wailing for forty-eight hours; I calmed them a little. The commanding officer, Dentzel, was kind enough to come with me to assure these ladies of all the care that we would show them and to pledge his support and help to them; I wanted to offer them money; I did not dare. The surgeons that I have left in Friedland will stay with them and will be useful to them; they have orders to have all the Russian troops on the ground gathered, to bring them together in a building and to help them as best they can. This operation is already underway thanks to the commanding officer, and we have seen the *chasseurs* who are to garrison the town bringing back several of these miserable victims of a ferocious war on wooden planks and ladders. In most of the houses and under all the roofs and eaves, some of these people are lying in the street or on the ground. Some wounded French officers have withdrawn to the town: there will be enough surgeons to dress them. We left Friedland at half past four. We travelled until eight o'clock, following or preceding the equipages and columns of troops who were heading for Wehlau, where, it was said, His Majesty was due to spend the night. When we arrived at 5 short leagues from the point of departure, we saw the Guard, the cavalry and some regiments of infantry stopped and preparing to bivouac. We could have gone further; but we did not know precisely where the general headquarters would be and, besides, it was important to us that we allowed our caissons time to arrive. Therefore, in spite of the crowd, which is always bothersome, and despite the barrenness of the area, where everything was to be lacking, we dismounted and took a barn, writing 'Ambulance' on all the doors. The Guard soon took the straw from the roofs of the neighbouring barns and houses; we did the same for our own purposes, but it was necessary to defend our barn, for they were constantly trying to climb onto its roof. I showed myself and sent away those who were taking the straw, as well as the ones who were collecting wood, who came in turns to tear down two large buttresses supporting a wall face of our poor lodging. I saw the Secretary of State and the Intendant-general pass by. I spoke with them, offering them a place in our covered bivouac, but with no guarantee of a drink, which made them laugh; we did indeed have something to give them, for at my supper I drank, over two tartines[2] of butter, two good cups of excellent red wine. We spread out our straw to lie down, numbering twenty-five or thirty; they wanted to choose a good place for me, and accordingly I was put next to a rotten corpse that I could smell all night and from which I could not move away because I could not see, and I feared that I would be even worse elsewhere, for it stank everywhere. This barn was a sheep shed with a layer of dung more than a foot high. I was fully dressed; I had kept my tail and my tie. At midnight, I could no longer stand it: I was burning and my head and neck were sore from leaning against a very hard bale of hay. I rose, removed my clothes, undid my tie and tail, put my saddle blanket under my head as a pillow and returned to bed, hardly able to support myself, so sleepy or numb was I. The stench of death lingered with me for a long time.

In the hamlet where we bivouacked, there was neither drinking water nor an inhabited house: our men were lacking everything. I saw young soldiers drinking foul pond water and devouring rotting meat and sprouted potatoes, for which they went to look in the newly disturbed land that they came across. The army is hungry: if the enemy could keep it in this region for a few days, it would die of misery.

Our carriages arrived before midnight. Tomorrow we will need them. The night is mild and excellent.

16th – I slept well on my straw and beside my dead body, which I chose not to disturb, nor uncover; sleep has restored me well. While I was savouring the sweetness of it, those who were taking the straw from the roofs were at work on ours; fortunately, the straw from it seemed too old for them. They were content to tear out the parts that had been placed at the end of the winter

---

2. Slices of bread, typically with butter or jam.

to fill in a few holes, which means that our premises could still be used as an ambulance if we were to fight within range.

When I rose at five o'clock, my young friend prepared two tartines, a glass of my good red wine and (would you believe it?) a cup of coffee: judge, dear reader, if I had a good breakfast. I dressed and groomed myself, and at six o'clock we left for Wehlau. His Majesty stayed the night there, or at least not very far away. It is a small town, near to which passes the River Alle. Over the river there is a bridge that is still burning; the army is waiting in magnificent meadows and beautiful countryside for another to be built, a little further upstream, opposite a fine castle where the Emperor is with his generals, having crossed on a boat. We dismounted in a meadow near the river and the new bridge; we unbridled the horses and went around the surrounding area, looting where we could, and my surgeons brought back dried fruit, rose-hip or blueberry jam, powdered coffee and utensils. We made the fire by a stream, on the other side of which I am writing all these details, resting the notebook against my knee, so that I remember them one day and to make me feel more exquisitely the price of peace. Not that today we are unhappy. The soup is being made; yesterday we bought a good fat hen from a soldier; our surgeons have a lamb that has just been skinned and the weather is as fine as anywhere. I shaved in the middle of the meadow (the sun is not yet showing). My little mirror was positioned against my hat, placed on top of my rolled-up clothes to raise it up; I drew water from the stream in a bad earthen dish and, after scraping thoroughly with my blunt razor, I borrowed *M.* Le Vert's, which finished the job well. I washed in the stream, the water from which does not flow on a bed of gold, far from it: the whole country is low and marshy.

The heat is extreme and there will be a storm. We are firing on the right and left, but only very sporadically, and the enemy has not resisted the construction of our bridge, the completion of which the whole army is awaiting. It seems that we will go to Tapiau this evening and that we want to squeeze the enemy into this small area of country that surrounds Kœnigsberg and which, blocked by us from the direction that we are following, will become their prison or their tomb. I gave a botany lesson to our surgeons while waiting for dinner and for the bridge to be ready: a leader must take advantage of everything while on campaign to arouse emulation and to educate. There are no distinctive plants in this country. Wormwood grows everywhere.

I had *M.* Mayot extract the left eye of a young *chasseur*, out of whose orbit it was all in the form of a large blood clot. This wounded man had been hit, he said, by a musket ball to the temple. I judged that this foreign body, which had indeed entered through the angle of the coronal, had stopped in the orbit and had pushed the organ out. When this was removed, we found a rather large biscayan that had embedded itself in the internal angle of the eye, breaking everything in its path and ahead of it; its extraction was difficult. This poor young man will recover, if he is well cared for.

We had a good dinner, but the bridge is not complete: it is said that it will not be ready for a few hours. While I was eating on the grass and in the middle of a small willow bush covered with my clothes and handkerchiefs to keep me cool, a young soldier looked at me with a kind of bashful avarice: I offered him my soup, which he ate with a pleasure that amused me. He thanked me well. The sun set two hours ago; it is hot and there is no other shelter than the one I have made for myself; it is only modest, but the sun cannot enter it. It is said that two corps of our cavalry and part of the reserve have passed the Pregel by swimming or at a ford, with water up to their waists. The enemy can be seen on the right bank and we can hear a few cannon shots: it is a pity that the bridge is not ready; the troops are restless, and so are we.

I do not know where we will sleep, or what will become of us. I do not think I have ever been hotter in France; I am sweating blood and water. Here, the rye is in the ears and tall; the wheat is still budding and the oats are beginning to come up. The Emperor worked this morning for more than an hour at the bridge over the Pregel, with his axe in his hand; from there he sought shade in the surrounding area, drank a glass of red wine and had something to eat. He then swam across the river, his horse being up to its back in water; at present, he is in the town. Of fifteen soldiers who were going to this town and who crossed the river in a boat, nine were drowned; they were from the 32nd Infantry of the Line.

It is a pleasant thing to see a hundred thousand men marching on foot, on horseback, in carriages filing past, with a ravine to pass and hurrying to get there first, arguing, insulting each other, threatening each other with their sabres, sometimes fighting each other. From the depths of my little shelter I am enjoying this curious spectacle; I have seen the *cuirassiers* stopping the artillery by using their sabres against the horses' noses and the officers of the artillery and baggage train shouting to the soldiers driving the horses to crush the cavalry. Then a general arrives, strikes one, using his sabre against the other. They are continuing to pass, and I see all this without any dust, or obstacles, or fatigue, for I am sitting down, with my notebook in my hand.

## 1807 (continued) – Friedland and Tilsit

But what horrible heat! Everyone is sweating, wiping their heads; there is not the slightest wind and no shade. The months of June and July are extremely hot in this area; nature balances this by bringing longer winters and the early onset of autumn; moreover, the harvests are very plentiful in these regions.

At eight o'clock, the bridge was still not finished and we were unable to enter the town, except by crossing the river, almost by swimming. I decided to retire to a large house a quarter of an hour away. I found it already ravaged by all kinds of people eating and drinking all around; we were about to arrange ourselves there when General Nansouty and seven other generals came to lodge there, so I chose a room for myself and placed our surgeons in a kind of large kitchen, where they have fared very well. A huge ham and a 12lb loaf of bread intended for the generals took a wrong turn and entered my room by mistake, from where, out of an excess of kindness and tenderness, I did not want them to leave; we found their company very pleasant and we ate it with them unpretentiously.

At ten o'clock, the bridge collapsed and more than 12,000 cavalrymen flooded into the unfortunate house. I made my bed on straw and a good feather quilt, and after saying a final word to the dear ham and drinking lemonade made from a shrivelled old lemon and enhanced with a glass of red wine, I fell asleep.

17th – It was not until five o'clock this morning that I began to hear any noise: I had been surrounded by the horses and bivouacs all night, but my sleep was so deep that I heard nothing. We rose, saw to our horses and equipages, and set off for Wehlau, where the Emperor and the main headquarters had spent the night. In order to reach the town, we had to cross the River Alle at a very deep ford, which the horses had to swim across in some places. It had been said that there were many wounded in the town; there were only eight or ten, for whom I left a surgeon there. On my way from my lodgings to those of *M.* Le Vert, His Majesty shouted to me from his window: '*M.* Percy, come up here.' He asked me many questions, treated me with particular kindness, allowed me to walk beside him for more than a quarter of an hour, and appeared to be very cheerful and in perfect health. He informed me, with the enthusiasm and pleasure that one has in telling good news to a friend, that 150,000 English rifles had been found at Kœnigsberg, to where they had just been shipped; that the surrender of this place would re-equip the army perfectly; that the Battle of Friedland had been fought on the same day as that of Marengo; and that there was not much left to do now. We spoke of the wounded, the wounds, the industry of the soldiers, the good meals they can occasionally make, the bad ones they make most often, and then he remarked that he needed a lot of food; that everyone in the army, starting with him, ate or had an appetite four times greater than usual, which is easy to explain because of the fatigues that one experiences, the little sleep that one enjoys and the losses caused by sweating. I add that, since the extremely coarse bread that we eat is hardly nourishing, it is necessary to eat more often. Finally, the Emperor said some very kind things to me about the way in which our service was performed. I praised the skill and the precious practice of our surgeons, who alone do everything or can do everything; I took care to recommend to him this class, which is so important and so devoted, and to make him feel how dangerous it would be, in peace, to disperse it and reform its members. Against custom, I took leave of His Majesty without waiting for him to send me away, saying, as he usually does: 'That's good.' In my profession, I am always supposed to be very busy and, indeed, I can be forgiven for having sinned against a custom of etiquette.

I sent the principal surgeon Capiomont to all the lines and places where he will be able to place wounded and surgeons, in order to put the service in order and to provide me with accurate notes of what is happening behind us. We left at ten o'clock. Wehlau is a small, rather nice town where there was plenty of affluence and commerce, but our people have laid waste to it: wine, beer, sugar, everything has been looted from the houses and cellars, which one enters from the outside near the front doors of the houses. To leave the town we must cross the river again; I crossed it on a long boat that is taking the place of a bridge for people on foot, and our horses were led by hand over the ford, which is as deep as the other. The country is beautiful, and the road that will lead us to Memel, for that is where we are going, is unusually well looked after and maintained. We met Russian prisoners, two-thirds of whom were well-dressed soldiers and the other third were Tartars, Kalmyks – devils, indeed. I have never seen anyone more ugly in my life; they are black and smoky, with a fur cap on their heads and clothes made of black sheepskin. His Majesty stopped after two hours in a castle on the road by which the V Corps is marching. We also stopped and took a rather poor house, where my hussars (I am referring to my young surgeons) soon provided me with dry hay, curdled milk – that I found delicious – potatoes, a goose, etc. The country is good and the army will live well here. The army's route will henceforth be from Kœnigsberg, via Braunsberg, Elbing, Marienbourg, etc., to Berlin; all the other routes and hospitals not part of this line will be moved in this direction, although Marienwerder will remain.

It is extremely hot, but there is some wind. I shout to our soldiers: 'Children, run after vinegar rather than schnapps and mix it with your water.' Wherever I can find vinegar, I put it in large tubs and they drink it as they pass by.

After waiting several hours in our village, we set off again, leaving a good old woman of 82 – blind in one eye, toothless, but active and intelligent – in the poor house where we were staying. Her children and grandchildren fled when the French approached; she remained, unable to follow them, or persuaded that we would take pity on her old age, or not paying much heed to the life that she will soon leave. We took good care of this good old woman; we entertained her and protected her. The soldiers had already killed four of her little pigs; we saved two of them with the sow and the male. It was nearly six o'clock when we left: we are not following the road to Tapiau, as we had thought; at least the centre of the army is marching on the Memel[3] in a straight line. The Emperor, who has dined well and had his siesta in the small castle of the village, is passing at the moment.

We arrived at nine o'clock, in a village called …, where His Majesty has found a good farm and will sleep there. We are arranging ourselves in a large house that has been absolutely ravaged; we are taking the straw from one roof and, in an hour, beast and men, everyone will go to bed.

18th – I slept excellently on my straw, in a corner of the room that I had appropriated, swept and cleared, as the whole house is soiled with excrement and the debris of broken furniture. Our horses have fared quite well. My men, caisson and carriage are not coming; there is no talk yet of leaving. The weather is extremely hot: it will rain; a few drops are already falling. This country is not salubrious; it is full of ponds.

We travelled 5 leagues through rather beautiful countryside and found some fairly good villages, in which the soldiers have committed all kinds of brigandage. His Majesty stopped for half an hour on a hillock, both to observe his Foot Guard and to give it time to arrive, having allowed it to make soup; from there he went to a village on the right, where he also stopped for a while. As for us, we made our way to the next village and arranged ourselves in a rather nice house, in the middle of a garden, near the road. We were already sweeping and laying claim to it when the quartermaster of the court came to earmark it for the Emperor, who was to come to sleep in the village; he left us

---

3. Longin: Percy refers to the Neman under this name.

a room in it, where four of us are to sleep. It is pouring down; the bivouacs are in a bad way.

Shortly before the arrival of the Emperor, someone came to tell us that black hussars could be seen within a cannon's range of us; a *chasseur* of the Guard, a correspondence officer, confirmed this report. Immediately we started to bridle the horses and our surgeons came to place themselves in a battle line in front of my lodgings, hoping to punish the Russians who would have the audacity to disturb us, but a reconnaissance that we had sent to look for them found, instead of Russians, French *chasseurs* who were out pillaging.

His Majesty arrived soaked to the skin and galloping at full speed. I recognized that the Lutheran church very close to us would be an excellent place to stay and that in its galleries we could sleep more than a hundred people. Our surgeons have veal, geese, mutton, etc.; we have a feast similar to that of a wedding. Fortunately, I found two good candles in the church. My caisson is not coming and I am finding that extremely difficult.

19th – It has rained and is still raining. The whole army is converging on the same point and is leaving immediately.

We marched together, at first with the III Corps; but having found, on the left, a rather beautiful path that seemed to deviate a little from the road, we followed it and strayed more than a league. The countryside is quite beautiful, although marshy everywhere. I saw rye 5ft high, beautiful hemp, superb fields of flax, many fields of potatoes. The villages are surrounded by trees; each house has its own pasture, orchard and shade. These people must be happy during times of peace; everywhere there are flocks of sheep, pigs and geese; there are many poultry. The surgeons of the Guard and our own stopped to collect supplies; everyone had their own hen and goose. We found several soldiers who were also stocking up on provisions, but with less consideration than us; they had taken bread, and in this country the bread is black, red, bitter and coarse. However, the inhabitants are good-looking, robust and tall; the unfortunates had almost all left with their children and their linen; we saw many returning with their packages, and some cowardly and ruthless soldiers made them set them down, in order to take the most beautiful effects. I chased one away, calling him the most despicable names.

We had to return to the road; a good peasant set us back on our way. It was then that we saw some infantrymen who were demanding that two trumpeters and two unarmed Russian uhlans, who were deserting, dismount; they also took their money. Seeing us run towards them, these deserters invoked our protection and the despoilers ran away at full gallop; they had the effrontery to tell Marshal Davout, whom they met, that these Russians had shot at them, and that they had treated them in their turn as enemies: a false report that I refuted.

Having made another league, and the road being busy with troops, we halted in an orchard. Our horses ate well there.

After three hours' march, we saw the town of Tilsit, a rather beautiful place where we shrewdly managed to find lodgings in a fairly good house, all full of hunchbacked young ladies who deafened us with their masculine and Prussian voices. As soon as I had set down my belongings, I went to see the Memel, at the end of our street; the bridge has been entirely destroyed and the Russian army is on the other side, bathing and trying to rest a little. The bridge was burned this morning; the enemy was withdrawing all night. Eight hundred French prisoners were brought to this town three months ago; the most able-bodied were then taken further; 200 of those who remained have died; today there are forty-nine of them in the fine cavalry barracks, near the gate opposite the river. I have just ordered a division of battlefield surgeons to serve this hospital, which is going to increase greatly in size. Most of these poor Frenchmen are phthisic as a result of the bad treatment that they have suffered at the hands of the Prussians, who have cravenly abused them, beaten them and deprived them of all help. There is not a bad word, threat or barbarous act with which the Prussians have not treated these brave people, while the Russians showed themselves to be generous, compassionate and affectionate towards them. Therefore, we now look favourably on the Russians and hate the Prussians as braggarts, and that is the opinion of the Russians themselves. The way of feeding our men is to give them all indiscriminately a bowlful of clear slop made with flour, water and salt; at the same time, they are given butter for the day. At dinner, they have a small piece of meat, which is usually veal, with some bread and a little wine. In the evening, they receive a large bowl of oatmeal or barley gruel: they are free to eat their butter in their soup or on their bread. They are given a straw mattress on top of a pile of logs, a pair of sheets and a good woollen blanket. The Prussians kept them confined to the hospital: Grand Duke Konstantin let them out and gave them money; in the town, they could work, but the Prussians took most of the fruits of their labour away from them. The French army hates the Prussians; this feeling has become almost universal.

20th – This morning, I went to the barracks and spoke with all our sick prisoners: the joy of seeing the army again and of being handed over to it has made a favourable impression on most of them. The *sous-aide* Gallette, of a battalion of the wagon train, was taken on the 10th, near Landsberg, while he was on his way to join me; he was with several officers, some of whom were wounded. The Prussians treated them horribly, but the Russians welcomed them and the Grand Duke Konstantin rendered them all sorts of services; he often joked with them and on the way he occasionally made his officers descend from their carriages in order to have our prisoners ride in them. Gallette saw the good *M.* Goercke, my colleague in the Imperial army, in Kœnigsberg. He received him well, talked with him for a long time and lent him money.

Yesterday and today, several distinguished Russians came to discuss an armistice; our Major-General crossed the river and went to the enemy camp with the same intention, but it seems that nothing has yet been decided.

I have just received more than 250 ministerial messages. It has been extremely hot today. My caisson has arrived.

21st – The weather is gloomy and the wind is westerly; it will rain. The army is bivouacking around, or rather behind, the town: it is hungry; how will it be fed for another eight days? Biscuits are arriving; there is no shortage of meat, but the French want bread and, however bad it is, they need it. I am well and my lodgings are good, although I am sharing them with a colonel of the artillery of the Guard (Dauguereau), whose servants are a great burden to our hosts. Besides that, this colonel is a very amiable man, who, like me, does not demand good food and prefers beer to wine. We each have our own bed in the same room. There is talk of peace, and already we are being assured that the preliminaries have been signed. We went to the banks of the river to see the Russian army. We found six hussars of this army, who were guarding a small boat, on which a Russian prince sent as an envoy had just crossed; one of them, a sergeant, speaks French well and displays a great deal of erudition. *M.* Béclard spoke with him for a long time. Our Emperor seems satisfied. The two armies are equally eager for peace. Everything will be alright.

22nd – The rain is cold and falling heavily; the troops are wet. The sick are arriving in droves. I have had buildings identified to house 300 more of them; the town is doing what it can to provide us with supplies. There is more talk than ever of peace, and it is certain that, having received and treated the Russian envoys perfectly, our Emperor sent Grand-Marshal Duroc to the Emperor Alexander, from whom he is yet to return. There is no doubt of peace.

I have sent the division of the *chirurgien-major* Baudry to Wehlau, Friedland, Heilsberg, Preuss-Eylau, etc. in order to initiate the service, to have the wounded Russians treated and to help the surgeons, perhaps too few in number, whom I have left in these towns. This division will meet with that of *M.* Tainturier at the ambulance of the Maison-Rouge, on the battlefield. The two will come to an agreement so that the evacuations will be carried out regularly and such that surgical assistance will not be lacking for the wounded.

I have worked all day and sent out more than fifty letters or parcels; I have received 280 ministerial messages, which I am distributing or sending. I learned today of the death of three of my colleagues: I am losing many of them. This is the sad consequence of the overcrowding of the hospitals and the state of misery in which they are abandoned. Wine is lacking everywhere; in some hospitals, only beer is available. There are no pharmacists or doctors: the apothecaries are miserable speculators who only appear when we capture cities and they hope to obtain quinine, opium and other expensive items there.

I have left my lodgings, where, since the departure of Colonel Dauguereau, I was well off, to occupy one still better, in which they seemed to me to be very mean. There are four women in the house, three of whom are pregnant, and yet the only man is in his sixties; the mother, a daughter (a maiden) and a young servant are all bearing a child. My move was soon completed.

23rd – It has rained a lot; it is still pouring down and the weather is so cold that I am tempted to light a fire.

The murmurs of peace are continuing; everyone is pleased to be returning to France. If unfortunately the army were to be ordered to cross the Memel to pursue the Russians and continue the campaign, I do not know what would come of it, so great is the desire to leave, so inclined to homesickness are we. Without exception, from His Majesty, or at least from the marshals, to the drummers, the whole army is asking to see France again.

The town where we are staying is called Tilsit: it is quite beautiful for the country; the streets are long and well-spaced and there are some pretty houses, but the cobbles are awful. They are huge stones or blocks of granite, such as one finds in the fields, which have been laid in a fashion next to one another, so that it is difficult to walk and one could hardly do so without breaking one's neck if one stopped paying attention for a moment. In the middle of the street there is a line of boulders, larger than the others, on which it is possible to walk by hopping from one to the other; I think that during the winter this sort of path is useful, because of the floods. The Memel is a beautiful river: it is two-thirds the width of the Rhine; its blue waters are always moving and flow rapidly; it does not appear to be deep, since the bridge that the Russians burned was on fairly weak piles with wooden spurs to protect them from the ice floes. The cavalry barracks built a few years ago in Tilsit are quite beautiful; it is a pity that behind it there are dark cesspools and foul ponds. The latrines are emptied into the pits, which are always full of rubbish, stagnant water and excrement. There is a fairly large trade in wooden planks here; besides that, the town is poor and has little trade.

The number of patients is multiplying in a very troublesome way for us, since we can neither evacuate them nor give them supplies. At half past seven the cannon was to be fired in celebration of the signing of the preliminaries, but everything is quiet and this has raised doubts about whether it has been signed. The bivouacs are suffering greatly. The weather is extremely bad.

24th – It has rained all night; it is very windy and the rain starts again sporadically. Everyone is telling their own story about the peace: yesterday it was certain, today it is very doubtful; they say that the court is sad and wistful. I have not seen anyone for three days: I am drowning in papers up to my braces; while the others can rest, I continue to suffer, and only the nature of the torments has changed. Writing is a very big one for me: no matter how much I tear up and burn the papers, I always have new piles of them on my table.

This morning they go so far as to say that last night they were on the point of sounding the drums to make the army leave. I do not believe any of it, but things do not seem to be moving very quickly; it is true that there is a conflict of interests and discussions; it is a case of saying: *sat cito, si sat benè*.[4]

We have many patients.

25th – It is still raining. This morning, big news! I have been brought the preliminary peace treaty, or rather the armistice signed by the two emperors; the public papers will make it known. It is a great step towards a solid and presentable peace.

But there is something else! A wooden building on rafts is being hastily built on the Memel, opposite the centre of the town; it is to be finished by noon and the two sovereigns are to meet there. Everyone is waiting; people come and go, wondering if it is true, if it is not a fiction. As we wait, the building is

---

4. 'Soon enough, if but well enough.'

being finished, covered with cloth, decorated inside, and on both sides of the river a boat is being repaired to take the crowned heads to the meeting.

At half past twelve, the banks of the river were lined on both sides with troops. The emperors climbed into the boats; that of Napoleon was decorated with greenery; it arrived first. His Majesty waited five minutes for Alexander, greeted him affectionately as soon as he was close, and hurried to welcome him as soon as he set foot on the raft. The Imperial Marshals and several important Russians accompanied their sovereigns. The meeting lasted an hour and a half. The two emperors were alone; at the end of the session, they received all the men surrounding the wooden house inside; while it was ongoing, Grand Duke Konstantin talked with the Grand Duke of Berg, making large gestures. We paid close attention to everything that was happening. At about two o'clock, the two sides separated. The emperors said farewell warmly; their boats sailed together for a moment, then one went to the right and the other to the left, putting the two sovereigns ashore, amidst cheering from the Russians on one side and the French on the other. Our Emperor appeared quite satisfied. It was truly a charming and interesting spectacle; the rain had ceased and the sun seemed to come out intentionally to enhance these two memorable hours.

It seems that Alexander and Napoleon are getting on well, respect each other and are well-matched; we are all joyful and are already counting the distance we have to travel to return to France.

This evening, it is assured that Alexander will come tomorrow with his Guard to occupy one half of the city and that our Emperor will stay in the other; everything has been arranged accordingly. What an event! Perhaps peace will even be concluded at Tilsit and will be signed by the emperors themselves, who will thereby set a great example to the universe and a great lesson to posterity.

I am being moved out, but with great consideration, for the Prince of Benevento, who is arriving tomorrow.

The weather is still terrible: the rain is continuing; the bivouacs are faring worse than ever. The distributions are going badly. They are being made to the Guard; yesterday they were given three rations of wine that I thought were intended for our hospitals in the town, where at the moment we have 600 sick. Seven or eight physicians, five of whom are principals, are scattered across the town, but it is our surgeons alone who run the service; none, except that of the reserve, has even set foot in our hospitals. Tomorrow I will force them to go to work, or I will have them expelled from the town. We have been provided with 400 vacant straw mattresses and a few shirts; we still have no blankets;

fortunately, we have been able to obtain some straw. Among our sick, there are 160 men of the Guard.

I sent twelve surgeons three days ago to go to all the places through which the army has passed, in order to gather the sick and wounded who escaped our first searches. They went to Wehlau, Friedland, Preuss-Eylau, Heilsberg, etc., providing help and assistance everywhere and reinforcing the surgical divisions already established in these places. Tomorrow the 7th Division of battlefield surgery is leaving to follow the same route; it will be accompanied by a *commissaire des guerres* and a principal director, who are taking food, brandy, wine, medicines, material for dressings, and are carrying 3,000lb, so that I can hope that in a few days, especially if we are given vehicles, the wounded will be transported away. Some of them, the poor amputees and those with fractures, will go to Heilsberg; others will go to Marienbourg and other good hospitals. The 5,000 wounded Russians who are gathered at Friedland will undoubtedly fall to the charge of their government, which will relieve us of the gruelling and distressing responsibility of feeding and treating them; there are many very seriously wounded men among them.

26th – I moved out this morning, and came to find my old hostesses, the hunchbacks. We are happy to have a shelter: the French now only have half the town; the other half has been given over to the Russians. It is quite a nice day; the sun is even hot and it was about time that this change took place, for the sick are increasing in number by the day.

We have some cases of dysentery, which would have made terrible progress if the cold rains, after such hot days, had continued; we are treating a lot of throat infections and the intermittent fevers are overwhelming us. Tomorrow we will evacuate on foot 250 sick people who can walk, and about 400 who need to be transported on four boats; these boats will go down the Memel to the Friedrichs-Graben (canal);[5] they will then reach the Pregel and thus arrive at Kœnigsberg. From this town, nearly 200 wounded and sick were evacuated to Dantzig by the Kurrische-Haff.[6] The surgeons have been ordered to board the boats and go in advance to the staging posts where they will have to stop to rest. It must be 50 leagues by water from here to Kœnigsberg. The 26th will

---

5. A canal system on the Curonian Lagoon; it indirectly connects the Pregel and Memel rivers, via the Deima and Matrosovka. Work started on the first canal between these two latter rivers in 1671.
6. The Curonian Lagoon.

be forever remembered as the day that the Russian Emperor made his entrance into Tilsit, where he is planning to spend a few days. A beautiful apartment has been prepared for him in the part of the city that has been assigned to him. At noon, yesterday's meeting was repeated, but the wooden house in the middle of the Memel was finished, well painted, well decorated inside and bedecked on the outside with green festoons; above the door on the Russian side was the letter 'A' in greenery; similarly, above the door on our side was the letter 'N' in greenery. All around the raft was a balustrade covered with draperies with garlands of oak and leaves, because we do not have any olive trees. Green trees shaded the house and the hut; the latter was intended for the marshals and the senior officers of the two sovereigns' entourages. The sight was charming. The Russians were in full dress; part of our Emperor's Mounted Guard was also there. At a quarter past noon, the boats, which had been decked out in white, as a sign of peace, and decorated with greenery, brought the emperors from one bank to the other, to applause from the two armies; they shook hands and greeted each other amicably. The King of Prussia, I am assured, was with Alexander and our Emperor embraced him. The latter had at his side the plaque of the Prussian order and those of our marshals who are decorated with it took it back today. The meeting lasted an hour and three quarters, like that of yesterday; they separated as they had done yesterday and each army received its emperor to a thousand repeated cries of '*Vive!*' and '*Vivat!*'.

Several French officers were allowed to pass through the Russian camp to see the Cossacks, the Kalmyks and other soldiers little known to us. These latter troops are badly dressed; they wear a sort of capuchin robe tied around the middle; most of them have beards; their eyes are small and slanted like those of the Chinese; they are armed with a bow and a quiver, which is useless nowadays. A considerable detachment of Alexander's Guard has arrived here: these are specially chosen men, from eight to nine inches tall at least,[7] and they look even taller because of their shako topped with a huge feather; they have white cloth trousers and ankle boots, like all the Russian soldiers, which is not the best footwear for men who are obliged to march.

At four o'clock, the whole of our Emperor's Guard, in full military dress, formed two lines from his lodgings to the port. Alexander came out at five o'clock, with his brother and two or three lords from his court. Our Emperor

---

7. Percy perhaps means 'feet' rather than 'inches'. However, he uses 'inches' in several places to describe height.

had gone to meet him; he gave him his hand and displayed a great deal of gallantry and, above all, cheerfulness. Alexander mounted one of His Majesty's beautiful horses and the shining procession went between the two rows of superb troops to our Emperor's house, where a great dinner had been prepared; the marshals who followed the Emperors dazzled with gold and embroidery and I do not believe that, even on a parade day in Paris, the Guard could look more beautiful. The Emperor Alexander is 30 or 32 years old: he is a handsome man; he must be at least 4 or 5ft tall; he is blond and has white skin; his face, without being very beautiful, has something distinguished about it; he is fat; his eyes are lively; he has a military bearing and is full of confidence. He smiles, greets and speaks pleasantly. He is wearing a simple, pale blue outfit with his decorations, and a large Russian hat with a black plume. His brother, Grand Duke Konstantin, is shorter, stockier; he has the features, and above all the nose, of his father Paul; he talks, moves a lot, laughs and frolics like a second lieutenant. He wears a square cap, a white pelisse and long stable trousers.

27th – We sent out our four boats carrying nearly 400 sick people with food for three or four days; a *chirurgien-major* and three *sous-aides* left with this great and beautiful evacuation. Two hundred patients have left to return to their regiments or to go on foot to Kœnigsberg. I dispatched surgeons everywhere, so that the sick and wounded can find assistance everywhere.

There was a fine manoeuvre by the Foot Guard; the emperors and the Grand Duke were present. I was curious to see them return: they came back at full gallop. The Guard outdid itself; Alexander was delighted. We are living in the greatest harmony with the Russians; everything is going very well. The King of Prussia is ill; it was indeed he who was seen entering the barracks yesterday. I saw *M.* Benningsen, who is not handsome. In general, the Russian Emperor's retinue is not superb. There is a lot of talk about our forthcoming departure.

28th – *Buona notte*. The sun came out in the morning, but it has still rained almost all day at more or less infrequent intervals; it even hailed. At one o'clock, a large room made from wooden planks was built, in which the officers of the Guard will entertain their Russian counterparts. The Guard of our Emperor has received a triple distribution to entertain that of His Majesty Alexander on its side. I believe it is this very evening that it is to be done. There is a great operation underway.

The King of Prussia passed the Memel, followed by a single officer; we had gone to meet him on the banks of the river, but he did not disembark at the point where we were expecting him, and he thus found himself left behind and waited, not without distress, for more than twenty minutes for someone to come at last to get him out of this awkward situation. Alexander was the first to arrive; he gave him his hand; they mounted their horses and went down to the home of His Russian Majesty, from where they went to see Napoleon, who came to meet them on the front doorstep. Poor William is very thin. He wears a blue uniform with two or three silver buttonholes on the collar and trims; he has a Russian-style shako with a black plume, which makes him look even longer or, if you like, taller. Overall, he has a sad face and looks so melancholic that everyone is inclined to feel sorry for him. Our Emperor treats him more with kindness than distinction; he did not receive the welcome and the delicate and gallant honours lavished on Alexander, but also the Prussians did nothing but foolish things.

I have written a statement of presentation of thirty candidates for an award. It is as follows:

> List of surgeons in the Grande Armée who have particularly merited, during the campaign, that His Majesty deigns to grant them an award.
>
> CHÉDIEU, *chirurgien-major*, the decoration of the Legion of Honour.
>
> GALLÉE, principal surgeon, -- -- .
>
> LAROCHE, *chirurgien-major*, the decoration of the Legion of Honour.
>
> LEPROUST, --      --      -- .
>
> BANCEL, the elder, --      --      -- .
>
> COLS, --      --      -- .
>
> LE ROY, --      --      -- .
>
> LECLERC, --      --      -- .
>
> LACOURNÈRE, PICARD, --    --      -- .
>
> CHARMEIL, *chirurgien-major*, to be named to the 4th Regiment of the Line.

| | | |
|---|---|---|
| LE VERT (Marcel), -- | -- | 24th -- . |
| DAMIENS, -- | -- | 34th -- . |
| BARRÈRE, -- | -- | 48th -- . |
| MULTON, -- | -- | 55th -- . |
| FAURE, -- | -- | 69th -- . |
| FOUILLOTTE, -- | -- | 95th -- . |
| BOYER, -- | -- | 15th Light [Regiment]. |
| LE VERT (J.-F.) -- | -- | 6th Foot Artillery. |
| ARBEY, -- | -- | 14th Dragoons. |
| VALLÉE, -- | -- | 4th Light Infantry. |
| BÉCOEUR, -- | -- | 4th -- . |
| PAJOT, LACCOLEY, -- | -- | 24th Light. |
| LEFEBVRE (Hippolyte), -- | -- | 55th -- . |
| GROS, -- | -- | 1st Foot Artillery. |
| DUBROCA, -- | -- | 64th -- . |
| CHARBONNIER, -- | -- | 64th -- . |
| CHARMOILLE, -- | -- | 65th -- . |
| MAILHES, -- | -- | 65th -- . |
| GOUPIL, -- | -- | 88th -- . |
| SONGIS, MARCHAND, -- | -- | 76th -- . |
| MACÉ, -- | -- | 34th -- . |
| CHOCARDELLE, -- | -- | 4th *Cuirassiers*. |
| DARRIBÈSE, -- | -- | 4th -- . |

There has been a cavalry drill. The two emperors and the King of Prussia attended it. The latter seems not to dare to ride next to the others; he almost always remains behind them and does not open his mouth; however, he is greeted and his colleagues are polite to him. On his way back from the manoeuvre, our Emperor saw me and greeted me with a smile; on his left were the Emperor of Russia and William. How much this knowing smile told me! It was noticed by everyone, and such a flattering distinction always honours the faction of which I am the leader.

Nothing is more beautiful as the little mare that was bought for me the day before yesterday: I have called her Memelée, in memory of the place where I acquired her.

29th – I have written a letter in the name of my nephew for His Imperial Highness the Grand Duke of Berg and a similar one for the Prince of Neufchâtel: I am asking them for the position of lieutenant-colonel for this absent-minded fool, who, instead of being with me and staying there, has gone to hurry to Warsaw. I also neatened my statement of presentation and, having dressed, I went to the Grand Duke of Berg, who welcomed me with a particular kindness and friendliness. I spoke to him about Wadeleux, before handing him my letter. 'By the way,' he said, 'what has become of him? Why did not he stay with me, as I told him and as His Majesty decided? He would have finished the war with us and that would have been very useful to him. The Emperor asked me again the day before yesterday for news of him; I did not know how to answer.' I attempted to excuse him and gave his so-called petition to His Highness, who read it attentively, exclaimed at the passage in which he mentioned the twenty-two wounds he had received in Egypt, and gave me his word that in the first light cavalry regiment that he would form, he would call my nephew to be its lieutenant-colonel. From there, I went to the Prince of Neufchâtel; there were many people there; he received me no less and very affectionately. I gave him my statement, inviting him to be our support to His Majesty and to render this last justice and this last service to the army's surgery. He reminded me that much had already been done for it, that the decree of 5 March had been very advantageous to it and that perhaps we should not show ourselves to be so demanding. I answered him that surgery, tireless in its zeal, in its devotion, in its work, should believe the generous benevolence of the Emperor to be inexhaustible. I made him understand that if necessary I would address myself, as on 1 March, to His Majesty himself, but that I preferred to have recourse to the intervention of His Highness and to owe him a new favour, which would have him seen as one of the greatest benefactors of surgery, etc. He promised that he would set my statement before the Emperor; it will be necessary to follow this up. In any case, I will always have a duplicate with me, in order to present it myself to His Majesty, when the occasion arises.

The wind is to the south-west, and the weather makes me go all strange; my vision is clouded, I am not firm on my legs. Looking around me, I feel as though I am dizzy; finally, I lack appetite and my ideas are not lucid. Yesterday I was already in this state, so I could hardly see our Emperor well and I only caught a glimpse of the King of Prussia.

I slept for two good hours having dined well; then, when I rose, I felt fit and fresh, with my eyes sharp and my sight very keen. I went to the field where the artillery was manoeuvring in front of our sovereigns; I walked around there for three-quarters of an hour and saw them coming back at a canter. This time, I had a good look at the King of Prussia and noticed him very well; he was riding beside our emperors. The weather has been fine; it has changed and I will be well.

My Memelée has been admired by connoisseurs, so kind and gentle is she.

30th – I am well and happy. The sun rose brightly and with a heat that, towards one o'clock, was almost unbearable. It is the wind from the south that prevails over all others: *Austri visum habitantes, caliginosi*.[8] Each time the southern constitution arises, it is as though I have a fine gauze before my eyes and my hearing is also a bit obtuse.

The *sous-aide* Bataille saw the Emperor Alexander this morning. He gave him a very beautiful ring, worth 3,000 *francs*; he coupled this gift with things that were flattering for French surgery. After he had given him the small red box containing the ring, a chamberlain took his hand and left a roll of 150 ducats in it, telling him that it was to reimburse him for his errands that His Majesty was offering him this money. It can be said that the emperor puts a lot of delicateness and kindness into everything he does. Here is a surgeon in sub-order who has been treated wonderfully. *M.* Willier, surgeon general of the Russian army, had given a favourable account of my colleague to His Majesty Alexander. My counterpart enjoys the highest consideration: he is only 32 years old; his name is French; however, he was born in Saint Petersburg. He is considered to be very talented. At the moment he has an erysipelas swelling on his left arm as a result of an injection in his finger; people are worried about him and it is clear from his sovereign's concern for him how much esteem and confidence he enjoys at court and in the army. However, he is poorly assisted and, in general, he has only a small number of educated surgeons around him. He has the rank of major-general; his salary is 10,000 roubles, not including very considerable rations and table and office expenses.

---

8. Loosely, 'those who live in the south wind have foggy vision'.

The 30th of June will be forever famous in the French, Russian and Prussian armies for the fraternal banquet that took place between the elite troops of these armies. In a very open meadow, within cannon range of the town, rustic tables had been prepared: they were planks fixed by stakes, arranged in such a way as to make a square, in the middle of which the musicians were standing. Soup, beef, pork, mutton, goose and chicken were not lacking; beer and schnapps, in special barrels, figured at the ends of each table. The *grenadiers* and foot soldiers of the French Guard, mingled with the Russian Guard, were standing, eating and drinking. The Russians, shy and unable to speak our language, did not dare to indulge at first; but, pressed by the advances and caresses of our people, they gradually became emboldened and by the end of the meal, they were all well. The feast, already well underway, was suspended to await a battalion of the Prussian Guard that was on the other side of the river, because the Russians were too few in number for our Guards, and moreover it was appropriate, since the King of Prussia was in the city and taking part in the agreement, that his people should participate in the feast. The *Gendarmes d'élite* and the mounted *grenadiers* set up tables on their side and entertained Prussia and Russia with the sound of fanfares. It was quite cheerful. In front of the camp of the *gendarmes* was a kind of white pennant, on which one could see the initial letters of the names of the three sovereigns: 'N. A. F.' This evening, one can no longer recognize the Guards: those of France have taken the caps of the Russians, who have taken theirs; they have exchanged clothes, shoes, and they go about like this in the camps and in the city, shouting: 'Long live the emperors! Long live the King of Prussia!' This latter cry is rare and very faint. The Prussians, who are generally bolder than the Russians, had a field day; admittedly, since they arrived last and there was significantly less food, they had to make up for it in drink. Everything else went well and, although drunk, everyone retired without any noise or scandal.

The Russian and Prussian officers were also given dinner. The feast was held under a huge tent or shed covered with ships' sails, the interior of which was decorated with garlands, festoons and bouquets. Each battalion of the Guard sent three senior officers to this meal, in order to establish the proportion with the foreign officers, who are not as numerous as ours. There was a great deal of joy on all sides, and this meeting must have given great pleasure to everyone.

The three sovereigns went on horseback to see the mounted *grenadier* corps; when they returned, they seemed very satisfied, especially the King of Prussia, who was seen laughing and standing next to our Emperor for the first time.

# 1807 (continued) – From Tilsit to Berlin

1 *Juillet* – Having donned my full dress, I went to the lodgings of His Majesty the Emperor of Russia, whom I had the good fortune to find alone with the Grand Duke Konstantin, his brother. They welcomed me with particular kindness; we talked together for a long time. The Emperor is a little deaf: when one has obtained an audience with him, it is the protocol for the resident chamberlain to warn you by saying that His Majesty wishes to be spoken to somewhat loudly. Unfortunately, this precaution had not been taken in my case, so I noticed that the Emperor often leaned over to me to hear me better. He asked me about the wounded in his army; he wanted to know if there had been many of them at the Battle of Friedland. The question was embarrassing; I got myself out of the difficult situation by responding that, when two brave armies come to blows, blood must necessarily be shed. I reassured him about the care that he feared his people would not receive, not for lack of generosity on our part, but because of the shortage of resources. We spoke of the ambulances of his army; I praised them, and, indeed, they are better organized than ours. I thought that their surgical instruments were produced in England: His Majesty disabused me of this idea and informed me that in his capital there were cutlers as good as those in London. The Grand Duke's ebullience is unmatched: he explains himself with a vivacity and gesticulation that one might ordinarily interpret very badly. I thought I saw in this prince a good heart, an ardent imagination, and a fiery and impulsive character.

His Majesty received my leave as graciously as he had accepted my visit and let me go, thanking me for the pleasure that I had given him.

2nd – The Grand Duke's doctor, *M.* Lindeshoem, came to find me at three o'clock; he told me how much he had been looking forward to making my acquaintance. I received him as well as I could. He is not staying in the town; every evening he crosses back over the Memel and stays on the right bank, where the prince's house is. He is a man of fairly good appearance, 36 years old, able to speak French well, and he explains himself with reserve and nobility; he has been with the prince, who is only 26 years old, for eighteen years; he has received the Order of Wladimir of the fourth class.[1] We talked together about *M.* Willier,[2] the surgeon inspector-general of the Russian army; he described him to me as a kind man, educated, honest, energetic and respected. He knew of the accident that had befallen him. The Emperor had spoken to me about it in the morning with the interest of esteem and of the greatest benevolence. This *M.* Willier is English. His Majesty had previously had a *M.* Willis, also an Englishman, as his doctor and surgeon, but he died nearly two years ago; *M.* Franck, from Vienna, replaced him at the court of Saint-Petersburg; his son remained in Wilna. The chief dentist of this court is young Saucerotte, from Lunéville, who does his work there perfectly. They pay well in that country: Willier has a large salary and is a third-class member of the Order of Wladimir, which means he wears the cross, which is its decoration, hanging from his collar, while for the fourth class it is worn on the buttonhole.

I could certainly go to see His Prussian Majesty, who will surely receive me well; I will see tomorrow. The weather is very fine; my health is feeling the effects of it and I am reasonably well. We are being assured that peace will be proclaimed on the 5th; already we are preparing to make our way back.

I know officially that we have 1,400 Russians in Friedland and 600 in Heilsberg. In the first of these towns, we found only forty Frenchmen.

The principal, whom I had sent on a mission along the whole line from Wehlau, Friedland, Heilsberg, Domnau, Guttstadt, etc., as far as Dantzig, has given me reassuring news. There are at this moment 1,409 patients at Marienbourg, 1,125 of whom are wounded; among the latter are 130 fractures and thirty-two amputations. There are still several limbs to remove: in the absence of a case of instruments, the *chirurgien-major* Affré is making use of an ordinary knife and a craftsman's saw. What shame! What calamity! Odious administration! I have just given an official account to His Highness

---

1. The Order of Saint Vladimir was established by Empress Catherine II in 1782 and had four classes.
2. The Scottish physician James Wylie, who served as a doctor to the Russian court from 1790 until his death in 1854.

the Major-General of all the details of the service from Friedland to Heilsberg, including these towns.

3rd – The weather is still fine; the heat is intense.

The wagon train continues to file past towards France; the Mounted Guard is also leaving; tomorrow the artillery of the Guard will set off; the *chasseurs* will leave this evening. At last we see with pleasure the arrival of the moment when we finally turn our victorious steps towards a country to which so many reasons call us back.

I wrote a great deal in the morning. My service is becoming much clearer; I have discharged 119 names from my control, seventeen of which are those of surgeons who have died or been killed. One of our *chirurgiens-majors* following the army, *M.* Kuhn, killed himself at Thorn with opium; before poisoning himself, he wrote to an aide-de-camp of General Jordy and asked him to take care of his affairs after he was no more. He had 30 *Friedrichs d'or* in his purse, very good belongings, and no bad business: we do not know what could have led him to commit suicide. In his letter, he said that this fate had been reserved for him since his youth and that he was fulfilling his destiny; moreover, he did not wish to be on earth any longer. Kuhn was blind in one eye as a result of ophthalmia; he was stocky, strong, fat and very flushed, and was said to be intemperate. He was Swiss: when we were together in Dantzig, he had explained to me his origins and the etymology of his name, which, in French, means 'bold'.

His Majesty the King of Prussia was kind enough to send me, through one of his aides-de-camp, a letter that had reached him on behalf of *M.* Goercke, first surgeon general of his army, to my address at the main headquarters. This good man *M.* Goercke is well-liked and well-respected by his sovereign and by all that is illustrious in Prussia. He has written the kindest things to me and has charged me with passing on to his wife in Berlin a letter included with the one he addressed to me, which I will look after with care, so flattering is it to me and so full of wise and sensible things. I replied at some length to this esteemed colleague. I had to carry my response to his gracious sovereign myself; I could have visited him at three o'clock, but it will be tomorrow and I am convinced that I will be well received by him.

Our emperors and king went to see a review of the cavalry on horseback. On their return at walking pace, against their custom, I found myself in their path; the Emperor of Russia did me the honour of greeting me with very amicable grace and said to ours: 'Ah! There is *M.* Percy.' Our Emperor was kind enough to greet me in his turn, smiling as usual, and perhaps they deigned to talk for a moment about their humble servant. Poor father Percy! If you were alive and could see your Pierre-François treated with such distinction by the most important rulers in the world, what would you say?

> *et in tenui re Majores pennas nido extendisse loqueris. HORAT., Epist. ad Librum.*[3]

I am far from being open to pride. I am far more susceptible to astonishment, and how could I not be surprised and almost ashamed of the reputation that I have acquired, of the universal benevolence accorded me, of the rank to which I find myself elevated, of the fortune that I have made; finally, of that which I am and that which one thinks of me? Heaven has blessed my work; I have fulfilled my duties and my role as an honest man and a zealous citizen. Without intrigue, without means unworthy of a sensitive man, I have been successful. Far from having the talents of the late J.-L. Petit, I had his simplicity and his love for our art, and, always while seeking the small things, the great things sought me out.

It is time to pack up and leave. Dysentery is taking hold; it is only killing a few of the sick, but it puts them in danger and leaves them so weak and meagre that they will remain unfit to return to France for a long time.

Tomorrow we are evacuating the 450 patients that we have in the hospital on four boats; the evacuation surgeons have their orders; they will be put in at Labiau and Tapiau, where we have staging posts to receive the sick for one night.

4th – *Ut sis nocte levis, sit tib cœna brevis.*[4] I more than observed this precept last night; thus, I slept wonderfully and rose this morning lively and fresh. It is getting hotter and hotter; the nights are an hour and a half shorter and the days are longer in the same proportion than in France; the sun had already risen and was very fierce at five o'clock in the morning.

I wrote and sent some dispatches. Three or four distinguished people came to take me away for half an hour each.

I went to see Grand Duke Konstantin to receive news of *M.* Willier, whom I was told had improved since the amputation of his gangrenous finger. I do not

---
3. Percy quotes from Horace's *Epistles*. The quotation means 'and of humble means, I spread my wings beyond the nest'.
4. Loosely, 'for a peaceful night, let your dinner be brief'.

understand how it was possible to decide to amputate, after a few days, a finger affected by necrosis, for at any rate, either the gangrene was confined, and so one could wait, or it was not, and in that case it was necessary to wait. But it is possible that the information I was given at His Imperial Highness's house was not very accurate. The Grand Duke was lunching, and I can attest that he eats a lot, very well, and for a long time. The Russians have a good appetite.

From there I went to see our Emperor. It was eleven o'clock; everyone except him was having lunch and I spoke for a long time with the usher of the study, the uncle of one of our surgeons, before I could be announced. Finally, a duty colonel arrived. His Majesty told me that he would receive me during his lunch. I waited while talking with Marshal Duroc, General Bertrand and other generals, who were asked to leave as soon as the meal was served. This service consisted of a fairly ordinary soup, cutlets, a plate of rice and, I believe, another dish. The Emperor, having been informed, entered and said to me: 'Good day, *M.* Percy! How are you?' He sat down at the table, saying: 'What a joy it is to eat!'

'Yes, Sire,' I replied, 'it is certainly a great joy when one has an appetite.'

'Personally, I devour food,' he continued. 'I have been ravenous for some time and, in general, we all eat well in the army.'

'One must also work in the army, Sire,' I allowed myself to add, 'and Your Majesty has done a lot of work for some time.'

'How do you find it?'

'Sire, one could certainly say that our language is poor; it does not offer me a single expression capable of describing what we all feel. Please accept that I speak to you in Latin: *Tu solus altissimus*.'[5] His Majesty laughed. He complained about the bad quality of the water in this country: indeed, it is bad, smells of mud and causes nausea.

'*M.* Percy, what is the best water?'

'It is that of Paris, Sire.'

'Oh! That's true,' said the Major-General, 'nothing is as good as the water of the Seine.' I meant more than that, and His Majesty understood me.

'I drink seltzer water; but I find it very strong, very sour ...'

'Sire, it must be sweetened by uncorking the bottles two hours in advance to release some of the carbonic acid gas.' He said to his butler on duty: 'Do you hear?'

---

5. 'You alone are the highest.'

'How are the wounded?'

'Sire, we have evacuated all those whom the transport should not harm too much to Elbing, Marienbourg, Marienwerder, etc., and a hospital of 1,200 beds has been opened at Heilsberg, in the great castle, for amputees or men with complicated fractures. There are 1,400 Russians still in Friedland, 600 in Heilsberg, etc.'

'As many as that?'

'Yes, Sire, and I believe that the Russian army has left us at least double that number.'

'Have you really had as many wounded as at Preuss-Eylau?'

'Yes, Sire, but in total, from the 5th to the 14th.'

'I believed so and have always calculated it that way. You have been over the battlefield of Friedland; you must agree that it is a terrible spectacle.'

'If one found only the dead there, the sight of a battlefield would not be so dreadful, but it is those unfortunate wounded whom one can neither help nor remove, it is these dying men whose torments must not be shortened, which break a sensitive heart.'

'That is true. Are you a child of the army?'

'More or less, Sire, my father was a military surgeon.'

'With which regiment?'

'With the Tallard-Infantry Regiment.'

'I have never been familiar with that regiment.'

'Sire, it has not existed for more than fifty years; I think that it was incorporated into the Beauvoisis Regiment.'

'And you chose the profession of your late father?'

'Sire, I was a *gendarme* of the King for a time, then a surgeon in the same corps, then a *chirurgien-major* in the cavalry; but I have only really been something since Your Majesty deigned to honour me with your trust and to shower me with your generosity.'

'There is a Prussian surgeon here who appears to be capable and who claims that French surgeons do not have an aptitude for dressings.'

'Sire, this man, whom I do not know, can only be a mediocre surgeon, since he judges the art only by accessories and mechanical means that are not at its core. It is true that the Germans are very fond of these small details that require neither ingenuity nor effort to understand; they overdress the art, like their clothes, like their furniture, like everything they do; they have shops and merchants for straps, ready-made bandages, compresses, wooden legs; they make large ribbons of thread that they call straps, but which, having two edges or selvedges, are difficult to apply, constrict, grip, hinder and have only the slight advantage of pleasing the eye.'

'Are the English better surgeons than the Germans?'

'Yes, Sire, and, if I were not afraid of appearing immodest, I would say that they are almost our equals concerning their knowledge and skill; they translate our works and we translate as many of theirs. There is much similarity between the surgical practice of the two nations. They have better instruments than we do ...'

'In what way? Do we not have instruments in the army that are as good as theirs?'

'We have some cases made by two skilful cutlers from Strasbourg; the others are absolutely worthless and we lack more than fifty.'

'Ah! Odious administration! How outraged I am about everything that happens in these administrations! ... Have any diseases taken hold?'

'Yes, Sire, it is now dysentery, but it is neither fatal nor contagious.'

'Dysentery? We must be wary. Is there rice in the hospitals? That is the cure. Incidentally, do we have any ourselves?' he said to the Grand-Marshal, who replied in the affirmative.

I took advantage of a moment's silence to thank His Majesty for the fresh favour he has done me by appointing me commander and asked him to be willing to take into consideration a statement of proposals that I had given to His Highness the Major-General for several of my colleagues, who had acquired great rights to his munificence and his kindness: it was concerning my list. I explained that I was asking for the cross for the ten most senior surgeons, the vacant post of *chirurgien-major* in ten regiments for ten others and the confirmation of ten *aides-majors* in the rank that I had provisionally conferred on them. His Majesty was good enough to promise me that this would be done. I had in my pocket the copy of my list; it was only a question of presenting it, which would not have offended His Highness the Major-General and, of course, I forgot. I had already handed over to the Major-General, in the presence of His Majesty, my unsealed reply to the letter from my good friend Goercke, about whom I had just spoken. Unfortunately, I forgot my duplicate and I do not know what this fault will cost me in worry and perhaps in regret: with a little more presence of mind my business would have been over immediately, but let us not despair yet.

## 1807 (continued) – From Tilsit to Berlin

Regarding the Russian wounded, whose number His Majesty found considerable, he said: 'After all, I prefer that it be these b... than our brave men. It is only a question of leaving them to their own and telling them to take care of them. What do you say, *M. Percy?*'

'I say, Sire, that nothing can better suit us than this measure, because indeed we are burdened with more than 300 Russian wounded and it is an additional problem and expense for us.'

After a few more remarks, His Majesty returned to his study, saying goodbye to me graciously, and I recommended to him the candidates on my list with insistence.

I had gone twice to see the King of Prussia, who was always absent. At four o'clock, I presented myself at his modest lodgings and, having waited for him for a quarter of an hour, I saw His Majesty arrive with Marshal Kalkreuth and another officer: they were returning from the other side of the Memel, I believe. The King went upstairs alone, leaving his two companions at the foot of the staircase; he entered the room where I was, without an entourage or guards, and said to me: 'Did you wish to see me, sir?'

'Yes, Sire, I took this liberty, placing the greatest value on the honour of presenting you with my respectful compliments.'

'You are, sir, the chief surgeon of the French armies?'

'Sire, I am to those of France what my friend Goercke, one of the most respected and most faithful servants of Your Majesty, is to those of Prussia.'

'Alas! ... Do you know *M.* Goercke personally?'

'No, Sire, but I love him no less for it; we write to each other often, and only the day before yesterday Your Majesty was good enough to have one of his letters passed to me.'

'*M.* Goercke is indeed an honourable man; I make a special case for him.'

'He deserves Your Majesty's goodwill and respect. He is an honest, wise man, with gentle mores.'

'Yes, and that is certainly how to describe him; he has very gentle mores and no-one has the love and virtues of his profession more than him; he has established a small school of surgery which has already provided some very good candidates.'

'Sire, I know the academy of Prussian surgeons; I have seen it, I attended one of its sessions, I have met and listened to the professors and the pupils: it is a fine institution, for which we are indebted to Your Majesty and your respected surgeon.'

'You have much more than this in France and the surgery of your armies enjoys a superb reputation and consistency; it shares in all the advantages of the military career, honours and promotion.'

'That is true, Sire. It is also staffed with the same men as the general staff and the officer corps, and it must be added that, if we have our share of the distinctions, we also have our share of the perils of war, the hardships and the fatigues.'

'Have you stayed in Berlin?'

'Yes, Sire: I spent enough time there to realize that Your Majesty was cherished and honoured there, and to grieve with all the good Prussians over the misfortunes and tragedies of your kingdom, to where the wishes and love of your faithful subjects call you back and where it will be consoling for the French to see you soon return.'

'Ah! I know that the good Prussian people are attached to me and pity me. We must hope that we will reach an agreement; the two emperors are here and, if yours leaves me an existence … '

This remark moved us both. I thought I saw tears spring to the King's eyes and, for my part, I am certain that I too shed them. What a stroke of bad luck! What a catastrophe! O human greatness!

I took leave of His Majesty, who led me to the door, signalling his esteem and a kind of gratitude.

I also saw Grand Duke Konstantin. So here I am in the midst of the potentates, and they are all are kind enough to think well of me and to treat me well.

*Principibus placuisse viris, non ultima laus est.*
*Epist. ad Scævam.*[6]

After dining, about six o'clock, we crossed the Memel and went to the camp of the Kalmyks and Tartar Bashkirs. I thought I may faint on the sailing boat that General Thiébault and I had boarded with six of our men; the river was rough. It had been a long time since I had been on the water; indeed, a little later, I felt sick to my stomach and it spelled the end of my dinner. Once we had set foot on the shore, we met some Russian officers and asked them to find us someone who could take us into the camps. They were kind enough to

---

6. Horace: 'To have gained the approval of powerful men is not the highest praise.'

accompany us there; besides, they had never themselves seen these kinds of savages who come from an area more than 800 leagues from Saint Petersburg, most of them near the Caucasus, and they were glad to enjoy this spectacle.

These Kalmyks are astonishing beings! They all look alike and one would think that they were all hatched from the same egg, officers and soldiers. They are generally quite short, not being more than 2 or 3ft high.[7] Their clothes consist of a blue jacket and large, broad trousers, also blue; they wear ankle boots and a fur cap. Their weapons are: first, a long lance like that of the Cossacks, but treated with better care and bearing a small blue and red pennon; second, a hussar's sabre; and third, a pistol. I could not help but laugh when I saw the sentry at the entrance to the camp: never had a more incongruous figure crossed my sights. They are all very brown-skinned and of a soot-like brown. Their naturally uncovered brows are enlarged by the cut of their fringe and the hair at the temples, which they often shave. They have small brown eyes, which the upper eyelid uncovers only incompletely; their cheekbones are prominent and very wide; they all have a rather small nose and the line of their profile is almost straight; and their mouths are nothing remarkable, but their lower jaw is wide and flares out. All this gives them an unusual and surprising appearance to us. They have made huts for themselves, where they sleep and in front of which they eat; it is a pleasant thing to see them crouching around their pot of soup made of barley, flour or something else; they live very badly and are no less well off. Their officers are well-dressed; they have silver stripes on their waistcoats and along their breeches, and they are well-armed. One of them, hardly 18 years old, showed us the point of a lance, remarking menacingly that it was sharp; then he made a gesture suddenly as though he were stabbing us with it, saying '*Hurrah Françouse!*' and laughing: the Kalmyks also have, as you can see, their jokers, but generally these people are not cheerful.

Further on is the camp of the Bashkirs. Here you could imagine yourself transported to China or Japan, as much for the outfits as for the appearances, the customs, the habits and the inclinations. The Bashkirs are, in general, of a good size; they are at least as smoke-coloured as the Kalmyks, except for a few exceptions; they have very small eyes, like the Chinese; their nose is squarer than that of their neighbours; their cheekbones are also more prominent than

---

7. This is an exaggeration, and says something about the way that Percy treats/analyzes the peoples he encounters.

ours and, in general, they have a sunken mouth and very good teeth. They wear on their ugly face a character of good-heartedness that is pleasing; they seem lively, alert, cheerful, welcoming and easy company; they received us with kindness and submitted themselves to whatever might have aroused our curiosity, except for a few individuals, who refused to allow us see their weapons and replied brusquely. It is the most enjoyable thing in the world to see this people. We found them eating or finishing cooking their supper, blowing out the fire, gathering around the pot or preparing food absolutely unknown to us. Some were kneading an extremely coarse dough in a small wooden trough to make *galettes* the size of a hat from it, which they then cooked at their hearth, first flat, then upright and turning them over in all directions: this unleavened bread, which none of us could eat, pleases them very much. They get this taste from the Asians, as well as most of their customs. Others were stirring a kind of flour and gruel broth without fat or salt with a wooden spoon made in their fashion. These people were preparing a cheese soup, and we only knew that that was what it was when we brought to our noses what was by all appearances a grey piece of clay that we saw being sliced into small pieces. Some Bashkirs laying in the hut, seeing that we were keen to guess what this strange mass might be that one of their friends was cutting into small pieces, told him to show it to us and have us smell it, which he did very willingly. These people eat only once a day, at about seven o'clock in the evening; they are abstemious and live more or less like the Kalmyks. They crouch in the manner of the Orientals. Their way of dressing is very varied; there is no regular or uniform costume among them; some have a European or Chinese-style pelisse or redingote, while others are covered with a mantle similar to that of certain savages; they are all in boots that they make themselves, for they sew, dress and embellish each other among themselves. The most striking thing about them is their hats, which are generally uniform. This cap is made of fox fur. It is enormous; the circumference is divided into four parts, one of which covers the collar, two the cheeks, and the fourth can be folded down over the face; it resembles the caps of some Polish Jews in size; when it is drawn back, it has this shape.[8] It seems that they take care of it and only put it on when they are on duty or in full dress; in the camp and in the hut, they have small pointed caps, like those of the Chinese and Japanese, and each of them has chosen the colour and the fabric that pleased them or that they might

---

8. Longin: Here in the manuscript are found two pen and ink drawings by Percy's hand.

have found. There are some of them made from woollen fabric, from painted cloth, damask or velvet; some of them wear a skullcap of leather or wool; others have a handkerchief around their head. There is not a single one who does not have his head covered, whereas the Kalmyks always have their heads bare. They are extremely modest towards strangers, to whose eyes they never appear naked or uncovered; they squat to urinate and never touch each other, which would make them impure. This is another trait of resemblance with the Mohammedan Asians. They are pagans; we asked to see their fetishes, but they pretended not to understand us, though our interpreter explained himself very intelligibly to them.

Each camp is a particular tribe, with its sheik whom it respects and fears. This chief is always a superb man, with a large beard, an embroidered black velvet bonnet, a scarlet simar without a belt and a Turkish, Persian or Indian sword. One of them has a dark red ribbon around his collar bearing a beautiful gold medal with the effigy of Alexander: we greeted him and he answered us with dignity; in his hut was a beautiful oriental carpet. We saw a Bashkir playing a long flute or, rather, a tin pipe made of two pieces welded together and pierced with seven holes, six at the top and one below. This pipe, as wide as the index finger at the top and the little finger at the bottom, has no mouthpiece, nor anything resembling a whistle. The Bashkir places the widest end of it on his lower lip, does not close his mouth, and plays by moving his fingers and no doubt by cutting the air or the wind that he introduces into this unusual instrument with the edge of the pipe; thus, the sound is piercing in a way that at first seems harsh and unpleasant, but that one then finds soft and melodious. The musician blows for more than two or three minutes at a time without taking a breath and always decreasing in volume; then he inhales strongly, which produces a loud and monotonous sound, after which the tune resumes its normal pace. This tune is steady, rhythmical, slightly wistful and resembles the *ranz des vaches*;[9] it gave us great pleasure. A Bashkir accompanied his friend's instrument with his voice, making a horrible grimace, restricting his breathing and drawing sounds very similar to those of the pipe from his chest; his face grew red and his jugulars were large and varicose. The duet did not lack charm. We asked for a dancer: a Bashkir around 30 years old – whose skullcap, decorated with American seeds and topped with a tip made of tin, we had already noticed

---

9. The echoing pipe tunes played by Swiss cowherders.

– was identified by his companions; it took a moment to persuade him, and then, having greeted us by removing his cap, as if asking for our lenience, he began to dance. The music became more intense, without changing tune, for I believe that these people have only one. The dancer, observing very well the timing of the music, which we could beat ourselves, displayed a lot of skill and a fair amount of charm: he made some difficult steps, one of which was very similar to what we call the *pas de Basque*. He fell on one buttock and rose again without losing the beat; he gesticulated, made faces, smiled, shrugged and lowered his shoulders, moved his hips, almost always tracing a circle. When the dance was over, he removed his cap for us again, while laughing like a good child; then we gave him, as well as the musicians, a few silver coins, and the dance began again. This amused me greatly. A crowd of Bashkirs surrounded us: it seems that dancers and musicians are not common among them.

The Tartars are armed with a very strong bow and a quiver full of well-made arrows: the tip of these arrows is made of steel and takes the shape of an ace of spades. They use these weapons adeptly: we saw several practising their shooting and aiming at two small pointed caps about 120 paces apart; they often hit them. They also have a sword, such as they have been able to obtain for themselves; there are some beautiful ones, and also some very poor ones; most of them are Turkish or Persian. The quiver, which is made of leather, is shaped like those of the Turks of the past. They have some very well-made coats of mail and Asian-style helmets that have cheeks and a train and carry a chain mail collar. This armour is very old and was not made by these peoples; they received it by means of conquests or trade, or took it from various arsenals. Nevertheless, when they are covered with it, they look very much like the ancient Parthians, such as Le Brun represented in his paintings of the battles of Alexander, and I am not far from believing that they are descended from this warrior race.

In our presence, some Russian officers bought coats of mail, bows and quivers, for the Bashkirs are the owners of their weapons and it seems that their chiefs do not forbid them from selling them. They like money and have hardly any of it, having arrived in the army only very late and having been unable to take the spoils. One of them asked to buy a watch from us, saying that he would pay what we wanted. *M.* Le Vert showed him his gold repeater watch, and the rogue turned it round and round, and, showing his bow and an arrow, made us understand that one day he would win one by these means; the watch was returned. These soldiers are on horseback; their mounts are small, very ugly horses, but are said to be excellent; their tack is truly baroque.

The Bashkirs are all Mahometans, and not idolatrous, as we had been told; they live in the area surrounding the Caucasus. The Kalmyks are their neighbours. Several tribes have remained unsubdued. They are constantly at war with them.

We finished this visit by going to see the camp of 2,000 thousand Cossacks situated a short distance from that of the Tartars. These warriors are generally handsome and well-built; they have a warlike appearance. They are all dressed alike. Their pikes, which do not have a pennon, are arranged in two lines and stretch as far as the eye can see, which creates a beautiful effect. Almost all of them have a mantle like that of the Cafres and Hottentots; the fur, which is on the outside, is very long; it is felt-like, thick and impermeable to the rain; they cover their hut with it and use it as a coat. Some of them with a lot of money ask to exchange French currency with Russian money; some of them proudly show the crosses that they have taken from our people. They are proud and haughty.

5th – We were waiting for the Queen of Prussia, but it seems that she will not arrive before tomorrow. We are always searching for news: the peace, it was said, was to be published today but the peace may not yet have been signed; we must wait. However, everyone is making arrangements to leave. Everything suggests that we will no longer be here on the 10th of this month. Amen.

6th – It is raining; it is oppressive and heavy, like when the sirocco blows in Italy; the south wind still prevails.

This morning we evacuated the fifty patients who remained. I saw the doctor of His Imperial Highness the Grand Duke again; he gave me fairly good news of *M.* Willier, whom he left yesterday, after having had an incision made in the palm of his hand, where there was a fairly large collection of pus. This is almost always what happens in this case, and, failing to make an incision in the palmar aponeurosis in good time, one can see the pus slip under the annular ligament and accumulate on the square-shaped muscle, which can form still more distant and deeper sinuses. *M.* Willier was certainly relieved after the operation; he slept for four full hours last night. He lost the two phalanges of the index finger of his left hand. In opening a gangrenous abscess six days ago, he twice pricked this finger, which he had used as a probe, and it was the following day, at four o'clock, in the morning, that he was awoken by sharp pains, which soon became excruciating. Everyone shared greatly in this accident. The three sovereigns showed in this situation how much they take notice of a skilful army surgeon. Yesterday I wrote a fine letter to this brave colleague.

The Queen of Prussia, who had been announced yesterday, arrived today. Our court went in full dress to pay compliments to her. Our two emperors went to her accommodation, greeted her, and each gave her a marshal to accompany her to Napoleon's lodgings, where there was a grand dinner. Her Majesty climbed into an eight-horse carriage at about seven o'clock; Marshal Bessières was at the right-hand door. The carriage went slowly enough, and the Queen was kind enough to show herself from time to time. The sovereigns took a different route and arrived before her at the lodgings; ours offered his hand to Her Majesty, said the most gracious things to her and led her into her quarters. She is still young, very blonde, white and, I believe, a little blanched; her features are pleasant; her various portraits capture her appearance quite well.

7th – Fine weather, but it was cold in the evening. Nothing new happened during the day. *M.* Kourakin, the Russian Minister Plenipotentiary, told a friend of mine that the peace was going to be signed, that it was being drafted and that there were no complications. I wish I could say the same for the success of my list; but the Major-General, all while making the right noises, seems to want to play me for a fool.

The Queen of Prussia spent the night beyond the Memel. She crossed the river again at four o'clock; everyone hurried to see her; our sovereigns are very gallant. At seven o'clock, she climbed into an eight-horse carriage to go to see our Emperor, accompanied by the Prince Major-General, and, the whole court having marched past under her windows, I saw her from very close. She is being treated perfectly and everything suggests that Napoleon has shown himself to be noble and generous.

His Majesty the Emperor Alexander presented a beautiful diamond ring to young Elie, *sous-aide*, returning from Kazan and the distant parts of Russia. He had been taken with the adjutant-major of his regiment near Mohrungen, six months ago; he is a fine man; he has suffered a lot.

8th – The weather is changeable. The peace is definitely signed. Everyone is leaving. My young friend Le Vert is leaving today with the messenger; I will not see him again until Metz. The Major-General presented a huge stack of papers for signing; my list was not among them. I saw him this evening:

## 1807 (continued) – From Tilsit to Berlin

he repeated his usual objections and made me understand that too much had already been given to the surgeons; that there had been jealousy; that this distinction should not be made too commonplace (it is high time!). Indeed, what did he not say to me? I answered defiantly to everything and reminded him that in his presence His Majesty had deigned to promise it all to me, to grant me everything and to allow me to lay at his feet my just gratitude and the tribute of my respectful sensibility. 'Yes,' he said, 'but His Majesty had not yet seen your request. In any case, I will present it to him; he will do with it as he pleases, refuse it, modify it, change it; it is his business. For my part, I am not of the opinion that we should grant all this to you.'

I am all ready to leave. *M.* Goercke sent a Prussian *chirurgien-major* to me yesterday, to find out if I was still in Tilsit and to come to see me there. He will arrive the day after tomorrow; I will not leave until I have seen him and embraced him.

9th – Superb weather. His Majesty is leaving the coming night. The III Corps will form the rearguard; I will take all my surgeons present in Tilsit; those of the aforementioned corps will run the service there.

That was how things stood at eleven o'clock; they changed around midday. The whole Guard of the Emperor of Russia, in very beautiful dress, arranged itself in a line almost opposite the lodgings of His Majesty. Shortly afterwards a battalion of *chasseurs* of our Emperor's Guard came to set themselves in a row on the other side of the same street. Our men's musicians played some beautiful pieces; those of the Russian Guard seemed to me to be more beautiful and more powerful; the tunes that they played gave me great pleasure. The Grand Duke Konstantin was on horseback at the head of the Russians; he had the grand cordon of the Order of Napoleon and was conversing familiarly with our officers, among whom was a captain of *grenadiers* who, being wounded and held prisoner, had received the most generous and delicate care from His Highness. The Emperor Alexander, also decorated with the grand cordon, came down from his house and appeared on horseback before his Guards, to whom he made a remark that was undoubtedly a salute, an expression that immediately caused a noise to erupt all along the line, which must have been the response to the salute. Soon after came Napoleon, with the grand cordon of Saint Andrew. He travelled the length of the Russian line, stopped at the head of the column, asked Alexander to bring the first *grenadier* out of the line and handed him his gold cross of the Legion, which the brave and superb man accepted with timidity and respect, not without kissing the hand that gave him such a beautiful gift, according to the custom of his country. Those watching were touched; I saw a Prussian bourgeois who was moved to tears by it. The two emperors climbed the stairs to the lodgings of the Russian Emperor, where the Grand Duke of Berg was waiting, also wearing the grand cordon of Saint Andrew, and where, after a quarter of an hour, *M.* Kourakin, with that of France, and *M.* Talleyrand, wearing the blue ribbon of that of Russia, arrived, making four red grand cordons exchanged for four blue. The sovereigns spent nearly an hour together, perhaps to ratify the peace treaty; then they separated, bidding each other fond farewells. The Russian monarch crossed the Memel with his brother and his Guards; the French Emperor did not leave Tilsit until three minutes past six. The King of Prussia did not appear; he had crossed over the water yesterday. The rain that began to fall in torrents dispersed the spectators; it has continued ever since, and still now (at ten o'clock in the evening) it is raining hard.

The chief equerry of Emperor Alexander fell yesterday with his horse on the terrible cobbles of the town and fractured his fibula. Our Prince Major-General informed me almost immediately of the accident, which he believed to be more serious; but I had the foolish reserve not to offer myself for the first aid that this lord needed. During the ceremony, the gentleman on duty to the Grand Duke Konstantin asked me to see the patient; we went together to his house; the leg was badly dressed and I found it between the two English-style splints with three buckled straps. This apparatus, which is very common among the Prussians, is rather crude; it does not prevent the leg from rolling; it requires that it be fitted with compresses and put in the state of a cylinder, and rarely does it favour coaptation. The surgeon who fitted this apparatus is called Morgen; he is a very famous man in this country, a great speaker, intriguing, bold and not without means.

I have packed my things to leave tomorrow, once I have seen *M.* Goercke. Everyone is already on their way to Kœnigsberg.

10th – I rose at five o'clock. The weather is fine; the sun is bright; it will be good for travelling. Tilsit is very empty and deserted now; there is not a Russian left there, except the wounded equerry, and one no longer sees any Frenchmen there. I will wait until noon for my good friend Goercke; if he has not arrived by then, I will leave. There will be rain again.

No Goercke. Noon struck and I left. The weather was quite fine and the path quite good, except for three or four dangerous passages that my driver, a local peasant, managed very well. We stopped at the village where the Emperor spent the night twenty days ago, and where they said they saw the Black or Death Hussars, a loathsome unit that does not frighten anyone, despite the skull and crossbones that they wear on their shako. I saw the house that I had stayed in again, but the beautiful clock was no longer there; everything was broken. Our horses would not eat. We travelled another 3 leagues and more. Having found in a beautiful village Major Christophe, of the 1st principal battalion, and this good man having made many insistent pleas to me to share his lodgings, we all dismounted there and had a good supper, a good shelter and I, in particular, a good bed. I drank Bordeaux and Chambertin wine and ate omelette and even crayfish; this put me in a good way. Our horses were treated wonderfully as well.

11th – I slept blissfully. When I rose, I found the coffee already served and the horses harnessed. After thanking my host, I climbed into the carriage in delightful weather; we crossed a nearby forest 3 leagues in length along a fairly good causeway, but uneven, because it is made of fir trunks; the ground is damp, peaty and foul-smelling. It is the same from Kœnigsberg to Tilsit; the plain is immense, sometimes quite fertile, generally hardly cultivated, interspersed with ponds and unpleasant streams. On our way we saw many blind people begging for alms; blindness is common in this country; they also lose their teeth early there, and there are countless hunchbacks. The inhabitants are poor; one finds them barefoot, both men and women; however, the men commonly wear sandals made from bark, which they fasten with hemp or even bark straps. There are some who protect their feet with leather that has holes all around it, and which they lace around their feet. All this gives the impression of poverty, but hardly any more so than in some of our provinces. The road is superb; there are places where it is well shaded by willows, lime trees and black (speckled) alders. I had a pleasant journey.

We arrived at Labiau at half past eleven, having always been moving at a trot, even with our caisson. We saw the Friedrichs-Graben. There were forty sick in this small town, who, for lack of boats, had not been able to be evacuated; they will leave tomorrow. Labiau is not a pretty town, but there must be some affluence there; I saw a food market that was well stocked with everything, and everything is sold cooked, even fried fish. It is the land of fish; that is all they live on – they are pescatarian; they sell salted and cooked salmon in slices and fricasseed eel in segments. If one has money, it is possible to buy a good dinner in passing. We had ours in a fairly good house that was home to the wife of a Prussian trumpeter, where, among a host of pictures, there was an engraving of the death of Louis XVI. Our magazines were given good hay, oats, meat and bread. Long live Labiau!

We set off again at three o'clock, in the fiercest heat. Beautiful countryside, superb road; it would not be possible to travel in a more pleasant fashion. At half past seven, we stopped in a village where 432 infantrymen were to be lodged; we chose a good barn, put the carriages into a sort of courtyard, then immediately put the horses out to pasture, arranged our straw to sleep on, had something to eat on the hoof, went for a walk and put on our nightcaps. At half past nine, we were lying on our straw; our horses will spend the night in the fields; we are all sleeping in the barn.

12th – I slept for seven hours uninterrupted. I had four bundles of straw under me, a small feather duvet, and I was in my sack with a good blanket. Our journey from the barn to Kœnigsberg was leisurely; the weather is beautiful and so is the countryside. The road is like a garden path; we are almost always moving at a trot and the time does not seem to me to drag, because of the beauty and variety of the places, the woods, the lakes and the houses that we continue to come across.

We arrived in Kœnigsberg at half past twelve. The town is situated on a slight elevation, but it is the position of the castle that must have seen it given the name of Royal Mount; it is, indeed, located on an area of high ground; one can only reach it by climbing. I am lodged in the home of a banker who has been in Riga with his children for several months and has left only a lady governess and a serving boy in his house. I was served a good dinner; I have good quarters; my servants and my horses are fine. I have already toured the town a little, having trimmed my beard, cleaned myself up and dressed, for today is Sunday and everyone is making an effort to look respectable. The ladies are pretty, of good blood and good health; they dress elegantly. I met thousands of them, each better dressed than the previous; they were trying to see His Majesty. I visited the Intendant-general and agreed with him on several essential points of our service. It has been extremely hot. The streets of Kœnigsberg are narrow, irregular and terribly badly paved; there are some nice houses, but in general the town is badly built and I have not yet seen a building or monument worthy of curiosity there.

13th – At daybreak I set to work and hurried through many pressing matters. I saw a small hospital in the reformed church: it seemed to me well managed. The town is endlessly long: to travel from my lodgings to those of *M.* Mouron, it takes three-quarters of an hour, and I sweated blood and water, so hot is the sun and terrible are the cobbles. I was unable to make any other visits. Several canals run through the city and the Frische-Haff is close by; the water in the canals is brown and almost stagnant; I cannot open my windows that give onto one of them without being poisoned; it is a swampy, mud-like odour that turns the stomach. However, they say that the health of the inhabitants does not suffer from these emanations. There are few regions where one eats more herrings than here: one even meets people in the street eating a raw herring without bread.

His Majesty left at five o'clock; he is going to Dresden, where he will stay for a short time. We will not leave Kœnigsberg until the 24th or 25th and will go to Berlin. We fear that we will be kept in Prussia for several months. I am sending surgeons everywhere: they are being paid at last and our young men have a lot of money. There are many to regroup. I will leave most of the Germans who took up service with us on this side. The French whom I will take will, in all likelihood, be retained; but I would like it to be decided that no-one will be re-employed before they have spent a year or two in a *grande école*, because they are in great need of training. During these two years, they would earn little or even nothing at all, which would cause a great number of individuals who are as poor in wealth as in spirit, and who in times of peace should not be part of it, to leave military surgery. I am well and doing wonderfully. *M.* Chappe, principal of the IV Corps, has just been made an officer by His Majesty during a review of this corps: it is a just decision. I have terrible bouts of impatience because of all the writing, but I must overcome them. I was dining and talking for a long time afterwards.

14th – I had a visit this morning from *M.* …, one of the principal or general surgeons of the Prussian army. I asked him if he would be willing to accompany me this evening to see *M.* Gerlach, the Nestor[10] and doyen of the Prussian military surgeons. This honourable old man, in his eighties, has only been retired for a year, having been unable, he told me, after he fell on his hip, to take part in the campaign; he has a superb mind; he retains all his memory and his cheerfulness. He was the teacher and predecessor of *M.* Goercke, whom he loves very much. His wife is old; she is not yet consoled of the death of her only daughter whom she lost two years ago. At the house of *Madame* Gerlach I met the wife of a Prussian commandant, who was the most beautiful woman

---

10. Nestor was an elderly king in Greek mythology esteemed for his wisdom.

I have ever met in my life. My visit pleased good father Gerlach and gave me great pleasure.

I was told that a young lady, convalescing from an adynamic fever and who had suffered a bout of illness, had grown almost six inches in ten hours. It was *M.* d'Albavie, among other observers, who swore to me that they had witnessed this event.

Here I am, deep in my writings. Sixty surgeons from Paris have arrived. They took two months to come, will take two months to return, and will each receive 50 *louis d'or* without having done anything: such are the economics of the war administration. We are going to march on Stralsund; I am sending the Baudry division in that direction; our Emperor wants to close this port completely to the English. It seems that we will also enter Copenhagen, because if the English have had a fleet in the port of this city, why should we not have an army within its walls? From all this it must be concluded that we are perhaps not yet close to returning to France; everyone fears that some kind of obstacle will again arise.

15th – Excellent night. Beautiful day. I went with the Prussian surgeon-general to visit some hospitals, which I found in good condition. The French did not establish them; they would be less good. We owe praise to *M.* Goercke, who presided over their creation. Those that have been set up in the churches have been well laid with wooden floorboards; the beds are new and standardized, and the supplies are not bad. The Guard has taken over the superb building of the military exercise hall: they found four beautiful rows of beds arranged on an excellent wooden floor; this hospital is very beautiful. Everywhere one finds forward planning and intelligence on the part of the Prussians. We make nothing good, nor clean, we who are roguish and glorious, as the respectable *M.* Coste says, because our administrations are staffed by thieves and brigands. Recently we were on the verge of shooting six directors; that would still not have been enough. A quarter of a league from the town, a cabin has been built out of planks, such as our hospital builders would never have constructed; the patients are faring excellently in this vast wooden shelter; air, cleanliness, facilities of all kinds; they lack nothing. One finds only physicians in the town of Kœnigsberg; the man in charge of them thought that he should show them all off at once, in the conviction that His Majesty, struck by this rare sight, would not fail to lavish decorations on these zealous public officials, among whom are some who are scarcely 19 years old. But these gentlemen will have to pay for the expenses of the journey, and His Majesty – who, before leaving, made the principal surgeon Chappe an officer of the Legion of Honour and Destouches, Petit, Godefroy, etc., members – did not even want to hear about the medical nomination list.

This morning, a man named H..., a *sous-aide* in the 44th Regiment of the Line infantry, where he murdered an officer and from which he was expelled, presented himself at my lodgings in a magnificent *chirurgien-major*'s uniform, with an Asian-style sabre, etc. I came down on him hard, kicking and punching, and hurt the ring finger of my right hand badly as I hit him. I forced this scoundrel, this extortionist, this corrupt official, to undress and chased him away in a vest; he is accused of all sorts of offences worthy of the galleys at least, and I preferred to treat him like that than to hand him over to the law. This scoundrel is from Karlsruhe; he has been to Saint-Domingue.[11]

At noon I saw His Highness the Prince Major-General, who spoke to me again about my request, which in his opinion was excessive, and who, to console me for not having paid enough attention to it, even though His Majesty had adopted it, promised to see half of it succeed on our return to Paris. I had a very good gala dinner at his lodgings; he showed me every consideration. I noticed in his objections to my list that, as the Emperor had rejected that of the physicians, mine could not have passed without adding to the disfavour that already besets this class of medical officer.

16th, 17th and 18th – These three days offered nothing remarkable. My health has remained good. I am content with my lodgings and, now that I know our fate, I am preparing myself to accept it. We will leave Kœnigsberg on the 25th; on 1 August we will cross back over the Passarge River again; by 1 October we shall have passed over the Oder again and on 1 November the Elbe. Therefore, it will be winter before we will return to France; certainly, there will still be some obstacle that will make us eat what remains of the bread of foreign lands. My wife was in Frankfurt on 5 July, on her way to Paris, where she has no doubt arrived: I am therefore at peace and can now wait for as long as is necessary.

It has rained a lot. The weather has turned. I will not speak of the harvest in Kœnigsberg: for more than 2 leagues around this place there will not be a single ear of corn; the horses have eaten everything. There are good strawberries there and I eat them every day. They distribute a lot of herrings here, which

---

11. The French colonial name for Haiti, which gained its independence in 1804, only a couple of years before Percy was writing.

the careless soldiers eat without having desalinated them, which makes their mouths dry and disposes them to scurvy; they are given wine, but what wine! They have bread, meat and are generally well. Only the IV Corps remains here and in the surrounding area.

The Major-General has left: it is General Lecamus who is now chief of the general staff.

It has been extremely hot since yesterday at noon. The magistrate is providing me with a carriage to run my errands *intra muros et extra*.[12] This morning I saw a lieutenant-colonel of the 76th Regiment of the Line, who, on my advice, was brought by hand from Domnau, where he had been since the battle on 14 June: his left leg is fractured in its middle part; the fragments of the tibia are overlapping and are exposed, but the leg is straight; the pus is of the desired quality, the communication between the two wounds is unhindered and everything is loose, which is to say that all the cellular tissue is void and drained by purulent weeping. The wounded man is safe: he will recover. I renewed the dressing, which was completely soiled, and I refrained from exerting extensions and counter-extensions to bring the bones back into contact. Here the best strategy is not only the enemy of the good, but it would become fatal: these limbs, fractured for a month, with part of the bones protruding, must remain in the state in which they are found, unless the shortening is too considerable. Blood flows from the wounds with the slightest movement; if one pulls at them, the result would be terrible haemorrhaging and a violent separation that would perhaps provoke trismus.

General Drouet, wounded in his left foot by a musket ball that had fractured the bone of the metatarsal that supports the second-to-last toe, suffered sharp pains throughout his foot during these days, although there was only a mild swelling and the wound, from which the musket ball has been superficially extracted, did not show any concerning change. Having found him yellow and without any appetite, I advised putting him on tamarind water mixed with emetics. It is the *chirurgien-major* Darbois, and his colleague Dubois, who are treating him. They have applied poultices and a small collection of pus formed on the dorsal surface, close and parallel to the wound; it was opened yesterday in my presence and the wounded man is faring well at present.

---

12. 'Inside and outside the city walls.'

I saw the hospital known as the Rosengarten. It is a superb cabin made of planks, with a second level, fitted with beautiful casements and extremely well arranged. In the wards on the ground floor, there are four rows of beds: it is too many. There are only two rows in those on the first floor, so they are more salubrious. The kitchen is also made of planks. The bookkeepers, the pharmacy and the administration are in a large and beautiful building. I tried the wine and other foodstuffs: everything is good. The bunks can be locked and are very simple; the bedding consists of a straw mattress, two sheets, a straw sack and a good woollen blanket.

19th – Today is Sunday: everyone is dressed well and either walking in the gardens or out on the water. The women are very elegant; everything in this town suggests good taste, affluence, gallantry and a concern for appearance.

I have written a letter to His Highness the Major-General to complain over the four crosses that he has agreed to grant to me, instead of the ten that I had asked for and that the Emperor had promised me. Here is what I am posting to His Majesty:

> 'SIRE,
>
> 'Before your departure from Tilsit, Your Majesty deigned to listen with kindness to the notes that I gave him on some of the *chirurgiens-majors* accompanying the general staff, whom I had taken the liberty of presenting to you through His Highness the Prince Major-General as a spokesperson in order to obtain the insignia of the Legion of Honour. The expectations, I would almost say the assurances, that he was prepared to give me that these chosen servants would be decorated aroused all of my gratitude and filled me with joy. However, Your Majesty has not made a pronouncement, and the objections of His Highness have made me doubt the success that you had, in some sense, allowed me to claim. It is possible that I have been indiscreet in asking too much of Your Majesty; in this case, I lay my respectful apologies at your feet. But, Sire, you have finished your glorious exploits by granting new benefits and additional favours to your army: will the *chirurgiens-majors* accompanying the general staff, whom you have seen on the battlefields and in the ambulances, and whose zeal and devotion you have praised, these public officials

who serve you with so much enthusiasm and warmth, be excepted from your munificence?

'Two of those whom you decorated on 5 March died a few days later, victims of hospital contagion, and the cordon of the Legion served only to adorn their coffins; they were the *chirurgiens-majors* Beauquet and Laurenchet. A third, Affré, is at risk of not surviving his unfortunate comrades for long. Please have these decorations returned to some of my colleagues and welcome the list that I have the honour of placing here before your eyes of those who are justly worthy of this honourable prize of merit.'

Nomination list for four *chirurgiens-majors* accompanying the general staff of the Grande Armée for admission to the Legion of Honour, a reward that they have earned by their services, their zeal, their talents and for whom the chief surgeon of the armies ventures to claim the justice and the kindness of His Majesty.

| CHÉDIEU, | Headquarters, | 30 years old |
|---|---|---|
| LAROCHE, | --- | 37 --- |
| GALLÉE, | --- | 18 --- |
| LECLERC, | --- | 18 --- |

It was excessively hot today. I dined at the lodgings of our resident general and then went for a walk in a public garden, next to the Finckenstein mansion; this garden, although not superb, is interesting because of its proximity to the canal, which in this part of the city is wide and on which elegant boats carry, to the sound of instruments, pretty women and whole families. From this garden, one can see a rather elegant bridge that crosses the canal; one can also enjoy several rather pleasant views. People drink and eat in this place and lemonade mixed with wine seemed to me to be the most common treat among the German strollers.

20th – The weather is extremely hot. We will leave on the 24th or 25th: I will therefore be able to observe the progress of the harvest and the degree of maturity of the rye in the country.

I saw several wounded in the town, whose dressing I oversaw. A Russian major, a kind and sensitive man, who had had his thigh amputated by *M.* Willier on the evening of 14 June, has been brought all the way to Kœnigsberg. The scar is quite advanced; the sides of the wound have been united lengthwise using strips of cloth, but the scar is no better contained and there will be exfoliation of the femur; a ring of bone some lines thick will separate from the cylinder. This officer, when I saw him the first time, had diarrhoea, which was exhausting him: I advised the *chirurgien-major* who was dressing him to administer ipecacuanha two or three times, which has improved his condition.

A French officer from the 24th Light Infantry, *M.* de Dreux, had his thigh fractured 6 inches above the knee by a cannonball that had just passed through two soldiers and came to rest on that thigh, leaving neither wounds nor contusions, and not even having torn his clothing. On the sixteenth day, after several more or less painful transports, a very sizeable phlegmonous swelling arose; an abscess formed externally and in line with the fracture. It was opened; from then on, no more tension, nor pain. Everything is going well; only the callus, or what one might call a callus, is swollen and very wide.

One of our surgeons, who became an officer in the 3rd Regiment of *Cuirassiers*, and who had been struck by a sabre and stabbed by a lance at Friedland, arrived in Kœnigsberg as a prisoner and we found him there. The most serious of his wounds is a sabre blow that has penetrated the elbow joint and cut the olecranon at its base; the arm is stiff, oedematous, and the joint is painful. This is almost always what happens following this kind of wound: often they leave an almost tumour-like, and in some way lardaceous, swelling of all the cellular tissue afterwards, which subsides with time and alkaline showers.

We will be obliged to leave *M.* Ristel-Huber, one of our *chirurgiens-majors* here because of an adynamic fever from which I hope nonetheless that he will recover.

21st and 22nd – Extremely hot weather; scorching sun; south wind; total dryness. Everything is being loaded onto ships, and there is an immense wealth of boats, grains, flour, wine, brandies, rum, rice, etc. in the port. The army will have some of it; the *commissaires* and storekeepers will have a lot more of it. What thieves! There was a serious question of shooting several of these gentlemen and some directors of the Warsaw hospitals convicted of theft, maladministration and corrupt practices of all kinds; peace suddenly changed the mood, and the Emperor, who wanted them to be executed, has forgotten this matter. These crooks stole nearly half a pound of meat from each patient every day, not to mention everything else: craven, barbaric, sinister murder, worthy of the cruellest death.

I will leave in Kœnigsberg, after the evacuation of the city, which will take place on the 25th, Béclard, *chirurgien-major*, Baltz and Charbonnier, *aides-majors*; Boileau, Henri Michel, Lecat, Beuquet, Merché, Poté and Hocquin, *sous-aides*. I am counting on there being hardly more than forty wounded who cannot be transported, as many of the officers lodged in the town as soldiers in the hospitals. We will give 500 *francs* per month to the *chirurgien-major* and 250 to the other surgeons, in addition to their salaries, with which they will be required to lodge and feed themselves. I fear that they will be very busy: there will be only one physician left, a feeble man who often only takes care of his own interests; at the first headache, he will abandon the service, which from then on will fall to the charge of our surgeons, some of whom will be victims. The list of names on the cenotaph will be long, since those who remain are from the very depths of the hospitals or still suffering the after-effects of a fever: we will excuse ourselves on the grounds that the physician had fallen ill after a few days of service and was forced to abandon the service to the surgeons, who, by this fresh example, will be shown to be very unsuited to fulfilling the two functions. I demanded that *M.* Béclard go to ask for a second physician from *M.* Desgenettes. One of our surgeons, *M.* Ristel-Huber, will remain ill in Kœnigsberg. We will also leave the *sous-aide* Fimet there.

23rd – Excellent night; the heat seems to be increasing, the sun is scorching. We are going to evacuate twenty boats filled with sick men. It would be desirable that those of the Guard could also be evacuated: they have been left to us without anyone to look after them, or to oversee their service. The other day I looked over the military exercise hall with *M.* Chappe, where the fifty-two of them are gathered: four of these brave people were about to die and the flies were eating away at their nostrils and the corners of their eyes, which is to say that they were depositing their eggs there by the thousands, without any charitable hand to swat them away. This sight distressed me. The stench of the hospital made me sick. I was outraged when I saw the disgusting food that was being distributed to these good people. Our surgeons complained and the wrongs will be remedied, but it will not be able to repair the damage that has been done already. The bookkeeper is a wretch who gets drunk three times a day; the poor patients are crying out; no *infirmiers*, no aid except that of the surgeons, who cannot do everything. The administrator-general, an upstanding and good man, never enters the hospitals: this is one of the sources of the heinous crimes to which they play host. But indeed, what service can one expect from a pack of crooks, rogues and bankrupts sent from Paris by His Excellency the Minister Director to be employed in our hospitals? Can one hope to find in such people any sentiment of humanity, piety and sensitivity that should distinguish hospital staff? They have come to the army to make money and, unfortunately, they can only succeed by murdering the poor sick. Oh ungodly breed! His Majesty knows them well; hence, he has not wanted to hear of any employee of the hospitals, those in charge or their subordinates, when it comes to decorations. Besides, it is the same story in almost all quarters: everywhere people steal with as much audacity as impunity; the officers steal; some *ordonnateurs* will leave Warsaw, Wloclaweck, etc. with half a million *francs* that they have plundered – they sell the magazine stores, they make deals with the suppliers, etc.

    My dear colleague Goercke, principal surgeon general of the Prussian army, arrived from the Memel especially to see me. He is an excellent man, 57 years old, with a happy face and very well kempt. He wears in saltire a large cross of Saint Anne of Russia with which Emperor Alexander has decorated him; this cross is set with diamonds and produces a very beautiful effect; the cordon is dark red, trimmed with yellow. I entertained my good friend and presented him to the Intendant-general. He is an extremely estimable man who has a love and even a fanaticism for his profession; one can say that he is the reformer and the patron par excellence of the surgery of the Prussian armies, which was in an abject state before him. In the past, under Bilguer, Theden and Schumacher, it obeyed the doctors; a certain Dr. Lothenius ran it for a long time as an arrogant and disdainful director. He knew how to rescue it from the degrading yoke under which medicine was crushing it; he made it an honourable profession, into which the best sons of the good bourgeois enter eagerly. It is *M.* Goercke who makes all the appointments, who commands, who organizes, who issues promotions, who has workers demoted. In the academy for military surgeons, many poor young men who have aptitude are raised at the expense of the king; once accepted, they practice in all fields, because the institution is medical-surgical. In Prussia, a *chirurgien-major* has the right to practise both functions throughout the kingdom, and it is they who benefit from the most trust in the garrison towns. There were, and still are, more than 2,000 surgeons of all ranks in the Prussian army; the bakers alone have sixteen of them. There are many senior surgeons. These men have golden embroidery, the others have it in silver; it is a simple stitched thread found on the collar, the lapels and the trims, with buttonholes composed of a similar thread. The uniform is all blue. The surgeons have no army grade, nor military integration. No one is more vain, nor more foolishly proud, than the Prussian officers, who are typically social outcasts from poor country seats. The king takes little interest in surgery, but leaves the good man Goercke to do it, without giving him much money, so that this worthy man has spent more than a hundred thousand pounds of his wealth to support his art and give it some splendour. He is highly regarded. The king having met him, when His Majesty returned from Tilsit, he said to him: 'My dear Goercke, I saw your colleague in the French army; he visited me; it is … He gave me great pleasure by the good things he told me about you and your academy. I have received no other satisfaction than that given to me by French surgery.'

24th – Still the same heat and the same dryness. *M.* Goercke did me the kindness of introducing me to all the Prussian surgeons present in Kœnigsberg. Among them were several *chirurgiens-majors* of the hospitals; they can be recognized by their white embroidery; the general surgeons have the same in gold on cornflower-blue serge like ours. We dined with father Gerlach and had a real feast there. This good old man speaks of Frederick II with nothing but affection: I saw him, when we were discussing the misfortunes of Prussia, kiss, with tears in his eyes, a ring that he always wears and which is decorated with a cameo depicting the great Frederick. This great man has left a revered memory, and all the servants who were his contemporaries still adore his image and glory in having lived in his time. The same cannot be said throughout the kingdom for the present king. They do justice to the queen and there is no one who fails to defend her against the calumnies to which she has been subjected. It is clear from the assertions of wise men well acquainted with the court that she has never ceased to be chaste and beyond reproach, and that anything that has been maliciously published about her liaisons with His Majesty Alexander is false and unproven. My friend Goercke, who is always in the family to care at times for the king, who has never given him the slightest gift; and sometimes for the queen, who at least compensates him by her gestures of affection; and often for the children, who call him father Goercke: this honest and truthful man swore to me that there has never been a word of truth in anything that has been said and reported about the love affairs of the Emperor of Russia and the queen. She is a good wife and mother; she is thrifty and her husband is miserly; nothing is sadder than their court.

There is nothing curious to see in Kœnigsberg. The faculty of medicine is dilapidated; the libraries of the university and the palace evoke pity; the palace itself is heart-rending. The famous Kant long baffled the minds of teachers and pupils: he must have been an ugly man, as his bust is almost hideous; the Russians have broken it or knocked it over.

We are leaving tomorrow. On the 25th, the Prussian garrison will take back possession of the city. Here is what was decided by our Emperor and agreed to, as to be expected, by the good King Friedrich Wilhelm: on 20 July, the French army will evacuate Tilsit; on the 25th, it will evacuate Kœnigsberg; on 1 August, it will cross back over the Passarge, on 20 August the Vistula, on 5 September the Oder, and on 1 November the Elbe, which will serve as the evacuation line.

25th – Yesterday I had arranged my few affairs, given orders and written the necessary instructions for the surgeons remaining in Kœnigsberg. I rose at four o'clock, thinking I would leave at five, but my men were not ready until half past six. My good friend Goercke came to embrace me again this morning. Last night there was a very thick stinking fog, which fell during the night. It was quite fresh this morning, but at noon the heat became almost unbearable and the horses suffered greatly.

At three o'clock, we arrived in Brandenburg, the old cradle of the House of Prussia, a rather miserable small town, or rather a long and sad village, where there is no trace of the residence of the former electors, to whom it gave its name, I believe. This village was crowded with troops forming the rearguard: we did not want to stop there. Two short leagues further on, we saw some trees on the right of the road, and we turned to that side to rest in their shade. I have never seen a more pleasant wooded area: it is a valley that can be compared to that of Tempé, at least when one is weary, hot, thirsty and hungry, and when one emerges from the dust and the sand. I travelled through this enchanted place, this English garden planted and designed by nature alone, with delight: it is a deep ravine, a rutted track, at the bottom of which flows a rural stream, silent and hidden mysteriously by the shrubs extending over its waters. In some places, it is only a thin trickle of water, which sometimes forms pretty little pools where the birds come to quench their thirst. These friendly hosts are extremely numerous and seem to amplify their birdsong when they see travellers arriving at their charming oasis. The trees and shrubs are strong and sturdy; the most striking flowers blend their varied and intense colours among their greenery. We saw pyramidal orchids 6ft high and covered with their beautiful blue bells. Large campanulas abound there. The meadowsweet spreads its fragrance far and wide. Nettles, with attractive blue flowers on one side and saffron-coloured flowers on the other, grow everywhere in this beautiful place; I have collected only two seeds from them, the others not yet being ripe. This flower is superb; I had already seen it on the road from Tilsit to Labiau, next to the lysimachia, but I have never come across it in France. The buphthalmum and the blue chicory have discs larger than I have ever seen elsewhere; there is violet lamium of the greatest beauty; we picked blossoming centaurea. I cannot express the good, the pleasure, that this pretty valley gave me. It is not even an eighth of a league long, and at its end I can see and almost touch the Frische-Haff, all covered with sailboats loaded with our sick.

We ate in a cool spot, lying on the grass and in the shade of an oak tree. After my dinner, I stretched myself out on a rug, or more accurately on a horse blanket, and slept for more than an hour. Our horses ate at least as well as I did in a nearby field of barley and vetch. Our boys ate well too.

We continued our journey under a most intense sun, which was reflected on us like a harsh mirror by the Frische-Haff. This lagoon was on our right and we travelled along its edge for 2 leagues. This track is bad, stinking, slow and very unpleasant. We stopped at an isolated building, which is called The Cavalier Inn; it was already full of soldiers. We opened an outhouse and swept it; we were shown to some straw and in a moment our bed was made. The carriages and horses, tied to the wheels, were arranged in front of our barn. We had supper while seated on the step of our large door. Nothing is better in this season than a well-ventilated barn: the houses smell terrible and are full of vermin.

26th – I rose fresh and ready. Warblers had been singing delightfully since three o'clock; I heard the first chorus of the morning birds; they were celebrating the break of day; an orchard adjacent to our barn was full of those pleasant animals that have always been the charm of my life. I am resting and refreshing myself while listening to the birds singing.

We left at five o'clock, all in good spirits, horses and men. The morning was pleasant; it was not until nine o'clock that the sun resumed its scorching heat. It is Sunday today; I noticed it upon our arrival in Braunsberg, where everyone was dressed for celebration. This town is very old. The French spent some time there during the winter; on 26 February, they evacuated it. We saw a tree around which a four-storey scaffold-like construction has been built; from the outside it gives the impression of a large green and square tower, with four casements on each side. The garden where this beautiful lime tree is situated is pleasant and very extensive; the old man who created the tree-house led us everywhere very nimbly for his age; naturally he had his *trinkgeld*. We dined excellently at the home of our host, a wealthy hemp merchant from Russia, who has a huge storehouse near the Passarge, the river that flows alongside Braunsberg and which carries large sailing boats.

We have a hospital with three surgeons, but with no staff or pharmacists; it is in the convent of the Recollect Franciscans. I found only twenty-seven patients there; thirty were evacuated yesterday by water.

We left at five o'clock, and at half past eight reached a hamlet of five houses, where we cleaned a barn and made our bed, as usual. Nothing could be better than that: I am going to sleep on my good straw.

27th – We left a little late; the sun was already high and strong; there was a lot of dust and plenty of bad road, except around 2 leagues from Elbing, where the beautiful new roadway begins, which will connect this town to Kœnigsberg one day. It could be said that it is a very beautiful road: wounded Prussian veterans take care of it; from time to time, there are benches and even grass amphitheatres where one can rest and take refreshment; we saw several terraces in the shape of a quarter-circle, very elegantly arranged and located opposite a fresh stream with a rather beautiful appearance. We would have done well yesterday to stop at Frauenbourg, a charming little town that we only passed through. It is impressive because of the mountain on which it is partly situated, and from which one can see an immense area of land and the Baltic Sea quite close. In the Catholic church there are two paintings, one very large, representing the Communion of Saint Paul, and the other smaller, with Jesus multiplying the loaves in the desert as its subject: they are, everyone assures, masterpieces. Quite close to the church is a house built by Copernicus, which served for a long time as the location of the hydraulic machine that he had invented and had built to bring water to the top of the mountain; the gearwheels still remain there.

We arrived early in Elbing, which is a very pleasant place. Today, and especially around three o'clock, the heat was as strong as ever; it was almost unbearable. I am lodged with the town's chief doctor and in some style. He is an old man who married, two years ago, a woman of 30, very bright and very obliging. After dinner this evening, we went for a walk in the doctor's garden, and I found it very large and quite beautiful; it will be my walk from now on, for we shall spend twenty days here.

28th – The weather has not changed; however, it seems that the heat will be less intense.

Elbing is situated between the sea, the Frische-Haff, and a large lake. The evenings are always cold and damp there. The inhabitants have, in general, bad teeth; my host no longer has a single tooth remaining and his wife has already lost several. The town is rather pretty; it is built like those of Kœnigsberg and Dantzig. In front of each house is a sort of terrace surrounded by a gallery where one can take in the fresh air and go for a stroll; to reach it, one must climb six or eight steps, because, in the event that the canal and the river rise, the town is flooded. It is rare for the cellars to be completely dry; also, at the basement window of most of the houses, one can see a pump ready to drain the water of future floods. Affluence, cleanliness and kindness prevail among the inhabitants. The French have been generally well received here. A lot of business is done in Elbing; the canal is covered with superb merchant vessels and lined with immense storehouses. We have three hospitals there: the first, no.1, is established in the gymnasium and contains 560 bunks; the second is in a vast seven-storey storehouse; the third occupies the building of the freemasons and can only hold 120 patients, who are faring very well. As of today, there are 600 wounded in these three hospitals; they are evacuated each day to Dantzig by boat; it is a convenient means, but one which receives little care and attention. This evening I saw four large boats, one of which was loaded with Russians sent back from Dantzig to Kœnigsberg; these unfortunates were reduced to bread and a little beer, without anyone to assist them. I had an order given to the town's regency to provide a surgeon and three Prussian workers to each boat that arrived and to provide linen, lint, medicines, vinegar, brandy, bread, cooked rice, cooked prunes and wine or beer, as far as its destination. Ours are hardly happier and the surgeons who accompany the sick and wounded suffer greatly. These men, seeing only them, blame them for their misery; often they act with such indignity that they become a threat and we have all the trouble in the world to make them understand that the surgeons are as much to be pitied as they are, since the administration neglects them too and does not give them a quarter of what they would need to fulfil their mission acceptably. Those who went with the boats that left during the night were unable to obtain vinegar, wine or brandy; they were not spared bread, but received little else. They had two workers with them: these workers were seen arguing with the surgeons about the right to take part in the distributions during the journey, a sad and miserable recourse without a doubt; but was it still necessary for an insolent clerk to ultimately deprive my colleagues of them? I said, once and for all, that he who dared to create such an obstacle would be either drowned or beaten to death, and I hope that fear will have more effect than the displays of reason and justice.

The heat has been extreme today and every year, in this season, we experience the same.

29th – Complete drought, heat of more than 26 degrees; one can hardly walk in the streets, so scorching hot are the large stones with which they are paved.

The main headquarters has orders to go to Berlin and already the Intendant-general has left; my colleagues are going to make their way in that direction; it is said that His Highness the Major-General has received orders to stop there instead of going to Paris. The IV Corps will remain here until the 20th. We will hasten our evacuations and I have already chosen the surgeons who will have to remain after the departure of the army and the surrender of the town to the Prussians. They are Thomas, *chirurgien-major*, already head of hospital no. 1; Pla, *aide-major*; Legay, Pavy, Pinet, Dulac, Soleillet and Vila, *sous-aides*. I believe that on 20 August there will hardly be more than 120 wounded or sick who cannot be transported. These surgeons will be treated like those that I left in Kœnigsberg.

They spin some absurd tales here. The one that is the least absurd, although it is a terrible lie, is that the Princess of Saxony has fled, not wanting to marry Prince Jérôme, because of the kind and sensitive woman that he has deserted. It is also said that we are going to fight the Austrians: another error. After the convents of nuns and Capuchin monks, I know of no place where so much nonsense is said and so much false news circulated as in a headquarters that is at rest.

They say that the thermometer has risen to 30 degrees in Paris: this evening it is 28¼ in Elbing. The troops who march in this burning weather are suffering tremendously; thirst torments them to such an extent that any water they encounter appears good to them; the dust inflames their eyes and their throat, dirties their lips and renders them unrecognizable. Dysentery is making progress, yet it is neither an epidemic nor contagious. Six grains of ipecacuanha, two or three days in a row, is the best remedy; a tincture of rhubarb and a few days without eating brings an end to new cases; rice water, in which a little cinnamon is infused, and which is sharpened with a little lemon juice or good wine, is also very successful; quinine in vino-aqueous tincture supports recovery.

Most of the young surgeons sent from Paris since 12 May have fallen ill. They are children of 19 who have no other vocation than to shirk the conscription, so almost all of them are already talking about returning home. Some of them came to me from Naples.

30th – The weather is still getting steadily hotter; we can hardly stand the heat; I think it is over 28 degrees today. Everything is drying out and becoming scorched in the countryside. The army is suffering a great deal.

This morning I saw the three hospitals, which contain about 1,200 patients. In that of the freemasons, there are twelve officers who have had a limb amputated and who have all almost recovered; the stumps are beautiful; the leg amputees only lack good crutches. They have rightly complained that since they were wounded they have passed through the hands of more than ten surgeons: nothing is more distressing for a wounded man who has confidence in his surgeon than to see himself taken away from him. No matter what I do, this harm recurs too often: it must be avoided as much as possible. Most of our surgeons from Paris are bad. As soon as they arrive, they ask for money; they are young men without fortune, sons of artisans who should be artisans themselves; indeed, they would be, without conscription.

31 *Juillet* and 1 *Août* – The heat is still the same, sometimes at 28 degrees and most often at 30 degrees. The inhabitants, accustomed every year at this time to a very intense heat, are surprised at the strength of the heat that prevails; they say that they do not remember having experienced one like it. I have given up on wool and taken to little vests of cotton; during the night I am naked, with my windows wide open, and still I am very hot, I sweat and hardly sleep. Our wounded are suffering greatly: the amputees have severe stabbing pains in their stumps and are prone to nasal bleeding; in general, the wounded are very sensitive to this temperature; the pus in the wounds smells worse and the pains are more intense. The wounded who have a fractured thigh or leg, unable to change their position, are suffering a lot; I had ropes placed above the beds of some of them.

We can hardly breathe, so intense is the heat and so extreme is the dryness. However, I am adapting quite well to this weather; the heat suits me and I am better in summer than during the winter.

I have been to see the large Catholic church, which is dilapidated and where I saw nothing of interest, except a confessional panel where a fanatical painter, guided by a clever priest, has depicted a large heart, in the middle of which there is an angel armed with a broom, who is scrubbing and cleaning the filth and who brings out a throng of imps with mischievous faces by the ears. These are the seven deadly sins that stand out in the midst of this crowd of personified vices: the devil of lust is seductive; the devil of drunkenness has not left his tankard or his glass. The spirit has done so much with the broom that the interior of the heart is clean, although certain little devils, venial sins, but familiar and habitual, have tried to hide in its folds and to escape the great cleansing. Such is the story of the confession.

3rd – For the moment, one cannot stick to anything, so excessive is the heat. I cannot sleep; we can hardly bear it; the thermometer at this time, at two o'clock, reads 30 degrees. Dysentery is making progress: our host, the town physician, has been summoned by several towns to give his opinion and to advise on the ways of halting this plague; already, in a single village, 3 leagues from here, more than thirty people have died. The army is still only slightly affected: wine is being distributed to the troops; it is the best protection; the new beer predisposes them to this disease by giving rise to diarrhoea. Our doctor is called Kobis. He told me that a disastrous epizootic disease was compounding the ruin of the poor inhabitants by taking away their livestock, which perish in great numbers from an eminently inflammatory peri-pneumonia. He attributes this disease to the excessive exhaustion that these animals have endured during the fatigues and the requisitions; the same cause has contributed greatly to the diseases, and particularly to dysentery, which plagues the houses of the poor inhabitants.

Two of our hospitals are built of wood and plaster; the heat is extreme there. The flies torment all our wounded and sick horribly. Every morning they are given a sprig of foliage to cheer them up and to drive away these bothersome insects; I saw in the hospital in the gymnasium, which is the largest, a branch of walnut tree on each bed and was afraid that the patients would be bothered by it, but that has not happened.

We drink a lot of good white wine and have coffee twice a day. The watery and slightly acidic drinks and the refreshing diet would soon kill us, as the heat is so conducive to ataxia, degeneration of the humours, excessive sweating and a kind of colliquative necrosis.

4th – The weather has finally cooled. We have had rain this morning, but only a small amount; the sun is covered; the weather is changeable; it is likely that we will have a storm. At noon, we will leave and say farewell to the town of Elbing.

We left at half past twelve. Harnessed to my small carriage I have three small peasants' horses, which have to be whipped, but which are going reasonably well. The road from Elbing to Marienbourg is superb during the summer; in winter it must be impassable; it cuts across the isle of the Nogat and crosses a marshland, full of ditches filled with water and covered with low meadows. It would be impossible to grasp the fertility of this island, so rich and so abundant in all things that even the most dreadful pillaging has not yet been able to deplete it after eight months. One has drawn innumerable livestock from it, which the *commissaire des guerres*, called Claude, who is in Marienbourg, has only taken for 2 quintals each, while the most meagre cow weighs 3½; thousands of horses have come from it, most of which were thoroughbred. Wheat, flour, oats, fodder, everything has been taken from this beautiful land, and yet one still finds something to live on there; the heavy cavalry has been stationed there to consume the last of it. What crops I have seen! The rye is nearly 6ft high; the barley is scythed and the ground can hardly contain the heaps of sheaves that have been collected there; the hay is piled up in the meadows. Since the brave farmers no longer have horses nor carts, it will perhaps be difficult for them to carry these rich foodstuffs away. The journey seemed very short in the middle of this beautiful countryside, where one finds charming villages.

We arrived in Marienbourg at five o'clock. I saw the hospital, which I found in the same state as I had left it two months ago. It is the same people who are administering it: a contemptible director, a bankrupt, a crook, a thief, a drunkard, worthy of being drowned or hanged, and a temporary commissioner, a detestable subject, without modesty, without restraint, plundering, stealing with as much impunity as audacity. These are, in general, the people who have been put in charge of the hospitals. *M.* Affré, *chirurgien-major* of the hospital in Marienbourg, does his duty well there: he is more assured than the commanding officers who have not dared to punish the two wretches to whom I have just referred; he stands up to them and only makes them more secretive.

The former castle of the Templars or Teutonic knights of Marienbourg, where the hospital is located, is a curious thing; the fortifications have been destroyed and this immense building has been converted into a wheat store for the shipping on the Vistula. In a sunken chapel, which has been protected for the use of the Catholics, is a vault into which we descended with a light and by way of a good stone staircase. There are fifteen or sixteen coffins there, containing just as many corpses, most of which are those of Jesuits dressed in sacerdotal habits. Only one belongs to a woman, still dressed in her beautiful clothes and with a cat at her feet, which must have been put there dead and perhaps stuffed, for it would not have been buried there alive. The arms and hands of this woman are well preserved; the head is in a state of mummification; the clothes, which are made of silk, are there in their entirety; the dress is decorated with a very beautiful lace, which could still be used. At the back of the vault are two Polish magnates in their national dress; that is, a large silk robe with a belt, ankle boots, etc. In general, this place, which is cool but very dry, has the conditions of the cemetery of the Cordeliers in Toulouse; the bodies decompose very slowly there, and even become mummified. I believe that the heads of the corpses we saw there must have been sprinkled with quicklime at the time of interment, for this is the only part that is destroyed; the other parts hold together, have retained their skin, still have substance, and the body, separated from the head, could be removed in one piece. The coffins, which are covered on the outside with silk, bear fairly recent dates; that of a Jesuit is dated 17 November 1785.

In the same vault, near the altar, there is a shaft into which one can descend via a good ladder that is never withdrawn. I did not want to go down it. This shaft leads to a chamber filled with coffins like the one I have just mentioned; but from this chamber one can descend into another deep shaft, at the bottom of which is a recess filled with bones. It seems that at one time this was the knights' sepulchre; however, no matter how much the sand was stirred up, no armour was found there, which they would have been pleased to offer me.

5th – We set off at seven o'clock, in already hot weather. I saw, as we passed through, the hospital of Dirschau, which I found in good condition. We arrived early in Dantzig, extremely hot and slightly uncomfortable because of the two glasses of dirty water that I drank on the way. I was well lodged.

6th – Almost no sleep, so hot has it been and so stifling are these damned feather beds. This morning I visited the hospitals. The one in the arsenal is excellent; I doubt if there has ever been one so good. Each ward, well lit and flagged, contains four rows of more than sixty uniform beds; it will be easy to establish stoves there for the winter. The hospital called Orangebaum is a large warehouse without windows, but it is very open and the patients are not badly off; next to it is the Red House, where they are faring horribly; further on is a rope-making factory, where there is a single row of beds under the tile roof and, as a result, in a furnace. The sick suffer terribly from the heat; it is urgent that we close these last two hospitals, in which the mortality rate is frightening. I am referring to the rate for those with fever, because there are no wounded in these detestable hospitals and, in general, very few of them die in the city of Dantzig. It is true that the surgeons do their duty well there, that they recognize their situation and neglect nothing to save their patients. For the last fifteen days, wet gangrene has given them much to do: they are fighting it successfully with mineral acids taken internally, as well as with quinine, bitters and wine; externally they use bitter decoctions, quinine rattles, fomentations of oak bark, the application of camphor vinegar, slices of lemon and powdered charcoal alone or mixed with cataplasms or some dry powders, especially that of quinine. Crushed charcoal applied on its own sometimes causes too much irritation; it is advisable to moderate its effect by mixing it with other substances; slices of lemon dusted with charcoal powder do a lot of good. There are, as many in the arsenal as in the other hospitals, 2,700 sick; every day twelve or fifteen of them die. In the suburb of Ohra, there are five buildings in which 400 patients with venereal diseases are being treated; later, when the 270 Russians who are in Fort Wasser have left, the venereal sufferers will be established there, which will be more comfortable and more decent for the public. Moreover, it is necessary to have the 800 patients who fill the rope-making factory, the Red House and those at no. 395 leave; they are not wanted there.

7th and 8th – It is impossible to sleep: the great heat is the reason, and on top of that there is a diabolical noise, which from half an hour to the next comes and goes repeatedly, making a hellish racket. I am naked for part of the day and still I can hardly stand it. I reviewed all my surgeons present in Dantzig: *sunt boni mixti malis*;[13] in general, they do their duty well and we are very pleased with them. I will leave tomorrow, without fail, for Schöneck, where I will perhaps reassemble my equipage. There is talk of war with Austria and peace with England.

9th – We are sweating blood and water. I was wet this morning when I awoke as though I had just had a bath; I had gone to bed at midnight, and at three o'clock I was already awake. My effects were ready in a very short time and yet we were only able to leave at six o'clock. There is no ice in Dantzig; one does not know the pleasure of drinking a chilled drink; admittedly, they hardly drink water there and refresh themselves with beer and wine, which they fetch from the cellar.

---

13. 'They are good mixed with bad.'

There are 10 leagues of countryside from Dantzig to Schöneck, and one passes through arid landscapes, uncultivated and without value, as well as sad villages. We stopped only to enjoy some fresh water, at a spring whose stream I discovered. What a delight! I had not drunk such good water in a long time. Schöneck is a small town of poor appearance, surrounded by an old wall and with vast potato plantations. We made dinner with our provisions and I do not think that I have ever drunk as much as I have today: it was as hot as an oven. At four o'clock, I saw the funeral of a Protestant woman pass by: the coffin, very well made and bordered by white muslin festoons, was carried on a large stretcher by twelve men dressed in black who were walking slowly and in time, while some children and two schoolmasters sang German hymns. I noticed that the Catholic Poles, furious and senseless, were laughing at the cortège and the singers; while the dead woman went mournfully to take up her final resting place, drunkards who had filled themselves with beer were fighting in and outside an inn, making appalling cries. The women, just as drunk as the men were, for on Sundays everyone gets drunk in Poland, were trying to separate the 'contestants', and the whole time the coffin was moving. Near this inn sat an old soldier of the great Frederick, who, because he lacked a few *pfennigs*,[14] was watching the drinking, but could not give himself this pleasure; I called to him and gave him the coins, saying to him: 'Soldier of Frederick, go and drink to his memory and to my health!' This good man did not know how to thank me.

I am no longer asleep and I fear that this night will be like the ten that preceded it.

10th – I was pleasantly mistaken and my night was not bad. The weather seemed to have cooled slightly this morning. We left at six o'clock. At nine o'clock, the sun appeared again with full force; everything is dry, everything is scorched; the sands through which we are travelling are as hot as those of Egypt. The countryside is dreadful, miserable. We stopped in a village that we believed to be Alt-Kischau; the horses were hard-pressed; they rested for three hours. This is Polish country; the men all have moustaches and seem to be good people. I made soup with a large stock cube, grehuse[15] and biscuit. Along the way we had picked peas; I had a large pot of them cooked with butter, water and salt. We had a good dinner. We had begun to treat ourselves

---

14. Pennies in German currency for more than a millennium, until the introduction of the euro in 2002.
15. It is unclear to what Percy is referring with this term.

to lemonade mixed with wine; we ended up using up our cask of red wine. One of our *cognias*,[16] unable to go any further, was sold for 2 *thalers* and four good coins. At four o'clock, we harnessed the horses again, and this time we found sandy paths, woods and barren plains, indeed the customary sight of misery exacerbated by the extreme drought. The poor Polish peasants will die of hunger this year. We know a few words in their language: *gleba*, bread; *voda*, water; *zara*, right away; *nierozoni*, I do not understand; *daubré*, it is good.

The roads are terrible for the horses. They sink more than 6 inches into the sand and, if they are loaded with bags, they stay there. The harvests provoke pity. The unfortunate inhabitants are burning parts of the forest to sow something there, and nothing comes of it. We arrived at eight o'clock, in a hamlet, on a small river turning a mill; they call this sad place Voitar. It is composed of barely twelve huts. Beyond the river, on the high ground, is a sort of bourgeois house, surrounded by large barns, but empty and deserted; we stopped there. The horses were well accommodated; we fed them with green oats. As for us, we stayed outside, since the house was revolting, full of poor, dirty, naked little children, and the mother of a recent newborn with puerperal fever. We had a large piece of beef and three good loaves of *kommißbrot*; the soup was skimmed and then the rest of our peas were cooked in the broth. We also obtained some crayfish, so that we had a good supper, sitting on the threshold of the room where we were to sleep and drinking water brought from far away in a barrel. We could not wait for the soup to be ready; no one ate any; so much the better for the poor family of Polish peasants. We had visited all the barns to choose a place to sleep, and preference had been given to a cowshed, which was only filled with a little rubbish. Rye straw threshed during the day will serve as our bed: everyone was very happy with the discovery.

11th – We slept beautifully and this morning we were as fresh as the weather, which already last night seemed to foretell rain with great certainty, since the clouds, very dark, were moving rapidly from north to south. We set off at five o'clock, and I had to use my woollen vest, which I was soon obliged to abandon, so fiercely did the heat return. I do not believe that Siberia, for all the horror and the appearance of the country, nor Egypt, for the sand, the heat and the deserts, are as detestable as the wild regions, equally unbearable to nature as to men, in which we are travelling. We do not meet any other living beings there; not a bird in the forests, not a fruit tree in the countryside. If it were not for a few miserable

---

16. Percy uses the terms 'cogni' or 'cognia' to refer to Polish horses.

fields of rye and buckwheat, where the ears run in long lines, but which at least attest that the hand of man has been at work there, one would think that we are in true deserts. I am sure that along a distance of 25 leagues we have not found a population of 200 souls. We travelled up to 4 leagues in the same forest without stopping and it was even hotter there than on the plain, the heat being hemmed in; the trees are all pines in these forests. We see only willow trees around the houses and far and wide in the countryside. Some of them are enormous; the ash and the so-called verne[17] tree are also becoming just as huge.

At eleven o'clock, having travelled very slowly because the wheels caught in the sand, we arrived at Kausabuta, the village where the post station is; there we had the horses refreshed. The servants found beer and we found sour cherries, with which we were able to take refreshment in a large garden, where there is a long path lined with cherry trees covered with fruit; these cherry trees have not been grafted; however, although they are wild stock, they yield fairly large cherries, although they are very sour and even bitter. The master of the house forced us to sit down to dinner; we found a superb family of nine children, three of whom were tall boys, two beautiful young girls who were graceful, musical and well-dressed. The mother is still very good-looking; the father is a very handsome man; they are Prussians. I only ate soup. At three o'clock, we returned to the carriage and, having crossed the most dreadful of all countries with difficulty, not being able to stand the heat any longer, cursing the sand in which we could hardly move, even at a slow pace, and pitying the unfortunates condemned to live in poverty on this thankless land, we saw the points of the small bell towers of Konitz, which we finally entered at half past eight, tired, fatigued and gasping from the heat and thirst.

The little town of Konitz is quite nice. We are lodged on the square in a beautiful house always reserved for the generals. One of the two girls, only 15 years old, is so fat that she weighs at least as much as I do; she has a bigger bosom than four wet nurses combined, which does not prevent her from being lithe and pretty in her own way. When I arrived, I found my caisson loaded with all my effects from Riesenbourg. There is a small hospital in Konitz: Bonjour and Karsten are looking after it; I found only twenty-five patients there.

12th – The small hospital is in the barracks, which was once a Jesuit convent; today it contains twenty-four sick people, who would be fine if they had wine, but the officer in command, Saint-Mars, does not want them to be given any,

---

17. Speckled alder.

claiming that it is of no value to them and that it would be more useful to give them schnapps in the morning and tamarind water in the evening. This man is a kind of crank, full of pretensions and having had the stupidity to send a sergeant of the *gendarmerie* to call me to go to see him: I sent both of them on their way and I would have been delighted if my refusal of such a ridiculous measure might have inflamed the commander in order to cool him down quickly. One day the Emperor, speaking of his enemies, said pleasantly: 'I have so many that soon I will no longer know them; firstly, the commanding officers of the towns behind our lines, the *commissaires des guerres*, the quartermasters and workers; then the Cossacks, the Kalmyks, the Bashkirs, the Russians, etc.' He was quite right, and this combination of enemies expresses perfectly the people about whom everyone in the army has to complain. Konitz is Catholic, except for a few houses. The churches there are so poor as to be pitiable: the Augustinians are dying of hunger there; there are only one or two Jesuits left; the convent is falling into ruin.

Dysentery is ravaging Riesenbourg and the surrounding area: a charming little daughter of this town's apothecary, with whom I was staying, died of it. The German doctors do not know how to treat this disease.

A lot of woollen cloth is made in Konitz.

13th – I slept for five good hours: it was nearly four when I awoke. We left at six; it was as hot as all these previous days. The road from Konitz to Friedland is sandy, but quite beautiful: one crosses a rather sad landscape where everything is being harvested, rye, barley and oats; it is pitiable, and in France one would refuse with scorn to gather such a miserable crop. We passed the old battlefield of the Teutons and the Swedes, who fought extremely ferociously 200 years ago: the Teutons were victorious; their grandmaster lived in a fortified castle at Schlochau, 3 short leagues from Konitz, where one can still see some very fine remains, including a well-preserved tower that overlooks the whole plain, which is large.

Friedland was once fortified; it is hardly as good as the one that became so famous for the battle of 14 June. I am well housed and fed as well as possible in such a small place. We will leave tomorrow at three o'clock in the morning, for the heat is killing our horses, while the new fodder and the lack of oats are also making them cough and grow thinner.

14th – We were lodged wonderfully and I am as well as I have ever been. I slept. We left at four o'clock and arrived at eleven in Jastrow, 7 leagues from Friedland, along 4 leagues of good road and 3 of sand that can hardly be passed. This town of 4,000 inhabitants is at the foot of an arid slope and set before a scorched plain, the appearance of which is frightening; they make rather fine cloth there. The heat is continuing; the horses are suffering greatly. We rolled around on the cool grass and I have not been able either to read or to write.

15th – The night was a little less hot than the previous ones: I slept from nine o'clock until half past two. We left at nearly four o'clock and took the road to Schneidemühl, instead of that to Deutsch-Krone, which saves us 4 leagues. Schneidemühl is a small town consisting of a large regular square lined with rowan trees, many of which have been badly damaged by the passage of the troops; it is scarcely populated by Jews. The commanding officer, a captain of the 55th Line Infantry, convalescing from having his right arm fractured by a biscayan at Eylau, gave me a good dinner, a great deal of oats and a carriage for tomorrow. Two leagues from here, on the Netze River, is a small town called Usch, where there is a hospice and a surgeon for the evacuations that pass through on boats. It is a pity to see the sick passing on this river, which flows into the Warta; those who can walk roam the countryside and feed themselves; the poor unfortunates who cannot leave the boat die of misery there. Almost all of them come from Nackel. here are no clerks, no employees, no *infirmiers*; the evacuation list is given to a non-commissioned officer who is being evacuated himself. Food is distributed as they leave and the convoy has to travel 25 leagues before it receives any more. Aside from that, everything is the same: the river is busy with boats loaded with flour and oats that are spoiled. We lack these foodstuffs everywhere; it makes no difference, the boats do not move and everything perishes there.

16th – It was pleasantly cool last night; I thought it would rain. I slept well and rose feeling in very good shape. At six o'clock, we left: it was cool to the extent that, not wearing a vest (I have not worn it for three weeks), I was forced to put my woollen blanket over my shoulders. I noticed several people, women and children, who had toes that were fused together and were so distorted that they could hardly be recognized. The distance from Schneidemühl to Schœnlanke is 6 leagues through dreadful sands; we made a mistake in leaving the town and travelled a full league in vain; it is impossible to go at anything other than a slow pace, since the resistance of the sand drags us back. The country belongs to His Highness the Prince of Neufchâtel, in whose name posts have been established everywhere announcing that he has taken its possession and asking for the respect of the landowners. The woods are beautiful; to the left there is a vast meadow, but in general the ground is arid and infertile.

The town of Schœnlanke is inhabited by wool carders and spinners; they make cloth sheets there. The little boys run after the French to offer them women: it is the same everywhere in Prussia; morals are lost there and debauchery is at its height. Tomorrow we will go to Filehne, 6 leagues from here, another empty, poorly built little town, which is very poor and already ruined. I am lodged with the apothecary and have been treated fairly well.

17th – It took me a lot of effort to rise this morning at three o'clock: I was sleeping so well! We left in cool and pleasant weather. It is only 6 leagues from Schœnlanke to Filehne, but the sand is deep and the road makes extremely hard work for the horses. The countryside is poor, except around two rather run-down villages that we passed. The heat has been bearable. On arriving at Filehne, we were taken to, and lodged with, the Count of Blankenstein, whose castle outside the town and near the Netze is very beautiful. We were received well there, but I could not take advantage of the good food as I was indisposed; it is the bad nights and the great heat that are making me ill. I saw the hospice in Filehne; it is pitiable. The evacuations on the Netze are organized terribly: no clerks, no supplies, no orders; these boats loaded with sick are like travelling tombs. We met two carriages with bundles of pharmacy supplies without a guide or a pharmacist; this is another place where there are flagrant abuses.

The day before yesterday I had inadvertently put three pillowcases in my saddlebags; I sent them back to our hostess in Schneidemühl, to whom they belong.

18th – Little sleep. The morning is quite cool. The road is sandy. At ten o'clock, unbearable heat, still the same dryness. To reach Driesen, one must travel 7 short leagues, with a long meadow covered with haystacks to one's right; the Netze is also on the right; the left is sand, mountains of sand, and desert. We arrived in Driesen at ten o'clock. Good accommodation. The commanding officer Favreau treated us to lemonade mixed with wine and with champagne in a charming English garden built in the grounds of the former citadel, which Frederick the Great had dismantled thirty-three years ago; this garden is delightful and in good taste. One sees some rather beautiful monuments there, including one of a woman crying over an urn; this statue is by someone named Baldon, a statue sculptor in Berlin. This pious monument was consecrated by the present master of the garden in honour of the former owner, who was its creator and who made the fortune of this kind and sensitive man. It is the young La Motte who is running the hospice.

19th – Left this morning in pleasant weather, without sunshine, but with frighteningly bad dust and sand. Arrived in Friedeberg[18] at ten o'clock, still

---

18. Percy calls this town 'Friedberg' and 'Friedeberg' interchangeably.

fairly fresh: it is only 6 leagues; bad countryside in places. Friedeberg is a fairly good town, with two old gates and a very old surrounding wall. Nine thousand souls live here. I am staying with the good Jew Moyse, with whom I stayed previously last December with Dr. Maugras. There is a beautiful lake at the gate of the town, the surroundings of which are good.

20th – The night was hot as usual: these damned feather beds cause me to sweat and become horribly hot; no mattress, even among the richest people; there is no country where one has a worse bed. We left at four o'clock, found more sand than ever, crossed the deserts of Arabia and arrived in Landsberg very early. We were lodged with the rich dyer with whom the generals are staying. We are faring marvellously there; it would be difficult to be better lodged and fed while on campaign. The small hospital in Landsberg is in a church near the entrance to the town: I found only twelve sick there; this morning there were 150, who were evacuated. This town has two old gates and a wall of stones 40ft high. The inhabitants have already suffered a great deal, yet there is still a lot of affluence; they make fabrics there.

21st – I had a very restless night. We left at five o'clock. Never had we found so much sand: there are 2 leagues of good causeway, which has been made recently, after which we fell back onto the sandy paths through the woods. Halfway to Kustrin, we were expecting to find a stopping place at Baltz, but everything on the road is ruined and pillaged. They wanted to send us to stay the night in Kammin, 2 leagues from the road: I preferred that we take refreshment in a hamlet, where we found good hay and good water, and continued on to Kustrin. We are lodged in the neighbourhood of Berlin, with a wealthy baker. My little mare is very ill; the heat has been unprecedented; everyone is falling ill; two of our servants have a fever. The dust, the burning sand and the sun that engulfs everything is enough to kill us all. There is a lot of dysentery and the mortality rate is frightening. The merchants selling coffins have plenty of business: it is a significant area of trade in this region, where even the poorest individuals have a coffin costing 8 or 10 crowns; one sees only small, very attractive coffins displayed like insignia.

22nd – The heat is fiercer still than yesterday. I went to see the hospital a quarter of an hour from Kustrin: it has been established in the vast grain stores of the King of Prussia; there is space to put 1,800 patients there, but at the moment there are only 1,000. The service is appalling; the courtyard is poisoned by latrines that empty into a pit that is overflowing and uncovered. At ten o'clock, I saw eleven corpses loaded onto a wagon that could not hold any more, a terrible spectacle for the patients who witnessed it, and disgusting for everyone. The loading was done at the foot of the stairs to the main wards; the corpses were bleeding and were emanating a dreadful stench. The wards are badly kept: all the patients are unhappy; there is an awful smell everywhere; the bed linen is dirty, and ten or twelve unfortunates have died on each mattress without them having been cleaned. There are no *infirmiers*, when such a big service would need 200. There is a shortage of more than 250lb of meat for the cooking pots. Having seen the meat cut, and the quantity having seemed to me to be extremely out of proportion with the day's activity, I wanted to know what had been put in the pot. The cook and all the kitchen boys replied that they had put in two hindquarters (50 or 60lb) and one front quarter (45lb), which made 160lb instead of 500. It is horrifying, and I burst into a tirade of threats and fits of indignation. The director is called Varocquier and the *commissaire* Dufresne, two truly contemptible people who enrich themselves at the expense of the poor sick; the bread is very bad; the head of the administration of food supplies is a man called Rosé, from Haguenau, a fraudulent bankrupt who came to the army to put his affairs back in order. This is what happens almost everywhere. His Majesty knows it, he swears, loses his temper, and the wrongdoing continues. I have threatened to expose the *commissaire*, who has made a reputation of probity for himself. As for the director, he should be hanged.

We have been just fine in Kustrin. Tomorrow we will leave at three o'clock.

23rd – I sweated last night and slept poorly. It was cool when we left: I was obliged to put on my redingote, but at ten o'clock, the heat returned as fiercely as yesterday. The road is very bad, always sand and desert, except in the area surrounding a small town and two villages that we encountered along the way. One end of the road is lined with acacias. In general, this tree is commonly grown in Neumark; one sees them everywhere, in front of the houses, along some paths and even in the woods. Rowans are even more common; they are found everywhere and are enormous in size. This tree, beautiful in flower, has superb fruit: this is its season; these small pears of a vivid and luminous red contrast marvellously with the beautiful green of the leaves. While terrible storms ravage Europe, and particularly France, not a thunderclap is heard here; no rain; few clouds. This is because there are no mountains and many canals, rivers and streams. It does not seem that the epizootic has made any progress in Prussia. I have encountered some very fine herds during the last fortnight; the cows are superb and the mutton is excellent; they also eat a lot of it at this time of year. Never have we seen so many flies; the horses are horribly tormented by them. Muncheberg, where we arrived at noon, is a rather ordinary town: the whole army has passed through there during November; the whole army, or very nearly so, will pass through it again, and yet the inhabitants are still holding out. In Muncheberg, there is a tower built in brick, which is very elegant and perfectly preserved; it dates from the twelfth century.

24th – Arrived in Berlin at one o'clock, in heat almost equal to that of an oven. The principal pharmacist insisted that the mercury thermometer, exposed to the sun, gave 45 degrees; in the shade, it showed 30. I am magnificently housed, on the main street, with *M. …*, in French *Esprit*; my private room is decorated with beautiful paintings, which had been hidden in the attic, and because of the confidence I inspired they were brought down to put them back in their place. There are also wax busts of charming women; nothing is sweeter than these portraits.

25th, 26th, 27th and 28th – Hot, scorching, unbearable weather; everyone is sweating night and day. Those who have spent time in Saint-Domingue assure us that it is less hot on this island. It rained during the night of the 25th to the 26th, with claps of thunder that I only heard while dreaming, so sleepy was I; this fairly heavy rain has done nothing to cool the atmosphere.

29th, 30th and 31st – The same weather, interspersed with a few showers. Dysentery is ravaging a part of Prussia; the towns of Kœnigsberg, Braunsberg, Konitz, etc. are plagued by it. Surprisingly, while we are losing few patients in our hospitals, where they are nonetheless so badly off, many people are dying among the inhabitants, to whom the doctors of the country dispense inflammatory remedies. The livestock are also dying from a dysentery of their own; the post-mortem investigation of several cows has shown their guts to be affected by phlogosis and in a state of mortification. The veterinarians are no more successful in treating their patients than the doctors are in curing their own. Inflammatory and disruptive medicine is in fashion in this area: there is not even a miserable case of gonorrhoea for which the best doctor in Berlin would not use twenty or thirty kinds of remedies.

Speaking of this city, which I have found more and more beautiful and where the park has so pleased me, I have not met Dr. Huffeland there: he is still with the king. I saw a fine collection of engravings and portraits of people of the art from Hippocrates to the present day at Madame Goercke's house. This collection forms three volumes in-folio; it pleased me enormously.

1 *Septembre* – The weather has cooled as a result of the rain. A fever is taking hold among our troops and surgeons that, after being elusive for a few

days, then manifests itself sporadically daily or three-daily. The attacks are long and painful; they threaten to become subintrant and would become so if we did not hurry, following an emetic and a purgative, to use quinine at a dose of ten-eighths of an ounce, or even an ounce and a half between two bouts. This sharp medicine stops the paroxysms and heals very well.

2nd until the 10th – The weather is almost cold; it has been necessary to wear our winter clothes. On the 6th, there was a white frost; the heat has finally passed, but the temperature has cooled too suddenly; this contrast causes illnesses. Dysentery and intermittent fever have made progress. I am not sleeping; however, I am going out a little, and I have already taken several walks in the park as I have been leaving Berlin, a charming forest, a place of delights, far more beautiful than our Champs-Elysées.

A quarrel arose between the adjutant to the *commissaires* Bourgoing and the *chirurgien-major* Gama: the latter was arrested by the former for a matter relating to his duty. I have recalled Gama from the 3rd Division of the I Corps, where the affair took place, and I have had an explanation on this subject from the Intendant-general; he has promised me that he would take care of the aforementioned matter and that I would be satisfied. We will see.

11th and 12th – Rain every day and cold weather. The French are bored with being away from home for so long.

The number of sick in the army has reduced to 16,000; it was 30,000 twenty days ago. The hospitals of Berlin are reasonably good; they eat bad rye bread there, which is detestable for the patients suffering from diarrhoea and dysentery.

Some of the *commissaires des guerres*, since His Majesty's departure, have decided to come out of their shell and take a tone towards the surgeons, whom opinion, the reality of the services and the benevolence of the master have placed far above them. I complained about this to the Intendant-general, to whom I believe I proved that a *commissaire* could be the head of a hospital, but never the head of the medical officers; there is still much to be said and done on this point.

17th – Until the 15th, the weather was cold; yesterday, the 16th, and today, the 17th, it has become milder. We are presuming that the winter will be very harsh.

# Appendix

## KEY TOPONYMS IN PERCY'S JOURNAL

An effort has been made to find modern equivalents for the places named in Percy's *Journal*; however, it has not been possible to source equivalent toponyms for some settlements.

| Toponym (in Percy's *Journal*) | Toponym (today) | Country (today) | Additional Comments |
|---|---|---|---|
| Aach | Aach | Germany | |
| Aalen | Aalen | Germany | |
| Aarau | Aarau | Switzerland | |
| Alle (River) | Łyna (River) | Poland / Russia | |
| Alsace | Alsace | France | |
| Allenstein | Olsztyn | Poland | |
| Altorf | Altorf | France | |
| Attinghausen | Attinghausen | Switzerland | |
| Auerstaedt | Auerstedt | Germany | |
| Augsbourg | Augsburg | Germany | |
| Austerlitz | Slavkov u Brna | Czech Republic | |
| Babiak | Babiak | Poland | |
| Baden | Baden | Germany | |
| Bâle | Basel | Switzerland | |
| Bamberg | Bamberg | Germany | |
| Bartenstein | Bartoszyce | Poland | |
| Bellinzona | Bellinzona | Switzerland | |

| Toponym (in Percy's *Journal*) | Toponym (today) | Country (today) | Additional Comments |
|---|---|---|---|
| Bergzaben | Bad Bergzabern | Germany | |
| Berlin | Berlin | Germany | |
| Besançon | Besançon | France | |
| Blindheim | Blindheim | Germany | |
| Blonie | Błonie | Poland | |
| Braunsberg | Braniewo | Poland | |
| Breslau | Wrocław | Poland | |
| Brieg, Brag, Brug, Brog (Rivers) | Breg, Brigach (Rivers) | Germany | The headstreams of the river Danube. |
| Bromberg | Bydgoszcz | Poland | |
| Bruck | Brück | Germany | |
| Brugg | Brugg | Switzerland | |
| Brünn | Brno | Czech Republic | |
| Bug (River) | Bug (River) | Belarus / Poland / Ukraine | |
| Burgau | Burgau | Germany | |
| Bürglen | Bürglen | Switzerland | |
| Calvar-Berg | Kalvarienberg | Germany | |
| Charlottenbourg | Charlottenburg | Germany | |
| Coire | Chur | Switzerland | |
| Colmar | Colmar | France | |
| Copenhague | København (Copenhagen) | Denmark | |
| Dantzig | Gdańsk | Poland | |
| Danube (River) | Danube (River) | Throughout central Europe | |
| Dessau | Dessau | Germany | |
| Dillingen | Dillingen an der Donau | Germany | |
| Dirschau | Tczew | Poland | |
| Dissentis | Disentis | Switzerland | |
| Domnau | Domnovo | Russia (Kaliningrad Oblast) | |
| Donaueschingen | Donaueschingen | Germany | |
| Donauwerth | Donauworth | Germany | |

# Appendix

| Toponym (in Percy's *Journal*) | Toponym (today) | Country (today) | Additional Comments |
|---|---|---|---|
| Dresde | Dresden | Germany | |
| Driesen | Drezdenko | Poland | |
| Elbing | Elbląg | Poland | |
| Elchingen | Elchingen | Germany | |
| Engadine | The Engadin | Switzerland | |
| Engen | Engen | Germany | |
| Ensisheim | Ensisheim | France | |
| Erbach | Erbach an der Donau | Germany | |
| Erfurt | Erfurt | Germany | |
| Eylau | Bagrationovsk | Russia (Kaliningrad Oblast) | Site of the famous battle in 1807. |
| Feldkirck | Feldkirch | Austria | |
| Filhene | Wieleń | Poland | |
| Finkenstein | Finkenstein am Faaker See | Austria | |
| Fluelen | Flüelen | Switzerland | |
| Fontainebleau | Fontainebleau | France | |
| Forcheim | Forchheim | Germany | |
| Francfort-sur-Oder | Frankfurt an der Oder | Germany | |
| Francfort | Frankfurt | Germany | |
| Frauenbourg | Frombork | Poland | |
| Freudenstadt | Freudenstadt | Germany | |
| Fribourg | Fribourg | Switzerland | |
| Frick | Frick | Switzerland | |
| Friedberg | Friedberg | Germany | |
| Friedland | Pravdinsk | Russia (Kaliningrad Oblast) | Site of the famous battle in 1807. |
| Friedland, near Konitz | Debrzno | Poland | Also known as *Preußisch Friedland*. |
| Frische-Haff | Vistula Lagoon | Poland and Russia (Kaliningrad Oblast) | A lagoon on the Baltic Sea between Gdańsk and Kaliningrad Oblast. |

| Toponym (in Percy's *Journal*) | Toponym (today) | Country (today) | Additional Comments |
|---|---|---|---|
| Geisingen | Geisingen | Germany | |
| Gengenbach | Gengenbach | Germany | |
| Gera | Gera | Germany | |
| Gmünd | Gmünd | Austria | |
| Graudenz | Grudziądz | Poland | |
| Grisons | Grisons | Switzerland | |
| Gundelfingen | Gundelfingen | Germany | |
| Gunzbourg | Günzburg | Germany | |
| Guttstadt | Dobre Miasto | Poland | |
| Halle | Halle | Germany | |
| Hambourg | Hamburg | Germany | |
| Haslach | Haslach im Kinzigtal | Germany | |
| Heidelberg | Heidelberg | Germany | |
| Heilsberg | Lidzbark Warmiński | Poland | |
| Hochstett | Höchstädt an der Donau | Germany | |
| Hoff | Hoff | Germany | |
| Hohenlinden | Hohenlinden | Germany | |
| Hornberg | Hornberg | Germany | |
| Hornhausen | Hornhausen | Germany | |
| Iéna | Jena | Germany | Site of the famous battle in 1806. |
| Jablona | Jabłonna | Poland | |
| Jastrow | Jastrowie | Poland | |
| Kammin | Kamień Pomorski | Poland | |
| Karlsruhe | Karlsruhe | Germany | |
| Kehl | Kehl | Germany | |
| Kleczewo | Kleczewo | Poland | |
| Klodawa | Kłodawa | Poland | |
| Kniebis | Kniebis | Germany | A mountain ridge in Germany's Black Forest. |

# Appendix 295

| Toponym (in Percy's *Journal*) | Toponym (today) | Country (today) | Additional Comments |
|---|---|---|---|
| Kœnigsberg | Kaliningrad | Russia (Kaliningrad Oblast) | |
| Kœnigsfelden | Königsfelden | Switzerland | |
| Konitz | Chojnice | Poland | |
| Kork | Kork | Germany | |
| Kostrzyn | Kostrzyn | Poland | |
| Kronach | Kronach | Germany | |
| Krumbach | Krumbach | Germany | |
| Kurrische-Haff | Curonian Lagoon | Russia / Lithuania | A freshwater lagoon separated from the Baltic Sea by a spit of land. It lies on the border between Russia and Lithuania. |
| Kustrin | Kostrzyn nad Odrą | Poland | |
| Kutno | Kutno | Poland | |
| Labiau | Polessk | Russia (Kaliningrad Oblast) | |
| Landsberg | Górowo Iławeckie | Poland | |
| Langfuhr | Wrzeszcz | Poland | Now a borough of Gdańsk. |
| Laufenbourg | Laufenburg | Germany | |
| Leczyca | Łęczyca | Poland | |
| Leipheim | Leipheim | Germany | |
| Leipzig | Leipzig | Germany | |
| Liebstadt | Liebstadt | Germany | |
| Limmat (River) | Limmat (River) | Switzerland | |
| Lobenstein | Bad Lobenstein | Germany | |
| Löffingen | Löffingen | Germany | |
| Lowicz | Łowicz | Poland | |
| Lucerne (Lake) | Lucerne (Lake) | Switzerland | |
| Magdebourg | Magdeburg | Germany | |
| Manheim | Mannheim | Germany | |

| Toponym (in Percy's *Journal*) | Toponym (today) | Country (today) | Additional Comments |
|---|---|---|---|
| Marienbourg | Malbork | Poland | |
| Marienwerder | Kwidzyn | Poland | |
| Mein (River) | Main (River) | Germany | The Rhine's longest tributary. |
| Mels | Mels | Switzerland | |
| Memel | Klaipėda | Lithuania | *See also* Niémen (River). |
| Memmingen | Memmingen | Germany | |
| Mengen | Mengen | Germany | |
| Mersebourg | Merseburg | Germany | |
| Mewe | Gniew | Poland | |
| Miseritz | Międzyrzecz | Poland | |
| Mohrungen | Morąg | Poland | |
| Molwitz | Małujowice | Poland | |
| Montagney-les-Pesmes | Montagney-les-Pesmes | France | The village in which Percy was born, in a house on the subsequently-named *Rue du Baron Percy*. A plaque on the house bears his name. |
| Mösskirch | Meßkirch | Germany | |
| Muncheberg | Müncheberg | Germany | |
| Narew (River) | Narew (River) | Poland | |
| Nasielsk | Nasielsk | Poland | |
| Naumbourg | Naumburg | Germany | |
| Neckar (River) | Neckar (River) | Germany | A tributary of the Rhine. |
| Netze (River) | Noteć (River) | Poland | |
| Neumarkt | Neumarkt in der Oberpfalz | Germany | |

| Toponym (in Percy's *Journal*) | Toponym (today) | Country (today) | Additional Comments |
|---|---|---|---|
| Neustadt | Neustadt | Germany | |
| Niémen (River) | Neman (River) | Kaliningrad Oblast | Also called the Niemen, Nioman, Nemunas, or Memel depending on the country through which it flows (including Belarus, Lithuania, and Russia's Kaliningrad Oblast). |
| Nogat (River) | Nogat (River) | Poland | A branch of the Vistula's delta. |
| Nordlingen | Nördlingen | Germany | |
| Nowemiasto | Nowe Miasto | Poland | Meaning *New Town*, Nowe Miasto is a common toponym in Poland. |
| Nowy Dwor | Nowy Dwór Mazowiecki | Poland | |
| Nuremberg | Nürnberg | Germany | |
| Oberhausen | Oberhausen | Germany | |
| Oberzell (Abbey) | Kloster Oberzell | Germany | |
| Ochsenfurth | Ochsenfurt | Germany | |
| Oder (River) | Oder (River) | Poland | |
| Offenbourg | Offenburg | Germany | |
| Offenheim | Offenheim | Germany | |
| Osterode | Ostróda | Poland | |
| Ostrach | Ostrach | Germany | |
| Passarge (River) | Pasłęka (River) | Poland | |
| Passenheim | Pasym | Poland | |
| Pelplin | Pelplin | Poland | |

| Toponym (in Percy's *Journal*) | Toponym (today) | Country (today) | Additional Comments |
|---|---|---|---|
| Petit-Bordeaux | Petit-Bordeaux, Villevaudé | France | Place of Percy's country residence, east of Paris. |
| Pfaffenhofen | Pfaffenhofen an der Ilm | German | |
| Pforzheim | Pforzheim | Germany | |
| Pfullendorf | Pfullendorf | Germany | |
| Pillau | Baltiysk | Russia (Kaliningrad Oblast) | |
| Plirchten | Plichta | Poland | |
| Posen | Poznań | Poland | |
| Potsdam | Potsdam | Germany | |
| Prasnitz | Przasnysz | Poland | |
| Praust | Pruszcz Gdański | Poland | |
| Prégel (River) | Pregolya (River) | Russia (Kaliningrad Oblast) | |
| Pultusk | Pułtusk | Poland | |
| Rastadt | Rastatt | Germany | |
| Reuss (River) | Rüüss (River) | Switzerland | |
| Rheinfelden | Rheinfelden | Switzerland | |
| Rhin (River) | Rhine (River) | Germany / Switzerland / France | |
| Rosenberg | Rosenberg | Germany | |
| Rosengarten | Rosengarten | Germany | |
| Rottenbourg | Rothenburg ob der Tauber | Germany | |
| Rottweill | Rottweill | Germany | |
| Saalfeld | Zalewo | Poland | |
| Saale (River) | Saale (River) | Germany | |
| Säckingen | Bad Säckingen | Germany | |
| Saint-Gall | St. Gallen | Switzerland | |
| Samter | Szamotuly | Poland | |

# Appendix 299

| Toponym (in Percy's *Journal*) | Toponym (today) | Country (today) | Additional Comments |
|---|---|---|---|
| Sans-Souci | Sanssouci Palace | Germany | The palace takes its name from the French 'Sans souci', meaning 'without worries'. It was the summer home of the Prussian King Frederic the Great. |
| Sargans | Sargans | Switzerland | |
| Saulgau | Bad Saulgau | Germany | |
| Schaffhouse | Schaffhausen | Switzerland | |
| Schleitz | Schleiz | Germany | |
| Schlochau | Człuchów | Poland | |
| Schneidemühl | Piła | Poland | |
| Schöneck | Schöneck | Germany | |
| Schorndorff | Schorndorf | Germany | |
| Schweinfurt | Schweinfurt | Germany | |
| Schwitz | Schwyz | Switzerland | |
| Seligenstadt | Seligenstadt | Germany | |
| Slupca | Słupca | Poland | |
| Soldau | Soldau | Poland | |
| Souabe | Swabia | Germany (region) | |
| Spandau | Spandau | Germany | |
| Stargard | Stargard | Poland | |
| Stettin | Szczecin | Poland | |
| Stokach | Stockach | Germany | |
| Stralsund | Stralsund | Germany | |
| Stuhm | Sztum | Poland | |
| Stuttgard | Stuttgart | Germany | |
| Tapiau | Gvardeysk | Russia (Kaliningrad Oblast) | |
| Thionville | Thionville | France | |

| Toponym (in Percy's *Journal*) | Toponym (today) | Country (today) | Additional Comments |
|---|---|---|---|
| Thorn | Toruń | Poland | |
| Tilsit | Sovetsk | Russia (Kaliningrad Oblast) | |
| Treuenbriezen | Treuenbriezen | Germany | |
| Trèves | Trier | Germany | |
| Triberg | Triberg im schwarzwald | Germany | |
| Tuttlingen | Tuttlingen | Germany | |
| Uberlingen | Überlingen | Germany | |
| Ulm | Ulm | Germany | |
| Unterzell | Unterzell | Germany | |
| Usch | Usch | Germany | |
| Varsovie | Warsaw | Poland | |
| Vieux-Brisach (le) | Breisach | Germany | |
| Villevaudé | Villevaudé | France | |
| Villingen | Villingen-Schwenningen | Germany | |
| Vistule (River) | Vistula (River) | Poland | |
| Waldshut | Waldshut-Tiengen | Germany | |
| Waldstetten | Waldstetten | Germany | |
| Wallenstadt | Walenstadt | Switzerland | |
| Warta (River) | Warta (River) | Poland | |
| Wehlau | Znamensk | Russia (Kaliningrad Oblast) | |
| Weimar | Weimar | Germany | |
| Wettenhausen (Abbey) | Wettenhausen (Abbey) | Germany | |
| Wettingen | Wettingen | Switzerland | |
| Wertingen | Wertingen | Germany | |
| Wilna | Vilnius | Lithuania | |
| Winterthur | Winterthur | Switzerland | |
| Wittenberg | Wittenberg | Germany | |
| Wloclaveck | Włocławek | Poland | |
| Wreschen | Września | Poland | |

| Toponym (in Percy's *Journal*) | Toponym (today) | Country (today) | Additional Comments |
|---|---|---|---|
| Wurtemberg | Württemberg | Germany | |
| Wurzbourg | Würzburg | Germany | |
| Zirke | Sieraków | Poland | |
| Zurich | Zürich | Switzerland | |
| Zusmarshausen | Zusmarshausen | Germany | |

# Select Bibliography

**Books**

Blaufarb, Rafe, *Napoleon: Symbol for an Age: A Brief History with Documents* (Boston, MA, 2008).

Bond, Brian, *The Pursuit of Victory: From Napoleon to Saddam Hussein* (Oxford, 1996).

Chandler, David (ed.), *Jena 1806: Napoleon destroys Prussia* (London, 1993).

Ducoulombier, Henri, *Le baron Pierre-François Percy, Un chirurgien de la Grande Armée* (Paris, 2004).

Forrest, Alan, *Napoleon's Men: The Soldiers of the Revolution and Empire* (London, 2002).

Gabriel, Richard, and Metz, Karen, *A History of Military Medicine, Vol. II: From the Renaissance through Modern Times* (New York, 1992).

Haller, John, *Battlefield Medicine: A History of the Military Ambulance from the Napoleonic Wars through World War I* (Carbondale, IL, 1992).

Harari, Yuval Noah, *Renaissance Military Memoirs: War, History, and Identity, 1450–1600* (Woodbridge, 2004).

Jones, Colin, *The Charitable Imperative: Hospitals and Nursing in Ancien Régime and Revolutionary France* (London, 1989).

Kuehn, John, *Napoleonic Warfare: The Operational Art of the Great Campaigns* (Santa Barbara, CA, 2015).

La Berge, Ann, and Feingold, Mordechai, *French Medical Culture in the Nineteenth Century* (Amsterdam, 1994).

Laurent, Charles, *Histoire de la vie et des ouvrages de P. F. Percy, composée sur les manuscrits originaux* (Versailles, 1827).

Lechartier, Georges, *Les Services de l'arrière à la Grande Armée en 1806-1807* (Paris, 1910).

Lynn, John A. (ed.), *Feeding Mars: Logistics in Western Warfare from the Middle Ages to the Present* (New York, 1994).
Muir, Rory, *Tactics and the Experience of Battle in the Age of Napoleon* (London, 1998).
Nosworthy, Brent, *Battle Tactics of Napoleon and his Enemies* (London, 1995).
Petre, Francis Loraine, *Napoleon's Campaign in Poland, 1806-1807: A Military History of Napoleon's First War with Russia; Verified from Unpublished Official Documents* (London, 1906).
Pigeard, Alain, *L'Armée de Napoléon (1800-1815)* (Paris, 2002).
Van Creveld, Martin, *Command in War* (Cambridge, 1985).
Van Creveld, Martin, *Supplying War: Logistics from Wallenstein to Patton* (Cambridge, 1977).

## Chapters

Bodinier, Gilbert, 'Les Guerres de l'Empire,' in Delmas, Jean (ed.), *Histoire Militaire de la France, Vol. 2* (Paris, 1992), pp. 343-370.
Fabre, A., 'Préface,' in Percy, Pierre-François; Jourquin, Jacques; and Longin, Émile (eds.), *Journal des Campagnes de Pierre-François Percy: Chirurgien-en-chef de la Grande Armée* (Paris, 1986), pp. 1-3.
Jourquin, Jacques, 'Avant-propos,' in Percy, Pierre-François; Jourquin, Jacques; and Longin, Émile (eds.), *Journal des Campagnes de Pierre-François Percy: Chirurgien-en-chef de la Grande Armée* (Paris, 1986), pp. 5-12.
Longin, Émile, 'Introduction,' in Percy, Pierre-François, and Longin, Émile (ed.), *Journal des Campagnes du Baron Percy, Chirurgien en Chef de la Grande Armée, 1754-1825* (Paris, 1904), pp. I-LXXVII.
Van Creveld, Martin, 'Napoleon and the Dawn of Operational Warfare,' in Van Creveld, Martin, and Olsen, John Andreas (eds.), *The Evolution of Operational Art: From Napoleon to the Present*, pp. 9-34.

## (Journal) Articles

Baker, David, Cazalaà, Jean-Bernard, and Carli, Pierre, 'Larrey and Percy – A tale of two Barons,' *Resuscitation*, 66(3) (2005), pp. 259-262.

Bourdon, Jean, 'L'administration militaire sous Napoléon I et ses rapports avec l'administration générale,' *Revue des Études Napoléoniennes XI* (January-June 1917).

Bowman, H. M., 'Review: *Journal des Campagnes du Baron Percy, Chirurgien en Chef de la Grande Armée (1754–1825)*. Publié d'après les manuscrits inédits par M. Émile Longin,' *The American Historical Review*, 10(2) (1905), pp. 417-19.

Caron, Pierre, 'Compte-Rendu: *Journal des campagnes du baron Percy, chirurgien en chef de la Grande Armée (1754-1825)*, publié d'après les manuscrits inédits avec une introduction par M. Emile Longin. Portrait en héliogravure et fac-similé d'autographe, 1904,' *Revue d'Histoire Moderne et Contemporaine*, 6(1) (1904), pp. 47-50.

Cénat, Jean-Philippe, 'De la guerre de siège à la guerre de mouvement : une révolution logistique à l'époque de la Révolution et de l'Empire ?', *Annales historiques de la Révolution française*, 348 (2007), pp. 101-115.

Dwyer, Philip G., 'Public Remembering, Private Reminiscing: French military memoirs and the Revolutionary and Napoleonic wars,' *French Historical Studies*, 33(2) (2010), pp. 231-258.

Dwyer, Philip G., 'Self-Interest versus the Common Cause: Austria, Prussia and Russia against Napoleon,' *Journal of Strategic Studies*, 31(4) (2008), pp. 605-632.

Harari, Yuval Noah, 'Military Memoirs: A Historical Overview of the Genre from the Middle Ages to the Late Modern Era,' *War in History*, 14(3) (2007), pp. 289-309.

Hutchinson, John, 'Rethinking the Origins of the Red Cross,' *Bulletin of the History of Medicine*, 63(4) (1989), pp. 557-578.

Millett, John D., 'Logistics and Modern War,' *Military Affairs*, 9(3) (1945), pp. 193-207.

Morgan, John, 'War Feeding War?: The Impact of Logistics on the Napoleonic Occupation of Catalonia,' *The Journal of Military History*, 73(1) (2009), pp. 83-116.

Rak, Julie, 'Are journals autobiography? A consideration of genre and public identity,' *Genre*, 37(3-4) (2004), pp. 483-504.

Richardson, R. G., 'Larrey – What Manner of Man,' *Society of Medicine: Section of the History of Medicine*, 70 (1977), pp. 490-494.

Wengert, James W., 'Jean Dominique Larrey (1766-1842): Surgeon of the Guard,' *Military Medicine*, 6(1) (1979), pp. 414-417.

# Acknowledgements

I would like to acknowledge the essential contributions of so many people who have improved the quality of this translation through their comments, suggestions, and knowledge. I am extremely grateful to Harriet Fielding, my editor at Pen and Sword Books, for taking a chance on my original manuscript and for being so patient during its completion and following the many rounds of suggestions and amendments. I also owe a debt of thanks to the many people who have read some or all of the manuscript to look for errors or inconsistencies, including my copy editor Tony Walton and the author Martin R. Howard, whose invaluable expertise of the medical and military practices of the period has filled many of the gaps in my own knowledge.

I would also like to thank my academic supervisors, who first nurtured my interest in Pierre-François Percy and who guided my historical research of the surgeon and his epoch, as well as my theoretical understanding of translation. They include, but are not limited to, Dr Tom Hamilton (Durham), Dr Vladimir Kapor (Manchester), and my lecturers in Manchester: Professor Maeve Olohan, Dr Anna Strowe, and Dr Rebecca Tipton.

Finally, I would like to recognise the help of my partner, parents, grandparents, and friends, all of whom provided feedback, guidance, and support. The time spent reading extracts from the book, listening to my thoughts and concerns, and offering encouragement has not gone unappreciated, and I love you all very much.

# Index

Administration, xxi–xxv, 2, 8, 10, 13, 94, 108–10, 152–3, 248
   *commissaire*, 5, 11, 20, 30, 42, 69, 83, 108, 284, 290
   corruption, xxiii–xxv, 267–9, 284, 286–8
   intendant–general, 72, 87, 94–7, 108
   Medical council, 31, 33
   *ordonnateur*, 61, 63, 98, 106, 124, 192, 219, 269
Agriculture, 7, 70, 75, 85, 160–1, 206–7, 215, 228, 278, 281–3
Alexander (Emperor of Russia), 235–6, 240, 242
Ambulance, 122–5, 211, 216–9
   corps ambulance, 2–3, 20
Amputation, 47, 66–7, 141–3, 176, 218–20, 243
Amputee, 276
Architecture *see* Culture, architecture
Army:
   misery, 103–105
Artillery, 176–80
Austria, 158

Baggage train, 55, 224 *see also* Provisions
Bandits, 44

Battlefield, 68–70, 100–101, 104, 116–7, 121–5
Berlin, 77–8, 289–90
Bivouac, 7, 12, 18, 100, 126
Braunsberg:
   tree, 272–3

*Cantinière*, 126, 215
Carriage:
   accident, 41, 93, 101, 140, 175, 198, 206
Corpse, 104–105, 136, 205–207, 213
Cossack, 255
Coste, 159
Countryside *see* Nature, countryside; Agriculture
Culture, 163, 172–3
   architecture, 34, 71, 91–2, 162, 188, 191–2
   clothing, 7, 84, 163, 172–3
   history, 34, 161
   religion, 51–52, 146, 275 *see also* Jews

Dantzig:
   arsenal, 192–3, 197–8
   canal, 192
   capture of a ship, 186–7

Index    307

entrance into, 191–2
　Napoleon's entrance, 197
fortifications, 178–80, 182–4, 189
hospitals, 193, 198
siege, 175–90
surrender, 188–91
trenches, 177–8
Desgenettes (physician), 159
Disease, 139, 185–6, 234
dysentery, 248, 275, 277, 287–9
epidemic, 111
epizootic, 277, 288
gangrene, 280
venereal, 34–5, 97

Émigré, 12, 45, 91–2, 181–2
Engineers, 184
Envoy, 68, 156
Evacuation, 36, 39, 55, 134–7, 201, 236, 268
poor organisation, 274–5, 286
Executive Directory, 1, 12, 29
Eylau:
Battle of, 120–5
church, 132–6, 167

Feudalism, 89, 92
Fever *see* Disease
Fire, 64, 67
Fishing, 184–5, 203
Frederick William III (King of Prussia), 236–7, 249–50
Friedland:
Battle of, 216–9
aftermath, 220–2
Percy's observations, 218
Funeral, 281

Garden, 118, 184, 201, 283, 286
General:
wounded, 46, 210–1, 218
Gerlach (surgeon), 261–2, 270
Goercke (surgeon), 88, 244, 249, 257–8, 262, 269–70, 289

History *see* Culture, history
Horse, 62, 168, 239
dying, 140
Hospital, 8, 42–4, 51–3, 59–62, 76, 89–90, 110–1, 141, 174, 202–203, 262, 265, 274, 279–80
fever, 170–1
inviolability, 40–2
Kustrin, 80–1, 278, 287–8

Illness *see also* Disease:
of Percy, 99–102, 106–108
Imperial Guard, 122, 152, 157–8, 218
*Infirmier*, 17, 128
Inhabitant:
misery, 208, 215, 282
Injury, 14–6, 19–22, 31–2, 43, 66–7, 79, 123, 179–83, 190–1, 199–200, 212, 218–20, 264–7

Jena:
Battle of, 66–7
Jews, 82–3, 87, 91, 93, 99–100, 145–6, 152–3
Jourdan, 1, 12, 14, 26–31
Journal:
provenance, xiv–xxi
translation, xxv–xxix
value to historians, xxi–xxv

Kalmyks, 226, 250–5

Larrey (surgeon), xiii–xiv, 54–5, 122–3, 129, 218
Legion of Honour, 186, 188–9, 237–8, 265–6

Marienbourg:
   Templar castle, 278–9
Medicine, 5, 200
Moreau, 40–2, 49

Napoleon, 154
   audience with, 88, 94–6, 126–7, 167–8, 219, 225–6, 246–50
Nature:
   birds, 147, 272
   countryside, 4, 23, 74, 82, 84–5, 176, 188, 207, 231–2, 271–2
   damselflies, 192
   plants, 11, 271–2, 288
Nurse *see* Infirmier

Opera, 78, 199
Orphanage, 76

Park, 73–4, 77–8, 86
Percy:
   audience with the monarchs, 239, 244–5
   biography, vi–x
   character, x–xiii
   wife, viii, 58, 263
Pillaging, 10, 28, 53–5, 64, 110, 114–5, 119, 202, 226–8, 278, 287
Prisoner, 49–50, 54–5, 132, 185, 229

Provisions, 8, 96, 130, 173, 229, 260
   cost, 192–3, 199
   surgical, 11, 15, 20–1, 27, 31, 44, 52, 56, 59–66, 98, 234, 243

Queen of Prussia, 255–6

Rastadt, 1
Rebellion, 37–8
Religion *see* Culture, religion
Retreat, 123–4
Return to France, 244, 259–90
Russians:
   behaviour, 132–3, 151

Sanssouci, 77
Soldiers:
   condition, 25, 74–5
   debauchery, 285–6
   presentation, 111
Starvation, 141
Supplies *see* Provisions
Surgeons:
   condition, 3, 9, 280
   corruption, 263
   praise and recognition, 31, 137–9, 154–7, 237–9, 248, 262–3, 265–6
   salary, 109
Surgery:
   battlefield surgery, 211–2, 216–7
   proposal for, 163–6, 194–6
   of Prussia, 169–70, 247–50, 269–70
   of Russia, 240, 243
   reform, 95–6, 144
   teaching, 156

Surgical instrument, 69, 131
   trephine, 3, 191

Tartar Baskhirs, 226, 250–5
Tilsit, 229–58
   banquet, 241
   departure, 257–8
   peace, 230–41
   procession, 235–6
   raft, 233, 235

Vanguard, 2–3, 52

Wadeleux (nephew of Percy), xv, 45,
   48–9, 87, 124, 239
Willier (Wylie, physician), 240, 243,
   245–6, 255, 267
Wine, 5–6, 42, 61, 84, 201
Women:
   soldiers' wives, 43, 53, 61
Wound *see* Injury
Wounded:
   convoy, 205
   Russian, 213
*Wurst*, xiii, 2–3, 5, 20–3